组织病理学教学与诊断图谱
双语版

主　编　陈　莉
副主编　王桂兰　何　松
编　委（按姓氏笔画排序）

卫颖泽　王建力　王桂兰　冯　佳
李春笋　杨其昌　吴雅昀　何　松
张丽丽　陆　鹏　陈旭东　陈　莉
季周婧　周家名　姜纯一　秦　婧
黄剑飞　缪小兵

科学出版社
北京

内 容 简 介

《组织病理学教学与诊断图谱》（双语版）由总论（第 1 ~ 5 章）和各论（第 6 ~ 19 章）两部分组成，内容包括了全身各系统器官常见疾病的组织病变，适当扩展与补充了反映当今病理学研究的热点和前沿问题，如组织中分子病理学检测技术显示的结果、电镜、共聚焦显微镜的亚细胞水平的观察等，共有 1000 余幅图片，均选自作者临床工作积累的和教材中的典型病理图片，并进行数字化处理，使图片分辨率更清晰，对每张图片配有中英文说明、语言精炼、内容扼要，便于初学者掌握要领，将有助于读者加深对病变基础知识的理解、学习、引证和参考。

本书适合本科临床医学各专业病理教学和来华留学生病理教学，以及临床病理医师进行病理诊断的参考。

图书在版编目（CIP）数据

组织病理学教学与诊断图谱：汉、英 / 陈莉主编 . —北京：科学出版社，2018.3
ISBN 978-7-03-056609-6

Ⅰ . ①组… Ⅱ . ①陈… Ⅲ . ①病理组织学－医学院校－图谱 Ⅳ . ① R361-64

中国版本图书馆 CIP 数据核字（2018）第 036204 号

责任编辑：张天佐 胡治国 / 责任校对：郭瑞芝
责任印制：吴兆东 / 封面设计：陈 敬

科 学 出 版 社 出版
北京东黄城根北街 16 号
邮政编码：100717
http://www.sciencep.com
北京中科印刷有限公司印刷
科学出版社发行 各地新华书店经销
*
2018 年 3 月第 一 版 开本：787×1092 1/16
2025 年 3 月第四次印刷 印张：18 1/2
字数：405 000
定价：198.00 元
（如有印装质量问题，我社负责调换）

前　言

　　病理形态的观察是病理学学习的重要部分，一张典型组织图片胜过许多文字的描述，它反映病变形态变化、鉴定疾病良恶性质、明确病变位置，是临床医师做出正确诊断的基础和依据。近年来免疫组织化学染色技术的普及、分子病理学技术的迅速发展，电镜、激光共聚焦显微镜的亚细胞水平的观察，极大地充实、扩大和丰富了病理学的内容，特别是精准医疗时代的来临、个性化的靶向治疗需要精准的分子靶向诊断，认识病变遗传学改变背景下的组织学特征和特异性基因的变化将是做出精准诊断的依据，是靶向性治疗的基础。本书的目的是通过提供典型、清晰的病变图像帮助读者更好地理解和掌握组织病理学知识。

　　《组织病理学教学与诊断图谱》双语版以编者长期从事教学、科研和临床工作所积累的资料和经验为基础，同时收集了部分经典的教学图片，其内容与编排顺序与我国医药院校病理教材相配套，由总论（第 1～5 章）和各论（第 6～19 章）两部分组成，内容包括了全身各系统器官常见疾病的组织学改变，并有适当的延伸，囊括了国家执业医师考试所需的病理知识，力争适用与全面，能满足广大学生扩大知识面的需求，满足教学改革和 PBL 教学的开展。图片中英文双语说明注重理论与临床结合，立足简明与确切，利于学生早临床、多临床和反复临床的要求，有利于提高医学生的临床实践能力。呈现的组织学病理图像力求清晰与典型，便于初学者掌握要领、加深对病变的理解、学习、引证和参考。作为一部病理教学与诊断的重要参考书，既适合本科临床医学各专业病理教学和来华留学生病理教学，也适合临床病理医师进行病理诊断的参考。

　　本图谱是在各位编者密切合作的基础上共同完成的，同时得到了南通大学杏林学院的支持与帮助，以及科学出版社的指导，在此一并表示谢意。限于编者水平，肯定不无缺憾，恳请读者批评指正。

陈　莉

于南通大学医学院病理学系

2017 年 7 月 1 日

目　　录

总　　论

各　论

总　论

第一章　细胞、组织的适应和损伤
Chapter 1　Cell and Tissue Adaptation and Injury

1-1　心肌萎缩 Atrophy of myocardium

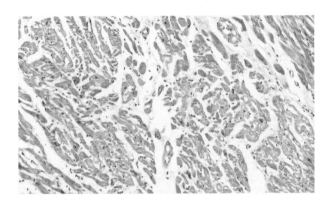

萎缩的心肌细胞体积变小，数目减少。胞浆深染，核浓缩，胞质内可出现脂褐素颗粒。

The atrophic myocardial cells show smaller volume or reduced number, with intensely eosinophilic cytoplasm and condensed nuclear chromatin. Lipofuscin can be seen in the cytoplasm.

1-2　心肌肥大 Hypertrophy of myocardium

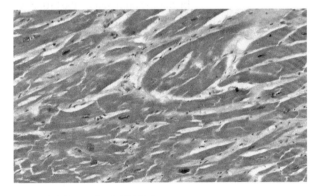

心肌细胞体积增大，细胞核深染，形状不规则；肌纤维增粗常有分支。

Myocardiocytes are enlarged and the nuclei are dark stained, varying in size and shape. Myofibrils are thickened with branches.

1-3　鳞状上皮疣状增生 Verrucous hyperplasia of squamous epithelium

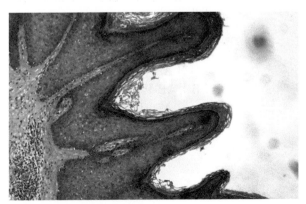

鳞状上皮向外形成乳头状突起，乳头表面角化亢进。

Squamous epithelium forms papillae outward and hyperkeratosis of the surface of the papillae.

1-4　子宫内膜增生症 Endometriosis

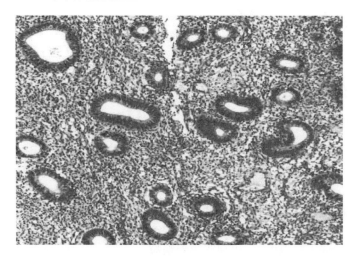

宫内膜腺体数量增加，部分腺体扩张成囊。腺体衬覆单层或假复层柱状上皮，无异型性，细胞形态和排列与增生期子宫内膜相似。

The number of endometrial glands increases with partial cystic dilation. Glands are lined by a single layer or pseudostratified columnar epithelium without atypia. The outline and structures of cells closely mimic the corresponding hyperplastic period of endometrium.

1-5　支气管鳞状上皮化生 Bronchial epithelium squamous metaplasia

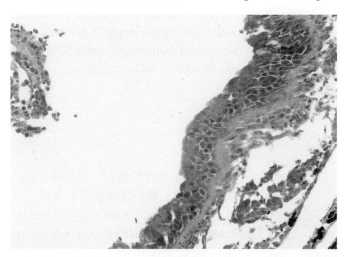

慢性支气管炎症，支气管内衬部分或全部纤毛柱状上皮发生鳞状上皮化生。

In chronic bronchitis, the bronchial epithelium（ciliated epithelium），partly or fully, undergoes squamous cells metaplasia.

1-6　胃炎肠上皮化生 Gastritis with intestinal metaplasia

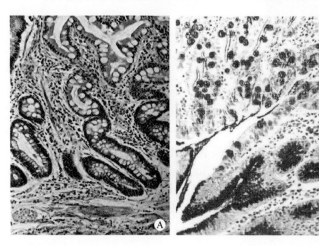

萎缩性胃炎的胃黏膜肠上皮化生。

Intestinal metaplasia of gastric mucosa in atrophic gastritis

（A）HE染色，10×20；
（B）AB-PAS染色，10×20。
（A）HE stain，×20；
（B）AB-PAS stain，×20.

1-7　混合瘤中软骨化生 Cartilaginous metaplasia，mixed tumor

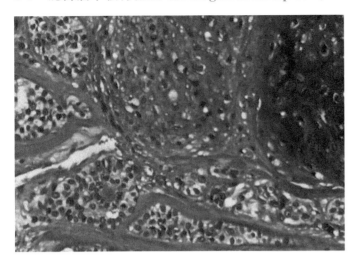

肿瘤中可见处于不同分化状态的上皮成分和间质成分。图右上方为软骨基质和软骨细胞，左下方为肌上皮细胞。

Various differentiatial states of epithelial or stromal components can be seen in tumor. The cartilage matrix and chondrocytes are at the upper right and myoepithelial cells are at the lower left.

1-8　骨化性肌炎中的骨化生 Bone metaplasia，myositis ossificans

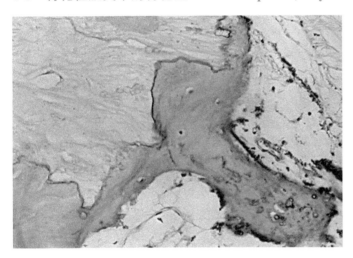

纤维结缔组织中骨化生。

Bone metaplasia in fibrous connective tissue.

1-9　肾近曲小管上皮细胞水变性（颗粒变性）Hydropic degeneration of proximal convoluted tubule of kidney（granular degeneration）

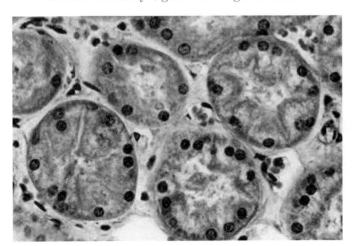

肾皮质区近曲小管上皮细胞肿大，胞质内出现嗜伊红染细颗粒。

The epithelial cells of proximal convoluted tubules in the renal cortex are enlarged，filled with eosinophilic granules in cytoplasm.

1-10　肝细胞水变性 Cell swelling，liver

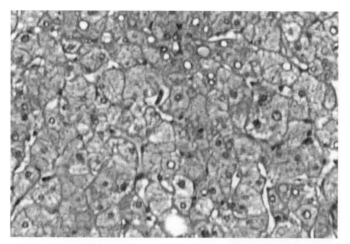

肝细胞明显肿大，细胞质高度疏松呈空泡状。

Hepatocytes are swollen, the cytoplasm is loose with the vacuolar appearance.

1-11　肝细胞脂肪变性 Fatty degeneration，liver cells

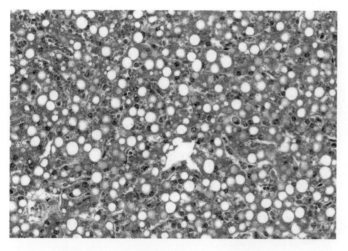

肝细胞内见大小不等的球形空泡（脂滴），大者可充满整个细胞而将胞核挤在一侧。

Various size vacuoles（lipids）accumulated in the cytoplasm of hepatocytes，and displacing nuclei to the periphery.

1-12　心肌间质脂肪浸润，Fatty infiltration，myocardial stroma

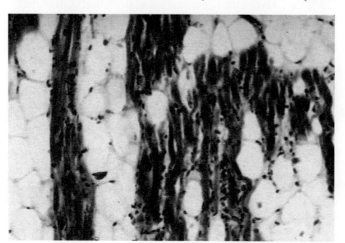

心肌间质见成熟脂肪组织浸润。

The mature fat cells are infiltrated in the myocardial stroma.

1-13 脾包膜玻璃样变性 Hyaline degeneration of spleen capsule

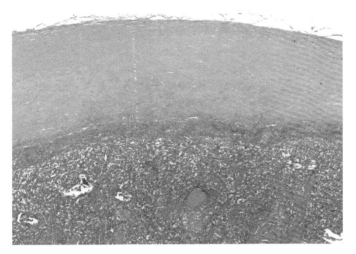

　　脾包膜呈均质、粉红色、玻璃样变，其间少有血管和纤维细胞。

The spleen capsule shows homogenous, pink, glassy appearance, few blood vessels and fibrocytes.

1-14 脾细动脉玻璃样变性 Splenic arteriole hyaline degeneration

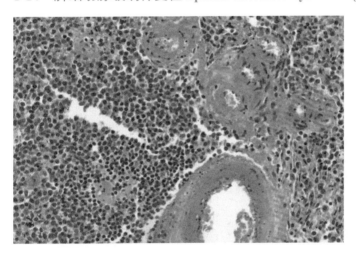

　　脾细动脉壁均质、粉红色、玻璃样变。

A homogenous glassy pink appearance in the splenic arteriolar wall.

1-15 淀粉样变性 Amyloid degeneration

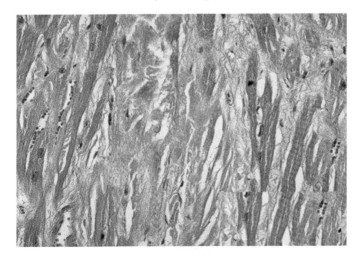

　　组织化学刚果红染色显示淀粉样变性为细胞间均质红染的物质。

Histochemical Congo Red stain for amyloid degeneration, as an intercellular pink homogeneous materials.

1-16 碳末沉着症 Anthracosis（Carbon）

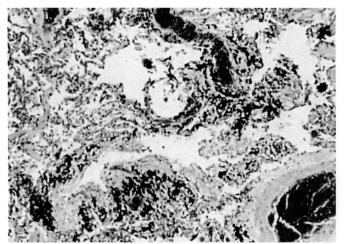

碳末色素在肺和淋巴结的巨噬细胞中积聚，与空气污染有关。

Accumulation of coal dust in the macrophages of the lungs and lymph nodes，which usually is associated with air pollution.

1-17 心肌细胞中脂褐素 Lipofuscin，myocardial cells

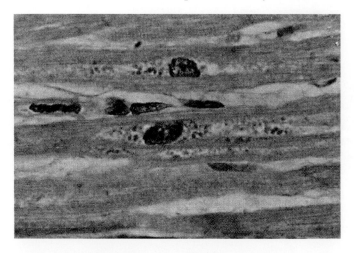

脂褐素呈棕黄色，聚集在核周区，常常与萎缩相关（"褐色萎缩"）。由脂质、磷脂和蛋白质等成分组成，提示其为细胞膜的多不饱和脂质的过氧化产物。

Lipofuscin is yellowish brown and accumulated in perinuclear area，usually associated with atrophy（"brown atrophy"）. It is composed of lipids，phospholipids and proteins，suggesting that it is derived from peroxidation of polyunsaturated lipids of cell membranes.

1-18 肺中含铁血黄素 Hemosiderin，lung

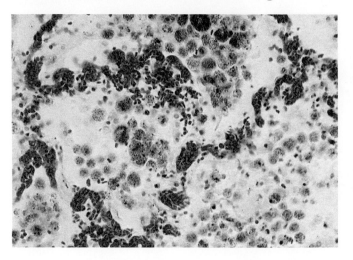

由铁蛋白微粒聚集而成。局部含铁血黄素沉着由大出血或小血管淤血后破裂引起。巨噬细胞吞噬血红蛋白，后者在溶酶体酶作用下转化成含铁血黄素。

It is formed by the aggregates of ferritin micelles. Local hemosiderosis results from massive hemorrhage or rupture of small vessels due to vascular congestion. Macrophages take up hemoglobin，and the latter transformed into hemosiderin by lysosomal enzymes.

1-19　肝脏胆色素 Bilirubin，liver

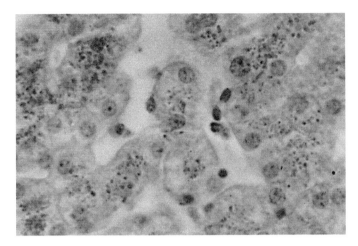

常由肝功能障碍、胆道阻塞或Dubin-Johnson综合征使胆汁肝外分泌受阻，临床常表现为黄疸。

Defect in hepatic excretion of bilirubin is caused by liver dysfunction，biliary obstruction，Dubin-Johnson syndrome，Clinical appear jaundice.

1-20　皮肤黑色素 Melanin，skin

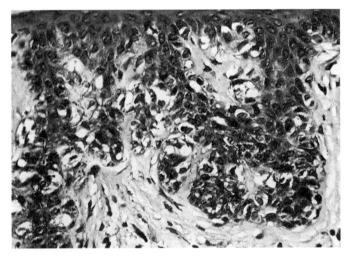

一种内源性、非血红素来源的、棕黑色色素。在黑色素细胞中，酪氨酸在酪氨酸酶的催化作用下氧化生成3，4二羟苯丙氨酸。

An endogenous，non-hemoglobinderived，brown-black pigment. Tyrosine was oxidized to produce 3,4 dihydroxyphenylalanine under the catalytic action of tyrosinase in melanocytes.

1-21　腹主动脉营养不良性钙化 Dystrophic calcification，abdominal aorta

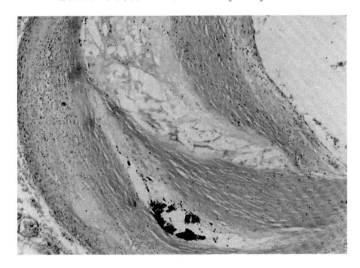

HE染色中钙盐常呈嗜碱性、无定形颗粒，有时成堆。

Histologically HE stain, the calcium salts show a basophilic，amorphous granular，sometimes clumped appearance.

1-22 肾凝固性坏死 Coagulative necrosis，kidney

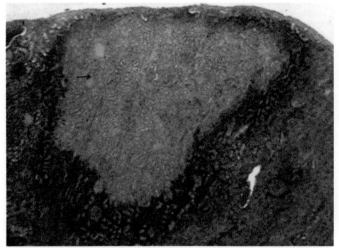

细胞结构消失但组织轮廓保存一段时间。

Cellular structure disappeared but tissue outline preserved for a span of days.

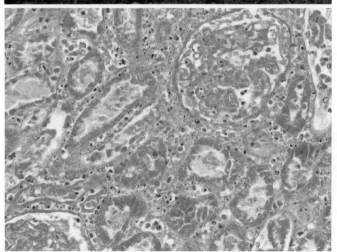

坏死区细胞核固缩、核碎裂和核溶解等改变，胞质嗜伊红染。坏死细胞外形和组织结构轮廓仍可保存，坏死周围有炎症细胞浸润及血管反应。

Pyknosis，karyonhexis，karyo lysis are seen in necrotic areas with eosinophilic cytoplasm. Tissue outline was reserved，inflammatory cells and hyperemia can be seen around the necrotic areas.

1-23 淋巴结干酪样坏死 Caseous necrosis，lymph node

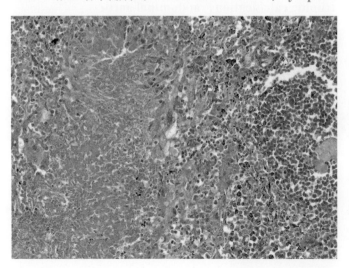

淋巴结结核结节中干酪样坏死呈无结构颗粒状红染物，不见坏死部位原有组织结构的残影，甚至不见核碎屑。

Caseous necrosis in lymph node tubercle shows unstructured eosinophilic granules. Previous tissue structure disappeared，even isn't seen nuclear debris.

1-24 脂肪坏死 Fat necrosis

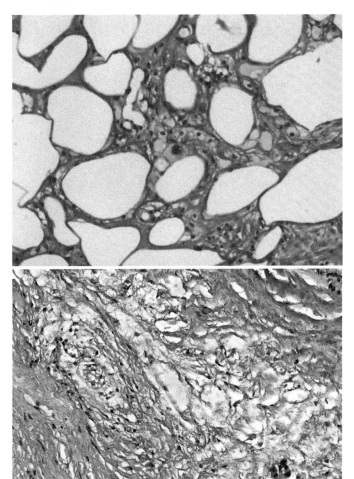

发生在乳腺脂肪组织内的脂肪坏死。脂肪细胞变性、坏死，细胞核消失，融合成大小不等的空泡。

Fat necrosis occurs in the adipose tissue of the breast, a adipocyte shows degeneration, necrosis and disappeared nuclei and finally are fused to form vacuoles in variable size.

急性胰腺炎（钙皂）
Acute pancreatitis（calcium soap）

坏死的脂肪细胞的轮廓模糊，胞浆内充满无定形的、弱嗜碱性物质（钙皂）。

Outline of necrotic adipocyte is unclear. The cytoplasm is full of unstructured, weak-basophilic materials（calcium soap）.

1-25 结缔组织纤维素样坏死 Fibrinoid necrosis，connective tissue

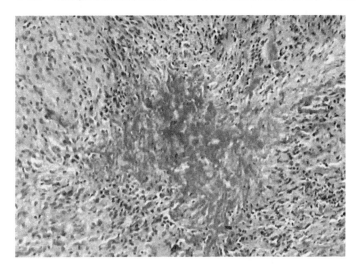

病灶界限不清，组织结构消失，为颗粒状、深伊红色、无定形状。

The tissue structure of the lesion disappears, with an ill-defined borderline. It is granular, deep eosinophilic, amorphous matter.

1-26 凋亡 Apoptosis

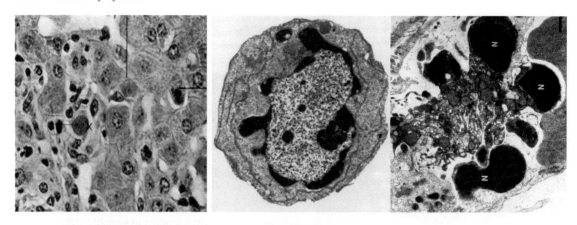

肝细胞中嗜酸性小体（eosinophilic bodies in hepatocytes）
电镜下凋亡细胞染色质边集和细胞出芽。
Under electron microscopy chromatin margination and bleb in apoptotic cells.

1-27 自噬 Autophagy

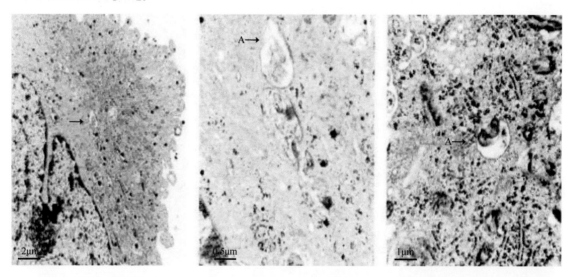

通过透射电镜观察的内皮细胞。细胞内存在双层膜结构包裹的自噬体，其电子密度较高，隐约可见遗留的线粒体脊痕迹。

Ultrastructure of endothelial cells observed under Transmission Electron Microscopy. There were autophagosomes presenting higher electron density，which was packaged by double membrane structure in endothelial cells，and indistinct legacy of mitochondria ridge remained.

第二章　损伤的修复
Chapter 2　Repair for Injury

2-1　肉芽组织 Granulation tissue

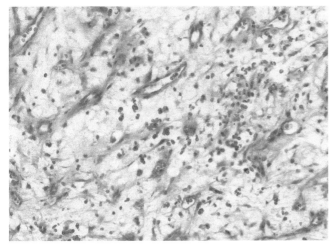

肉芽组织由新生的薄壁毛细血管、成纤维细胞和炎症细胞组成。新生毛细血管可形成实性细胞索或扩张，垂直于创面。

Granulation tissues are characterized by newborn thin-walled capillaries, fibroblasts and inflammatory cells. Proliferation of capillaries may form cord-like structure or dilatation, vertically arranged to the wounded margin.

2-2　创口愈合 Wound healing

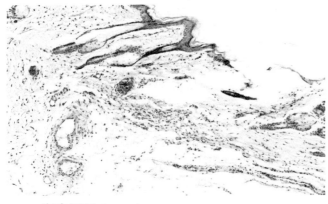

在创口愈合处可见肉芽组织和瘢痕组织。

Granulation and scar tissues in wound healing.

2-3　瘢痕组织 Scar tissue

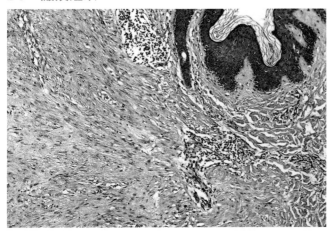

真皮中可见不规则的成纤维细胞增殖，伴小圆细胞浸润。

Overproliferation of fibroblasts are noted in dermis, associated with inflammatory cells infiltration.

第三章 局部血液循环障碍
Chapter 3 Local Fluid and Hemodynamic Disorders

3-1 肺慢性淤血 Chronic lung congestion

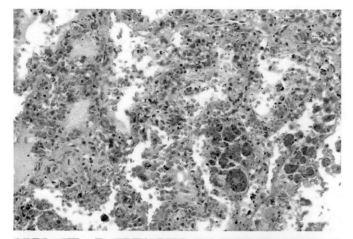

肺泡壁毛细血管扩张充血，肺泡腔内含粉红色水肿液及红细胞，可见大量含有含铁血黄素的心衰细胞。部分肺泡壁纤维化增厚。

The pulmonary alveolar wall capillaries are congested. The alveolar spaces are filled with pink edematous fluids and red blood cells, and many heart failure cells containing hemosiderin. Some pulmonary alveolar walls are fibrosis and thickened.

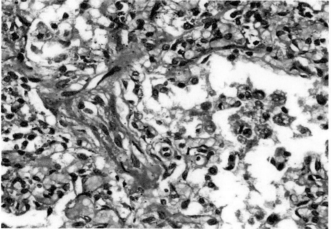

肺褐色硬化（早期）
Brown induration of lung（early stage）

肺泡壁纤维组织增生伴含铁血黄素沉着。肺泡腔内可见含有含铁血黄素的巨噬细胞。

Proliferation of fibrous tissue in the pulmonary alveolus wall with hemosiderin deposition. Some macrophages containing hemosiderin present in alveolar spaces

3-2 肝慢性淤血 Chronic liver congestion

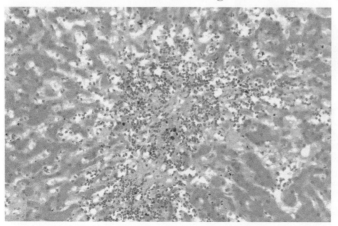

肝小叶中央静脉及肝窦扩张，明显淤血、出血。部分肝细胞坏死、萎缩。门管区肝细胞呈脂肪变性。间质纤维组织增生。

The central vein and vascular sinusoids are dilated with congestion and hemorrhage. Some hepatocytes show necrosis and atrophy. Portal area shows fatty changes. Stromal fibrotic tissues are proliferated.

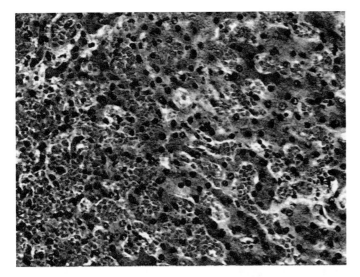

中央静脉和肝窦扩张充血，可以出现小叶中央肝细胞萎缩，变性，坏死。

Central vein and sinusoids are dilated and hyperemia，and the central zone shows atrophy，degeneration and necrosis of hepatocytes.

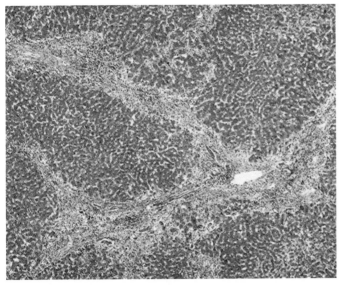

淤血性肝硬化。
Congestive liver cirrhosis.

3-3　脑出血 Cerebral hemorrhage

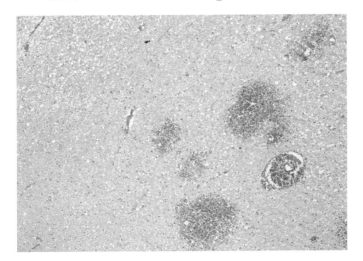

脑组织中可见片状出血区。
Several erythrocytes leak from the blood vessel and infiltrated in the brain tissue.

3-4 肺水肿 Pulmonary edema

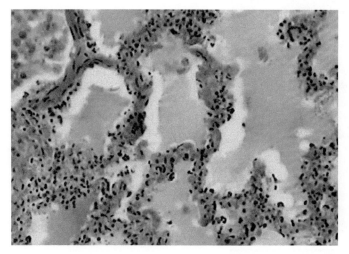

肺泡壁毛细血管扩张充血，肺泡腔内见大量的浆液性渗出物。

The capillaries in pulmonary alveolar wall dilatation and congestion, exudating serous fluid into the alveolar spaces.

3-5 血栓 Thrombus

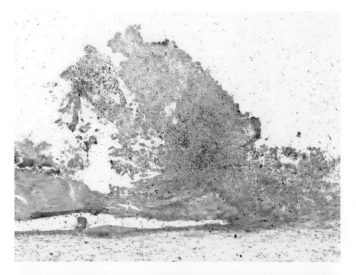

白色血栓（pale thrombus）

光镜下由血小板和少量纤维素构成，又称为血小板性血栓，也称血栓头。

Microscopically, platelets admixed with some fibrin form pale thrombus, and called platelets thrombi, that is the head of thrombi.

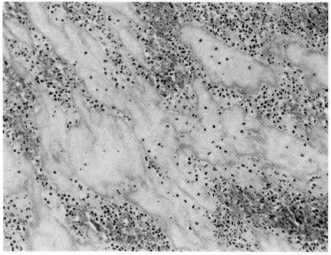

混合血栓（mixed thrombus）
（层状血栓 lamination thrombus）

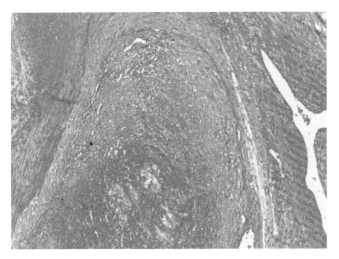

血栓中淡红色血小板小梁，呈分支状或不规则形的珊瑚状结构，小梁间有纤维蛋白网，小梁边缘可见中性粒细胞附着。在血栓与血管壁之间可见肉芽组织形成机化。血栓中裂隙覆盖毛细血管内皮细胞形成再通内有红细胞。

In the thrombus, the reddish platelets trabecula area, within them are fibrin networks. Neutrophils adhere to the edge of the trabecula between the thrombus and vessel wall, organization can be seen. There are some splits covered by endothelium in which blood flow could be reformed.

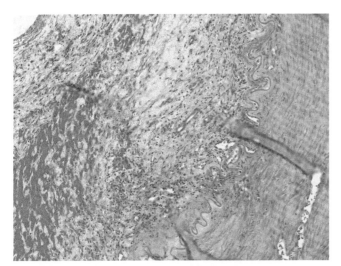

血栓机化（organization of thrombus）

肉芽组织从血管壁长入血栓并逐渐取代血栓。

Granulation tissue grows in the thrombus from blood vessel wall and replace the thrombus.

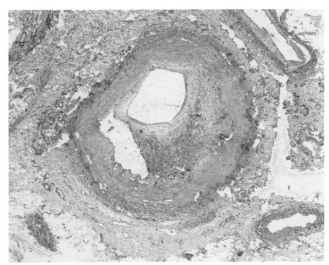

血栓再通（Recanalization of thrombus）

血栓内部形成新的血管相互吻合沟通，使被阻塞的血管部分地重建血流。

New channels across the thrombus were established and anastomoses, allowing the blocked vessels to partially reestablish blood flow.

3-6 透明血栓 Hyaline thrombi

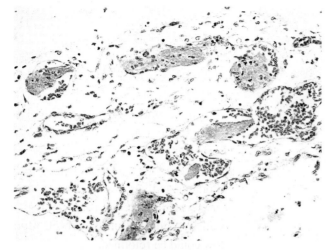

弥漫性血管内凝血（DIC）中可见毛细血管中有透明微血栓。

The capillaries are filled with hyaline microthrombi in disseminated intavascular coagulopathy.

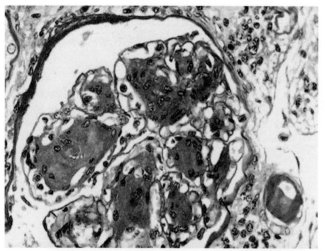

（DIC）肾小球透明血栓。

Glomerular hyaline thrombi.

3-7 肺血栓栓塞 Thrombus embolism，lung

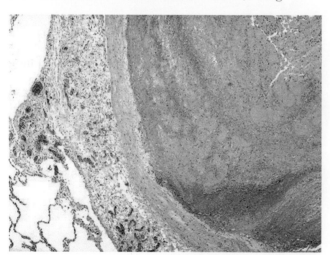

此为肺动脉分支中一肺部血栓的镜下观。

Here is the microscopic appearance of a pulmonary embolus（PE）in a pulmonary artery branch.

3-8　肺脂肪栓塞 Fat embolism，lung

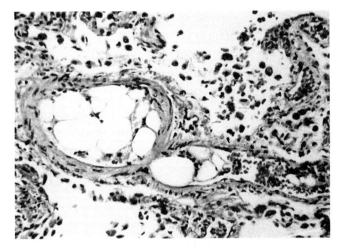

肺组织肺血管中有脂肪组织聚集。

The lung shows entrapped fatty tissue lodged in a pulmonary vessels.

3-9　肺瘤细胞性栓塞 Tumor cellular embolism，lung

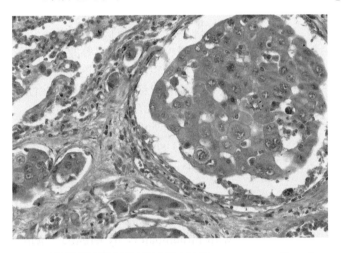

在肺组织扩张的毛细血管和淋巴管中见成团的深染的异型细胞（此即肿瘤细胞）。

Dark stained atypical cells（tumor cells）are seen in the dilated lymph vessels and capillaries of lung.

3-10　肠黏膜下静脉液体性栓塞 Fluid embolism in venous，intestial submucosa

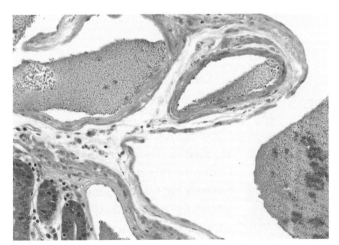

在肠黏膜下扩张的静脉和毛细血管中见有浆液性粉红色蛋白液。

Serous fluid（pink colored）is seen in the dilated capillaries and veins of intestinal submucosa.

3-11　肾贫血性梗死 Anemic infarction，kidney

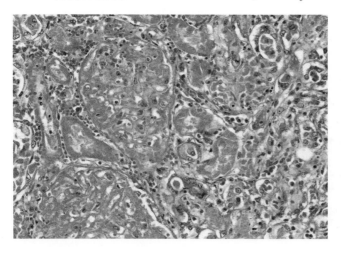

贫血性梗死灶（凝固性坏死）中可见核固缩、核碎裂和核溶解等改变，胞质嗜伊红染。梗死灶边缘炎症性充血、出血，有肉芽组织长入形成瘢痕组织。

Anemic infarct area （coagulative necrosis） shows necrotic cells with pyknosis, karyonhexis, karyolysis, and intensely eosinophilic cytoplasm. Inflammatory hyperemia, hemorrhage could be found on the edge of infarct area, granulation tissue grows and transform scars.

3-12　脾贫血性梗死 Anemic infarction，spleen

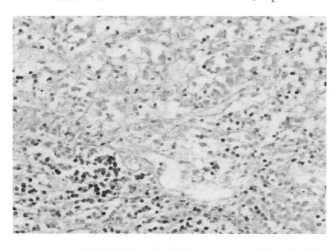

脾贫血性梗死区细胞坏死，核固缩、核碎裂和核溶解等改变，胞质嗜伊红染。脾组织结构轮廓尚保存。梗死边缘有肉芽组织长入和炎症性充血、出血，最终可形成瘢痕组织。

Anemic infarct area （coagulative necrosis） show necrotic cells with pyknosis, karyonhexis, karyolysis, and intensely eosinophilic cytoplasm. Spleen tissue structure still preserved. Granulation tissue grows on the edge with inflammatory hyperemia, hemorrhage, and scars formation.

3-13　肺出血性梗死 Hemorrhagic infarction，lung

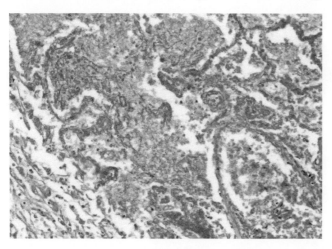

梗死灶内肺泡壁上皮细胞坏死，肺泡轮廓尚存。肺泡腔、小支气管腔及肺间质充血、水肿及出血。

Necrotic alveolar epithelial cells are seen in the infarcted areas. Tissue structure is preserved. Alveolar, bronchiolar spaces, lung interstitium interstitial spaces show hyperemia, edema and hemorrhage.

第四章 炎 症
Chapter 4 Inflammation

4-1 炎症细胞 Inflammatory cells

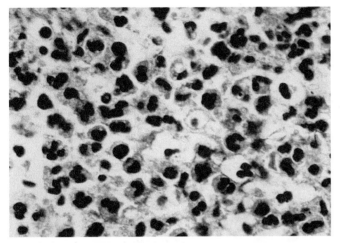

中性粒细胞（neutrophils）

中性粒细胞属于小吞噬细胞（10～15微米），胞核分叶状（3～5叶），胞浆中含嗜中性颗粒。在急性炎症分泌物中可见多叶核细胞和各种形式的变性中性粒细胞。

Neutrophils belong to small phagocytes, with lobulated nucleus and neutrophilic granules in the cytoplasm. Cells with multilobulated nuclei and various degenerated forms usually are seen in acute inflammatory exudate.

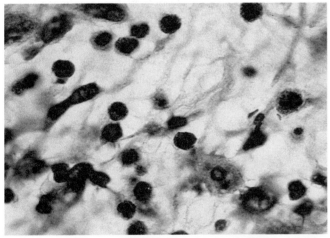

嗜酸性粒细胞（eosinophils）

嗜酸性粒细胞呈典型的眼镜样核（双叶），胞浆内含有强嗜酸性颗粒。

The eosinophils shows characteristic eyeglass-shaped nuclei (bilobed) and intensely eosinophillic granular cytoplasm.

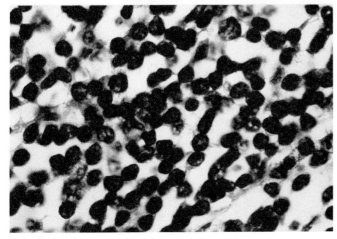

淋巴细胞（lymphocytes）

淋巴细胞核小而圆，深染，胞浆很少。

Lymphocytes have small round nuclei with dense chromatin and scanty cytoplasm.

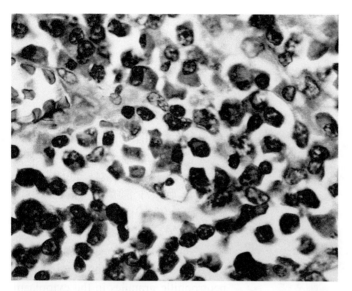

浆细胞（plasma cells）

浆细胞核染色质呈特征性的轮辐状排列，核偏位。胞浆丰富，核周浅伊红色空晕。有时胞浆内有免疫球蛋白Rusell小体蓄积。

The nuclei of plasma cells show characteristic cartwheel appearance of the chromatin and eccentrically located. The cytoplasm is abundant and faintly eosinophillic with perinuclear halo. Sometimes with accumulation of immunoglobulin forming Rusell body.

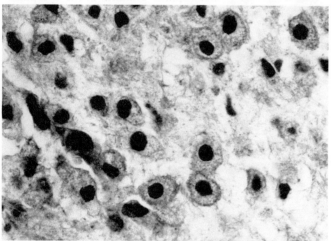

巨噬细胞（macrophages）

这些细胞胞浆丰富、泡沫状，核圆、居中。

Macrophages show aboudant fomay cytoplasm and centrally located round nuclei.

4-2　液体渗出 Fluid exudation

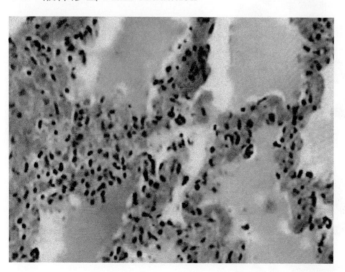

肺水肿（lung edema）

肺间质毛细血管淤血，肺泡腔内浆液渗出。

Lung interalveolar capillary congestion, exudating serous fluid into the alveolar spaces.

4-3　炎细胞渗出 Inflammatory cells exudation

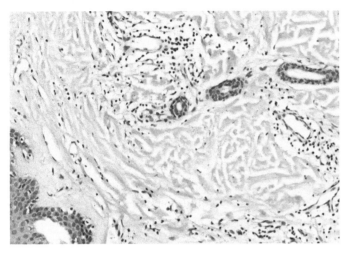

血管炎（vasculitis）

血管扩张充血，在血管周围炎细胞浸润。

Vessels dilation and hyperemia with inflammatory cells around the vessels.

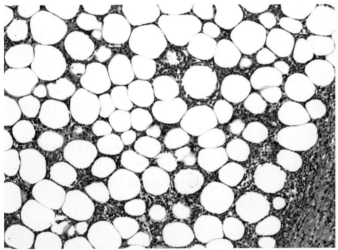

脂膜炎（panniculitis）

皮下脂肪纤维间隔内可见中性粒细胞和淋巴细胞等混合性炎症细胞浸润伴有脂肪坏死。病变晚期脂肪纤维间隔明显纤维化。

Mixed infiltration of neutrophil and lymphocytes are seen in subcutaneous fat fiber interval，with steatonecrosis. Later lesions show fat fiber gap fibrosis.

4-4　浆液性炎 Serous inflammation

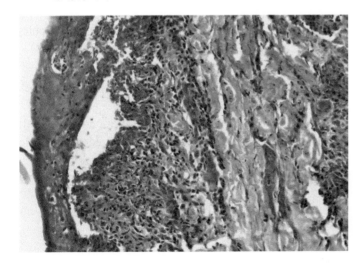

皮肤水疱（skin blister）

在表皮内和表皮下浆液性渗出物形成水疱。

Serous exudates in epidermis and subepidermis can be seen.

4-5 纤维素性炎 Fibrinous inflammation

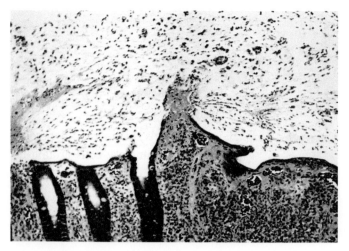

细菌性痢疾（bacillary dysentery）

假膜性肠炎（pseudomembranous colitis）

结肠黏膜表面纤维蛋白、坏死组织和中性粒细胞等渗出物形成假膜，伴肠壁炎性水肿。

Fibrin, necrotic epithelium and neutrophils form pseudomembrane in colon mucous surfaces, with inflammatory edema in colon wall.

4-6 化脓性炎 Purulent inflammation

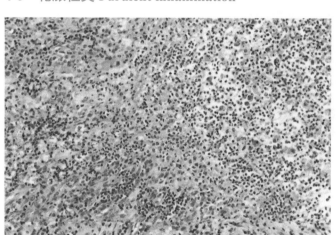

脓肿中中性粒细胞浸润与聚集以及细胞碎片。

There are neutrophils infiltration, accumulation, and necrotic debris in the abscess.

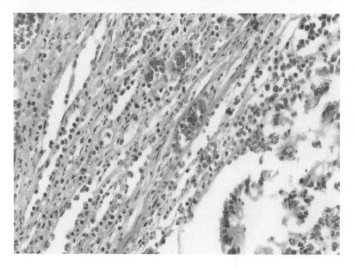

急性阑尾蜂窝织炎（acute phlegmonous inflammation of appendix）

阑尾壁全层充血水肿，肌纤维束相互分离，中性粒细胞弥漫浸润。

All layers of appendiceal wall show hyperemia and edema, musle fiber bundles are separate from each other, with diffuse infiltration of neutrophils.

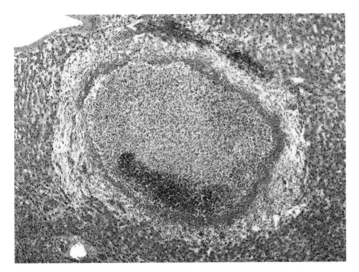

肝脓肿（liver abscess）

肝脏中可见一充满大量中性粒细胞的小脓肿灶。由大量中性粒细胞构成。

The liver shows a small abscess here filled with many neutrophils. Abscess is composed of a lot of neutrophils.

4-7　增生性炎 Proliferative inflammation

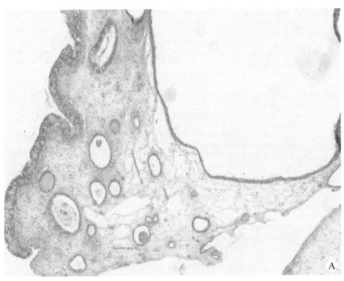
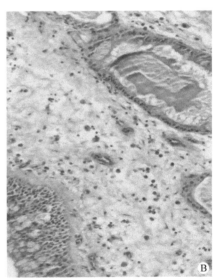

鼻息肉（nasal polyp）

A.鼻黏膜上皮细胞、纤维结缔组织、血管以及腺体增生伴有炎症反应。散在黏液腺增生，腺体导管可呈囊状扩张，导致潴留性囊肿形成。

A. Nasal mucosa epithelial cells，fibrous connective tissue，blood vessels and glands show hyperplasia accompanied by inflammation.There is proliferation of mucus gland，glandular duct shows cystic expansion，leading to retention cyst formation.

B. 鼻黏膜基底细胞增生、鳞化，偶见上皮的不典型增生。固有膜水肿，胶原纤维被冲散；数量不等的炎细胞浸润（包括淋巴细胞、浆细胞、中性粒细胞、嗜酸性粒细胞等）。

B. Basal cells of nasal mucosa show proliferation，squamous metaplasia and occasional epithelial dysplasia. Intrinsic membrane shows edema，collagen fibers are dispersed. Numbers of inflammatory cells infiltration（including lymphocytes，plasma cells，neutrophils，eosinophils，etc.）.

4-8　肉芽肿 Granuloma

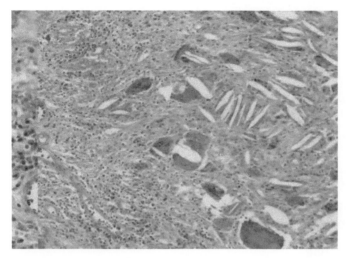

异物性肉芽肿（foreign body granuloma）

臀部肌肉组织中见多核巨细胞。多核巨细胞体积大，多核，细胞胞浆中易见异物（在此为脂质，呈针形及卵圆形裂隙）。

Multi-nucleated giant cells are observed in hip muscles. It is big and multi-nuclei, foreign bodies in cytoplasm with ovoid clefts.

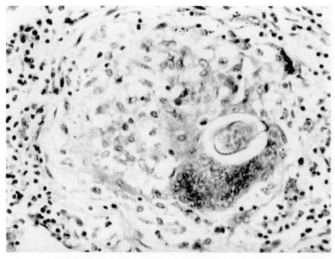

慢性虫卵结节（chronic egg nodule）

虫卵周围异物巨细胞和类上皮细胞，虫卵可发生坏死和钙化。

Eggs are surrounded by epithelioid cells, multinucleated foreign giant cells; eggs are often necrosis or calcification.

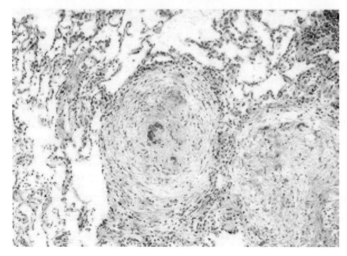

感染性肉芽肿（infecting granuloma）（结核结节tubercle）

低倍镜下结核肉芽肿呈圆形，境界清楚。

Tuberculosis granulomas of the lung have rounded outlines with well-demarcated in low light microscope.

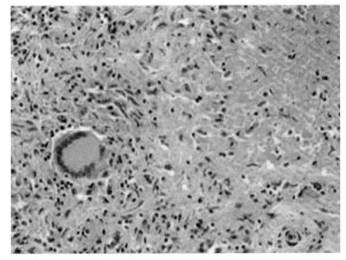

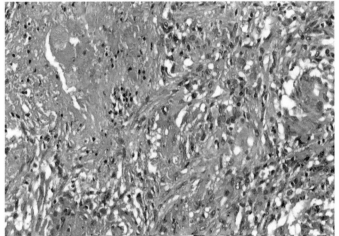

典型的肉芽肿结构，中心为干酪样坏死，周围为放射状排列的上皮样细胞，并可见Langhans巨细胞掺杂于其中，再向外为大量淋巴细胞浸润，结节周围还可见纤维结缔组织包绕。

The typical granuloma nodule is composed of caseous necrotic debris in the center, infiltrating by epithelioid histiocytes and Langhans giant cells in the surround and lymphoctyes at periphery. The proliferation of fibrous tissue surrounded this nodule.

4-9　肺炎性假瘤 Inflammatory pseudotumor，lung

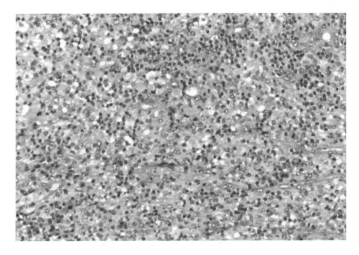

并非真正的肿瘤，由炎性细胞和纤维组织增生形成的肿瘤样病变。其中有成熟的淋巴细胞、浆细胞、巨噬细胞和黄瘤细胞（泡沫细胞）等炎性成分。

This disease is not a true tumor, only a tumor-like lesion composed of inflammatory cells and fibrous tissue hyperplasia. Imflammatory cells, including lymphocytes, plasma cells, macrophage, foam cells and so on.

第五章　肿　瘤
Chapter 5　Tumor

5-1　肿瘤细胞多型性 Pleomorphism of tumor cells

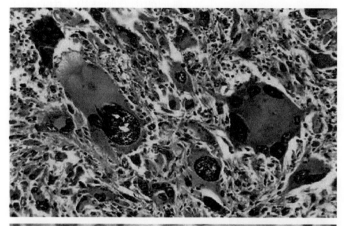

多型核和瘤巨细胞（pleomorphic nuclei and tumor gaint cells）

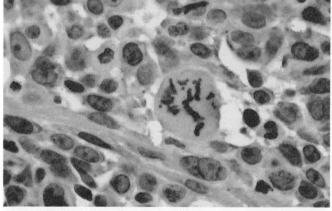

病理性核分裂（多极核分裂）〔Pathological mitosis（multipolar mitosis）〕

5-2　子宫颈上皮内瘤变 Cervical intraepithelia neoplasia（CIN）

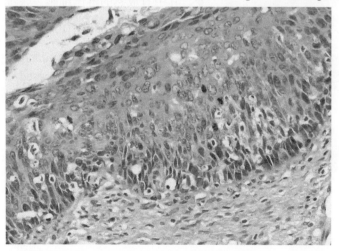

鳞状上皮细胞增生并伴有异型性，细胞大小和形状多形性，核浆比值增高，核大深染，核分裂增多，细胞排列紊乱、极性消失等。但异型细胞仅在上皮层内。

Squamous cells show hyperplasia with atypia. Cell is pleomorphism with size and shape diversity, nuclear plasma ratio increases, large, and darkly stained nuclei, mitosis figures increase, arranged disorder, polarity disappear. But atypical cells are located only in the epithelium layer.

5-3 皮肤鳞状上皮乳头状瘤 Papilloma of squamous cell，skin

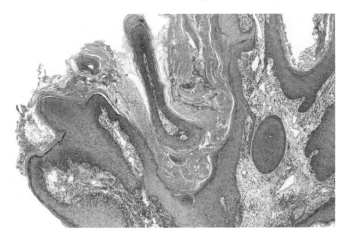

上皮性肿瘤形成乳头状突起。乳头由表面被覆增生鳞状上皮及其血管和结缔组织间质的轴心构成，间质与上皮的关系有如手指与手套的关系。

Epithelial tumor forming papillary-like projections. Papillary surface is covered by hyperplastic squamous epithelium，vascular and connective tissue constitutes in the axis of papillary.

5-4 皮肤鳞状细胞癌 Squamous cell carcinoma，skin

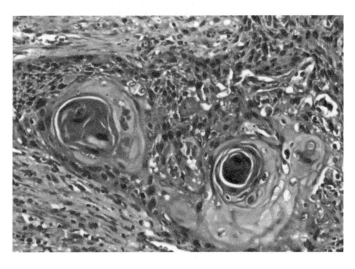

高分化（well-differentiation）

异型增生的鳞状细胞，浸润性生长形成癌巢，癌巢中央角化形成角化珠（或称癌珠）和癌细胞间有细胞间桥（即具棘细胞分化特征时在细胞间出现的平行排列短丝状细胞间连接）。

Atypically hyperplastic squamous epithelia with invasive growth form some cancer nests can be seen. Keratin pearls（or cancer pearls）are in the center of nest. The intercellular bridge can be seen.（The parallel short filamentous connection appear between cells with prickle cells differentiation）.

5-5 基底细胞癌 Basal cell carcinoma

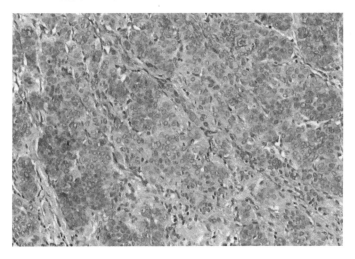

基底样细胞大小一致，胞浆较少，但核深染，核膜较厚，核有一定异型性。该细胞增生成巢，巢周细胞栅栏状排列，而中心部细胞排列较杂乱。

Basal cells show the same size, less cytoplasm，nuclei dark stain，nuclear membrane is thicker and atypia. The hyperplastic cells form the nest. The peripheral cells of nest show palisading arrangement，while the central cells messly arranged.

5-6 膀胱尿路上皮（移行细胞）癌 Urothelium（transitional cell）carcinoma，bladder

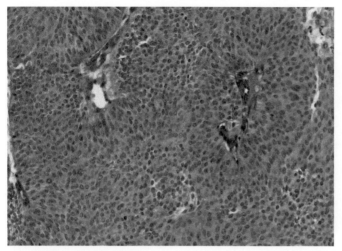

移行细胞癌呈乳头状，细胞层次超过8层，细胞排列明显紊乱。根据细胞层次、核分裂像、癌细胞浸润、出血坏死分为Ⅰ～Ⅲ级。

Transitional cell carcinoma grow papillary-like with more than eight layers. Cell polarity is disorder. Depending on cells atypia，mitosis，infiltrating in the lamina propria and hemorrhagic necrosis，it is classified to grade Ⅰ to grade Ⅲ.

5-7 腺瘤 Adenoma

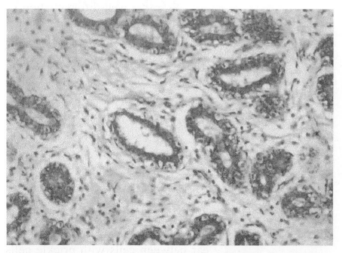

乳腺纤维腺瘤（fibroadenoma of breast）

腺上皮细胞增生和大量纤维结缔组织增生，共同构成瘤的实质。纤维组织围绕腺管增生，腺管大小不等，数目增多。

Glandular epithelial cells proliferated accompanied by large amounts of fibrous connective tissue，which together formed the parenchyma of the tumor. Hyperplastic fibrous tissue around the glandular canal. The number of gland ducts increase accompaning with vary size.

5-8 腺癌 Adenocarcinoma

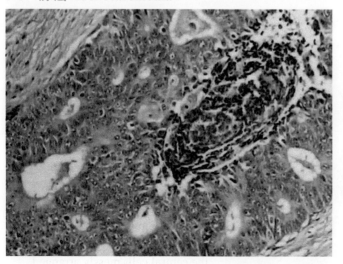

肿瘤细胞排列呈腺管状结构，异形腺体背靠背，共壁，明显的细胞异型性，核分裂多。

Tumor cells are arranged in an irregular duct-like structures，atypical glands back to back，co-wall，cellular atypia，a lot of mitotic figures.

5-9　肉瘤样癌 Sarcomatoid carcinoma

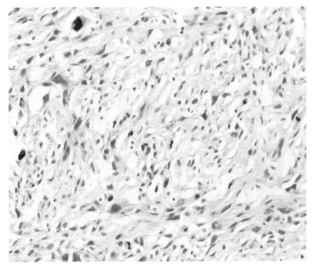

分化差的癌（poor-differentiation）

浸润性生长的癌细胞呈梭形，出现较多的病理性核分裂。

Atypically spindle cancer cells invasively grows. Tumor cells show more pathological mitosis.

5-10　癌肉瘤 Carcinosarcoma

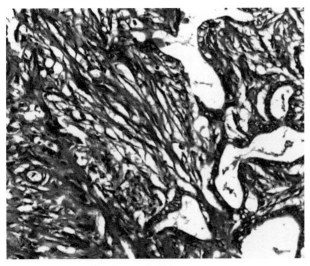

肿瘤由上皮性癌和间叶性肉瘤成分组成，最常见的成分是鳞癌、腺癌、大细胞癌，肉瘤常为梭形细胞，如纤维肉瘤、恶纤组软骨肉瘤，骨肉瘤或横纹肌肉瘤等，有时主要为间质性肿瘤仅小灶性上皮癌。

Tumor is composed of carcinoma and sarcoma ingredients, showing biphasic appearance. The most common component is squamous cell carcinoma, or adenocarcinoma and large cell carcinoma; sarcomatoid component is usually spindle cells, similar to fibrosarcoma or malignant fibrous histiocytoma, chondrosarcoma, osteosarcoma or rhabdomyosarcoma, etc. Some of the main components constitute malignant stromal tumors, only showing small focal epithelial carcinoma.

5-11　混合痣 Mixed nevus

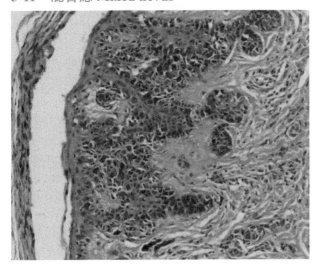

同时见皮内痣和交界痣。其中皮内痣的痣细胞主要在真皮层内，故称为真皮内痣，简称皮内痣。交界痣：色素性痣细胞位于真皮与表皮交界处。痣细胞大多为上皮样痣细胞。痣细胞可累及毛囊、皮肤及汗腺等。

Intradermal nevi and junctional nevus are seen. The nevus cells mainly locate in the dermis, it is referred to as intradermal nevi. In junctional nevus: pigmented nevus cells are located dermis and epidermis junction. Most of nevus cells are epithelioid. Nevus cells can affect hair follicles, skin and sweat glands.

5-12 黑色素瘤 Melanoma

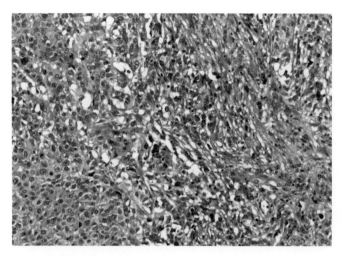

恶性黑色素瘤细胞可含黑色素，细胞异型明显。免疫组化显示Malan-A阳性，有大于10%的肿瘤细胞呈现强的胞质染色。

Malignant melanoma cells contain melanin, cellular atypia is significant. Immunohistochemical Malan-A positive Stronger cytoplasmic expression is found in more than 50% of tumor cells

5-13 肺软骨性错构瘤 Cartilaginous hamartoma, lung

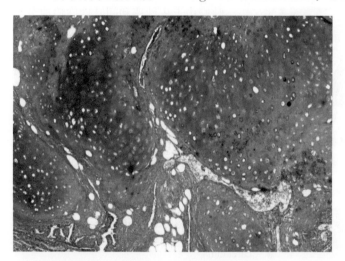

肺组织中，肿瘤组织由分化成熟的软骨组织构成，表明这种情况实际上是一种异常发育的状态。错构瘤都是良性的。

In lung, the tumor is composed of cartilage with matured-differentiation which indicates an abnormal developing state. Hamartomas are all benign tumors.

5-14 畸胎瘤 Teratoma

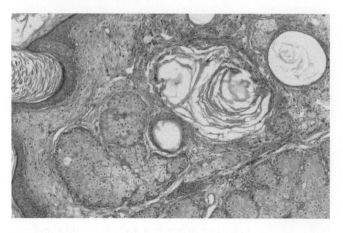

肿瘤由三个胚层的各种成熟组织构成。常见皮肤、毛囊、汗腺、脂肪、肌肉、骨、软骨、呼吸道上皮、消化道上皮、甲状腺和脑组织等。

Tumor is composed of a variety of mature three germ layers tissues. Commonly including: skin, hair follicles, sweat glands, fat, muscle, bone, cartilage, epithelium of airway and digestive tract, thyroid and brain tissues.

5-15 肿瘤转移 Tumor metastasis

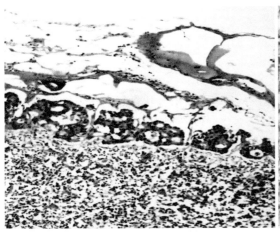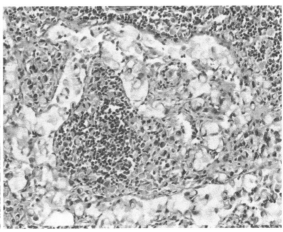

淋巴结转移（lymphatic metastasis）

转移肿瘤细胞（腺癌）首先见于淋巴结包膜下或边缘窦内，最终累及整个淋巴结，而后突破包膜浸润局部组织或继续沿淋巴系统扩散。

组织学表现为扩张的淋巴窦中含有癌细胞团（此例为胃印戒细胞癌淋巴结转移）。

Metastatic tumor cells（adenocarcinoma）are first seen in the subcapsular space or marginal sinus，and eventually the whole lymphnode，then infiltrate its capsular to the local tissues，or continue to spread the lymphatic system.

Histologically showing dilated lymphatics sinus containing carcinoma cell emboli.（here gastric signet-ring cell carcinoma metastasis in the lymph node）.

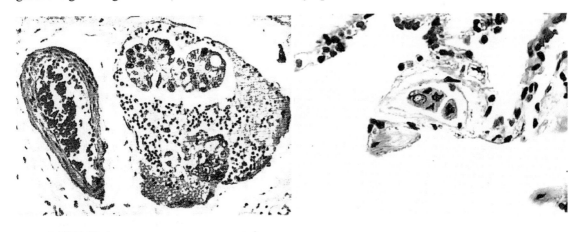

血道转移（hematogenous metastasis）

肿瘤细胞穿透静脉的薄壁，聚集形成栓子，运行于血流（此例扩张的静脉内有腺癌栓）。

Tumor cells penetrate the thin wall of a vein，are broken off，and are carried away as emboli.（here the dilated vein has some embolus of adenocarcinoma.）

5-16 纤维瘤 Fibroma

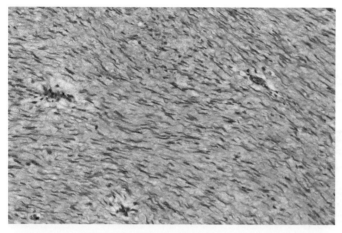

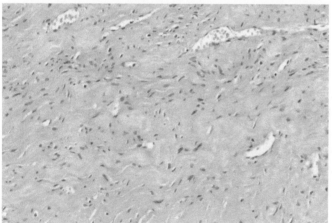

由分化良好的梭形细胞组成。梭形细胞核小。核分裂像难以见到，瘤细胞呈席纹状或血管外皮细胞瘤样排列。有时胶原纤维束粗大如绳状，平行排列伴有透明变性、其间梭形细胞散在分布，具有特征性。

Fibroma is formed by well-differentiated spindle cells. The nuclei of spindle cells is small. Mitotic figures are less. Tumor cells have storiform or hemangiopericytoma-like arrangement. Sometimes collagen fiber bundles are thickened, arranged in parallel with hyaline degeneration. Spindle cells are scattered in between.

5-17 纤维肉瘤 Fibrosarcoma

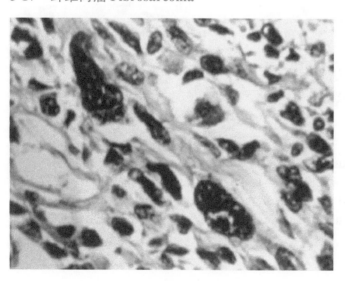

由形态一致的梭形纤维母细胞样肉瘤细胞组成。瘤细胞束状交织排列，典型病例可见鱼骨样或"人"字形结构。分为成人型和婴儿型。

It is composed of the spindle fibroblast loid sarcoma cells morphologically. The tumor cells are arranged in bundles and a typical fishboneloid structure. Divided into adult and infant types.

5-18　脂肪瘤 Lipoma

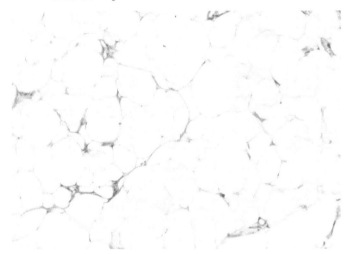

瘤细胞分化好与正常脂肪细胞相似，可由间质血管分隔成小叶状，肿瘤有纤维性包膜。

Well-differentiated tumor cells are similar to normal fat cells，which were separated by stromal vascular lobules. Tumor presents fibrous capsule.

5-19　脂肪肉瘤 Liposarcoma

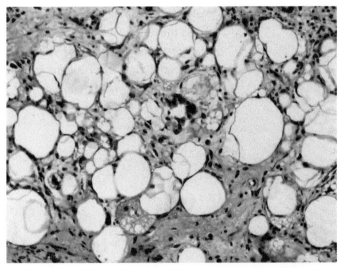

脂肪瘤样脂肪肉瘤（lipoma-like liposarcoma）

高分化脂肪肉瘤（well differentialed liposarcoma）

肿瘤由纤维组织分隔成大小不等的小叶；肿瘤细胞主要由成熟脂肪组织和少量散在的脂肪母细胞组成。

It is separated by fibrous tissue into varying size lobules；the tumor cells are mainly composed of mature adipose tissue and a small amount of scattered adipoblasts.

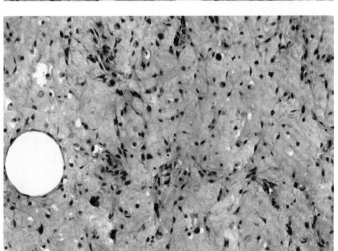

硬化性脂肪肉瘤（sclerosing liposarcoma）

高分化脂肪肉瘤（well differentialed liposarcoma）

致密胶原纤维化区域穿插于脂肪细胞和不典型的细胞及空泡状脂肪母细胞之间。

The region of dense collagen fibrosis is interspersed between adipocytes and atypical cells，vacuolated adipocytes.

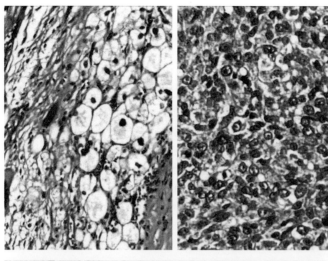

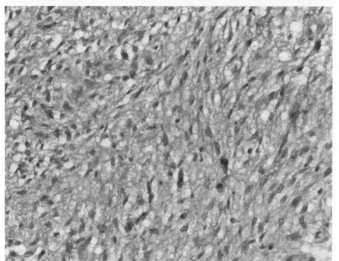

去分化脂肪肉瘤（dedifferentiated liposarcoma）

肿瘤由分界清楚的分化和去分化两种成分组成。前者多为分化良好型脂肪肉瘤（左），后者为恶性纤维组织细胞瘤样（右）或纤维肉瘤样，也可含有异源性成分。

The tumor consists of two distinct components of differentiation and dedifferentiation. The former was well differentiated liposarcoma（left）, the latter was malignant fibrous histiocytoma（right）or fibrosarcoma, and may also contains heterogeneous components.

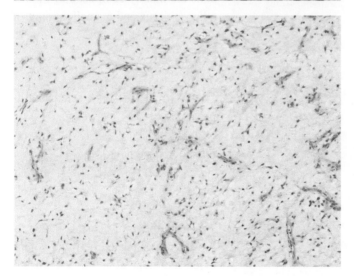

黏液性脂肪肉瘤（myxoid liposarcoma）

明显的分支状毛细血管，不同分化的脂母细胞和大量的黏液样物质。

A prominent branching capillary, differentiating lipoblasts and an abundance of myxoid material.

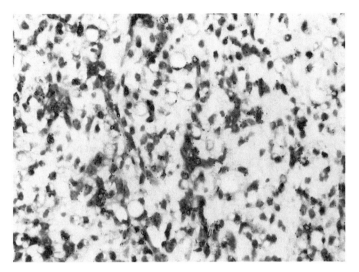

圆细胞性脂肪肉瘤（round cell liposarcoma）

一致性圆形和椭圆形原始非脂肪性间叶细胞和小的印戒样脂肪母细胞混合存在。

The consistency round and oval primitive mesenchymal cells mixed with small signet ring like lipoblasts.

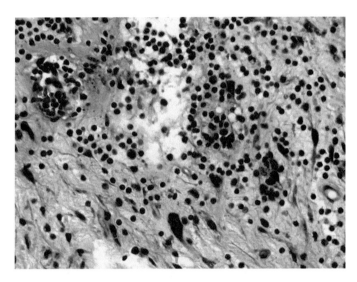

炎症型脂肪肉瘤（inflammatory liposarcoma）

多位于腹膜后；在脂肪瘤样型脂肪肉瘤或在硬化性脂肪肉瘤内含有数量不等的淋巴细胞和浆细胞浸润，常形成结节状的聚集灶，有时脂肪成分可被炎症背景所掩盖。

It located in the retroperitoneal region, lipomaloid liposarcoma or sclerosing liposarcoma contain vary amounts of lymphocytes and plasma cells, and often make focal nodular accumulating, sometimes tumor components may be covered by inflammatory background.

5-20　平滑肌瘤 Leiomyoma

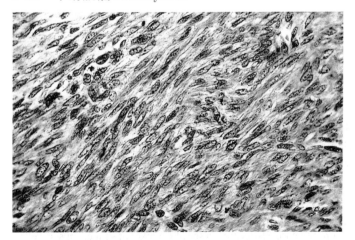

平滑肌瘤中见梭形肿瘤细胞，核呈雪茄烟样，未见核分裂。

Spindle tumor cells with nuclei of cigar shape are seen in leiomyoma. Mitosis is absent.

5-21　平滑肌肉瘤 Leiomyosarcoma

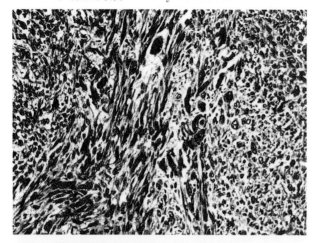

平滑肌肉瘤，由大小不等的长梭形细胞构成。瘤细胞多平行排列呈束，纵横交织，胞浆丰富、红染。胞核多为长形而两端钝圆，棒杆状，核两端胞浆内可见空泡，核被挤压。瘤细胞异形明显，间质可黏液变性。

Leiomyosarcoma is composed of varying size long spindle cells, arranged in parallel bundles, intertwined, showing eosinophilic and plenty cytopalsm. Nuclei vary in size, stained darkly, mostly elongated and rounded at both ends, stick rod, vacuoles can be seen in the cytoplasm of both ends of the nuclear, nuclear is squeezed. Tumor cells show obvious atypia, mucoid degeneration appears in the stroma.

5-22　横纹肌肉瘤 Rhabdomyosarcoma

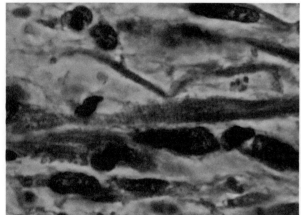

肿瘤细胞呈圆形、卵圆形或梭形，核大、深染，核仁明显，核浆比增高，核分裂易见，部分胞浆嗜酸性，肿瘤细胞弥漫成片分布。

The tumor is composed of round, oval or spindle cells with enlarged, hyperchromatic nuclei, prominent nucleoli, increased nuclei-cytoplasm ratio, visible mitotic activity and focally eosinophilic cytoplasm, diffusely distributed into sheets.

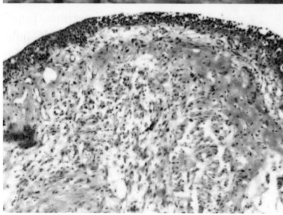 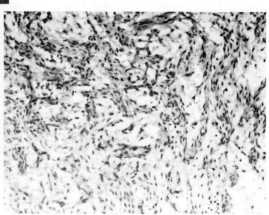

胚胎性横纹肌肉瘤（embryonal rhabdomyosarcoma）

肿瘤由成肌性原始间叶细胞组成，肿瘤细胞呈星形、蝌蚪样、梭形，胞浆浅嗜双染，中位椭圆形核，肿瘤细胞分布于疏松黏液样组织中。免疫组化染色显示横纹肌特异性标记 Myogenin核阳性。

The tumor is composed of the primitive mesenchymal cells of myogenesis. The tumor cells show stellate, tadpole or spindle morphology, sparse, amphophilic cytoplasm and central nuclei, distributed in loose myxoid tissue. Immunohistochemical stain shows nuclear positive for Myogenin, a specific marker of striated muscle cells.

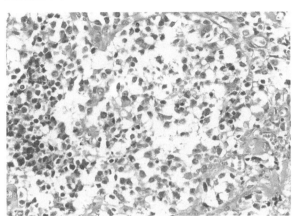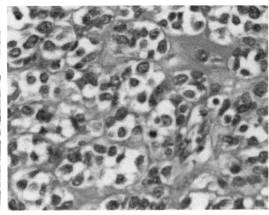

腺泡状横纹肌肉瘤（alveolar rhabdomyosarcoma）

肿瘤细胞呈圆形，类似淋巴瘤细胞，被纤维血管间隔分隔成清楚的巢状结构。

The tumor cells are round and similar to lymphoma cells, separated by fibrovascular intervals into the distinct nested structure.

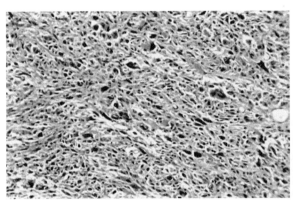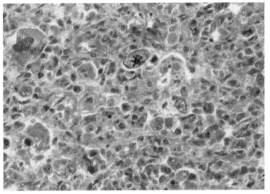

多形性横纹肌肉瘤（pleomorphic rhabdomyosarcoma）

瘤细胞多为发育后期的横纹肌母细胞，多形性十分明显，核分裂多，有大梭形细胞、带状细胞、各种奇异的瘤巨细胞（如蝌蚪状细胞、网球拍状细胞及蜘蛛状细胞）等。胞浆较丰富，呈深伊红色，有时可见到横纹。

Tumor cells are mostly rhabdomyoblasts in late development stage. Pleomorphism is very obvious. Tumor mitotic figures are common. There are large spindle cells, ribbon cells and varying bizarre tumor giant cells（such as tadpole-like cells, tennis racket-shaped cells and spider-like cells） and so on.Cytoplasm is rich, intensely eosinophilic, sometimes the stripes can be seen.

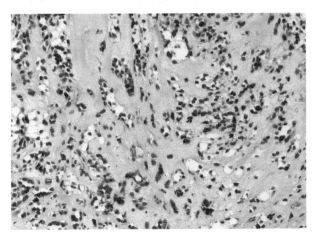

硬化性横纹肌肉瘤（sclerosing rhabdomyosarcoma）

肿瘤中大量间质明显玻璃样变和黏液变。

The distinct hyaline degeneration and myxoid degeneration of strom present in tumor.

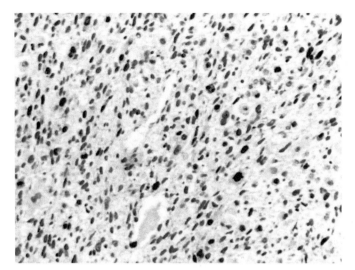

免疫组化结果显示横纹肌特异性标记Myogenin核表达阳性。

Immunohistochemistry is nuclear positive for Myogenin, a specific marker of striated muscle cells.

5-23 滑膜肉瘤 Synovial sarcoma

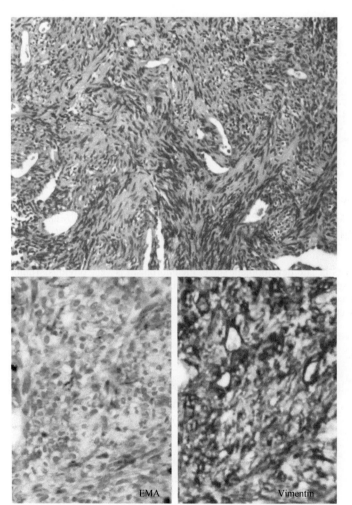

肿瘤完全由梭形细胞成分组成。梭形细胞成分相互交织密集呈束状，或呈血管外皮瘤样结构，局灶可见致密透明变的纤维化区。免疫组化显示EMA和Vimentin阳性。

The tumor is comprised solely of the spindle cell components. The spindle cell components, consists of interweaving fascicles, displays a prominent haemangiopericytomatous pattern, and focal areas of dense hyaline fibrosis. Immuno- histochemistry shows EMA and Vimentin positive.

5-24 血管瘤 Hemangioma

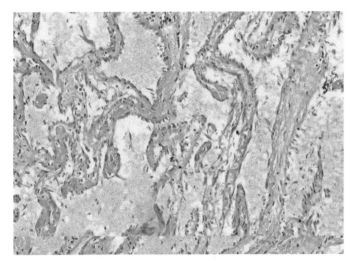

海绵状血管瘤（cavernous hemangioma）

由囊性扩张的薄壁血管构成，在扩张的血管内，有时可有血栓形成，或机化，或钙化而形成静脉石。

Cavernous hemangioma is composed by cyst-dilated thin-walled blood vessels. In the dilated blood vessels，sometimes thrombosis，organization or calcification forming vein stones can be seen.

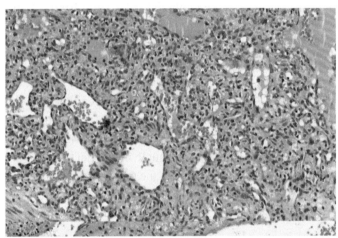

毛细血管瘤（capillary hemangioma）

毛细血管瘤由管径一致较小的小动脉构成。

Capillary hemangioma is composed of smaller arteries of the same diameter.

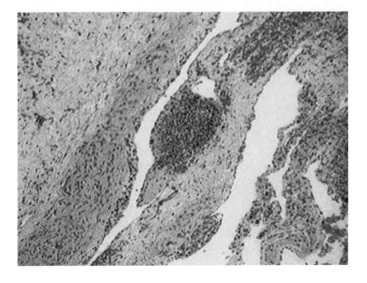

淋巴管瘤（lymphangioma）

5-25　血管肉瘤 Angiosarcoma

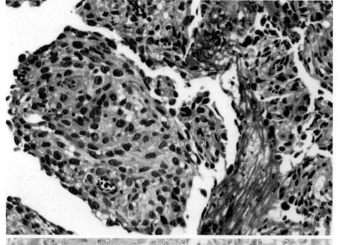

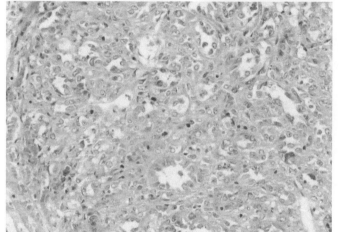

血管肉瘤为血管内皮细胞发生的恶性肿瘤，即恶性血管内皮瘤。肿瘤由不同程度异型性的内皮细胞构成，常形成不规则的相互吻合的血管腔。瘤组织因出血明显，常有含铁血黄素沉积。肿瘤细胞呈上皮样，胞浆淡染，核圆或卵圆形，大小不一，核仁明显。肿瘤组织内见裂隙样腔隙。

Hemangiosarcoma is the malignant tumor deriving from vascular endothelial cells with different atypical degrees, the endothelial cells often form irregular vessel lumen. Tumor tissue show obvious hemorrhage, and hemosiderin deposition. The tumor cells are epithelioid with pale stained cytoplasm, round or oval nuclei in various size and prominent nucleoli. Slifler cavities are visible in the tumor tissue.

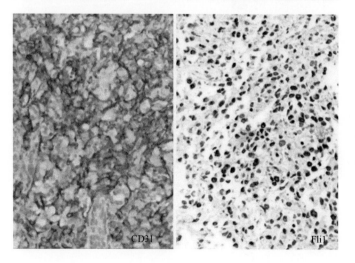

CD31　Fli1

免疫组化结果显示血管内皮标记CD31胞膜阳性。Fli1核阳性。

Immunohistochemistry is membrane and nuclei positive for CD31 and Fli1, respectively, two markers of vascular endothelium.

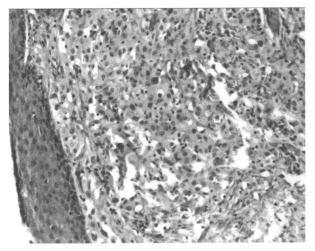

卡波西肉瘤（kaposi's sarcoma）

肿瘤呈片状分布，由明显异型的梭形细胞和血管组成，伴有红细胞漏出。

The tumor is arranged in sheets, composed of prominently atypical spindle cells and vessels with significantly red cells leakage.

5-26　恶性纤维组织细胞瘤 Malignant fibrous histiocytoma

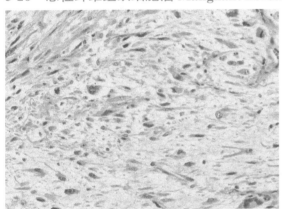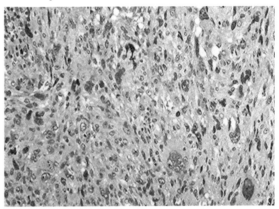

以"席纹"状排列的梭形细胞和异型性的巨细胞为主要形态特点的多形性未分化肉瘤。各种炎症细胞可以混杂于肿瘤中，可伴骨化生或软骨化生。

Plemorphic undifferentiated sarcoma has the main morphological characteristics of spindle cells with atypia arranging in "Dutch" like and giant cells. A variety of inflammatory cells can be seen in the tumor, and may be associated with ossification metaplasia or cartilage metaplasia.

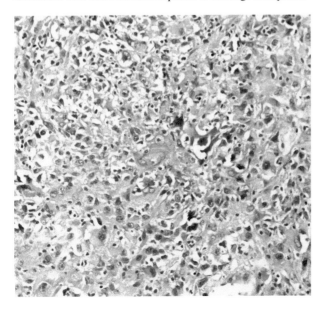

多形性恶性纤维组织细胞瘤（plemorphic malignant fibrous histiocytoma）

细胞及细胞核有明显多形性，常伴有奇异型肿瘤巨细胞，并混合有数量不等的梭形细胞和圆形组织细胞样细胞；常有编席状结构和间质慢性炎细胞浸润；梭形细胞最常表现为纤维母细胞、肌纤维母细胞或平滑肌样细胞。

Cell and nuclear have pleomorphism, which often accompanied by bizarre tumor giant cell, mixed with a mounts of spindle cells and round histcytes; and often has weaving mats pattern and interstitial chronic inflammatory cell infiltration; spindle cell is most often identified as fibroblasts, myofibroblasts and smooth muscle like cells.

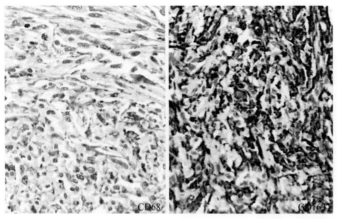

免疫组化Vimentin、AAT、ACT、CD68、CD163表达阳性，有时Desmin、Actin、keratin也呈阳性。

Immunohistochemistry，Vimentin，AAT，ACT，CD68，CD163 expression are positive，sometimes Desmin，Actin，keratin are also positive.

5-27 腺泡状软组织肉瘤 Alveolar soft part sarcoma

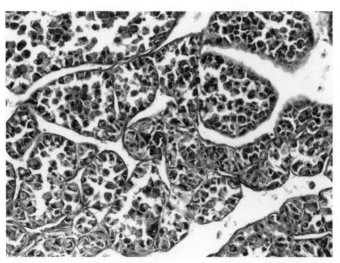

肿瘤细胞排列成实性巢或腺泡状结构，之间有薄的窦状血管分隔。肿瘤细胞为含有丰富嗜酸性颗粒状胞质的大圆形或多角形，空泡状核，核仁明显，巢中心细胞缺乏黏附性，并有坏死。

The tumor cells are arranged in a solid nest or alveolus structure，and separated by sinusoids thin wall blood vessels. The tumor cells were large round or polygonal with rich eosinophilic granular cytoplasm，vacuolated nuclei，prominent nucleoli，lacking of adhesion but having necrosis in the nest centre.

5-28 上皮样肉瘤 Epithelioid sarcoma

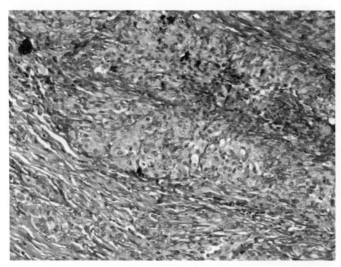

嗜酸性上皮样和梭形细胞混合呈结节性生长；细胞核有轻度异型性，核空泡状并有小核仁；肿瘤结节常有中心坏死，形成假性肉芽肿

The eosinophilic epithelioid and spindle cells are mixing with nodular growth；mild nuclear atypia，nuclear vacuoles and small nucleoli；tumor nodules often have central necrosis，formating of pseudogranuloma.

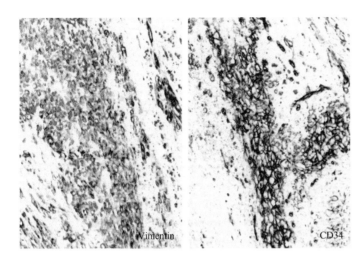

免疫组化，Vimentin和上皮标记物阳性，如CK8、 CK19和（或）EMA，半数病例免疫组化CD34阳性

Immunohistochemistry，Vimentin and epithelial markers were positive，such as CK8，CK19 and（or） EMA；half of the cases is CD34 positive.

5-29　透明细胞肉瘤 Clear cell sarcoma

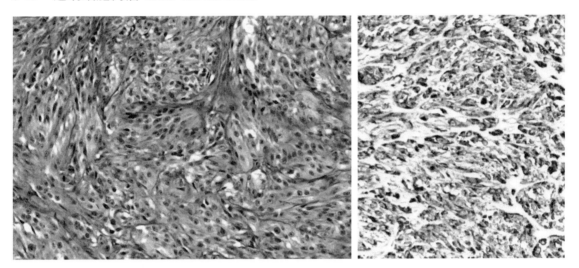

具有黑色素细胞分化特点的软组织肉瘤，肿瘤呈巢状或束状；瘤细胞为多角形或梭形，有丰富的嗜酸性或透明胞质；纤维组织间隔包绕肿瘤细胞巢。右图：免疫组化HMB45（＋）。

In soft tissue sarcoma with the characteristics of melanoma differentiation，the tumor cells were polygonal or spindle with abundant eosinophilic or clear cytoplasm，nests or fasciculate growth；the fibrous tissue interval is surrounding the tumor cell nests. Right picture：Immunohistochemistry，HMB45 is positive.

5-30 黏液瘤 Myxoma

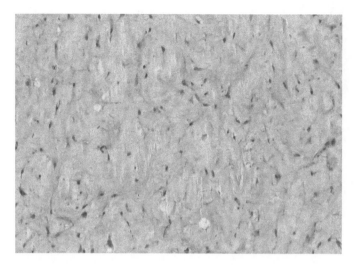

肿瘤由大量黏液、星芒状及梭形细胞构成，细胞境界不清，无多形性表现，亦无核分裂像。

Tumor is formed by much mucus, stellate and spindle-shaped cells, The cell boundaries are unclear, no polymorphous appearence, no mitotic figures.

各　论

第六章　心血管系统疾病
Chapter 6　Diseases of the Heart and Blood Vessels

6-1　冠状动脉粥样硬化 Coronary atherosclerosis

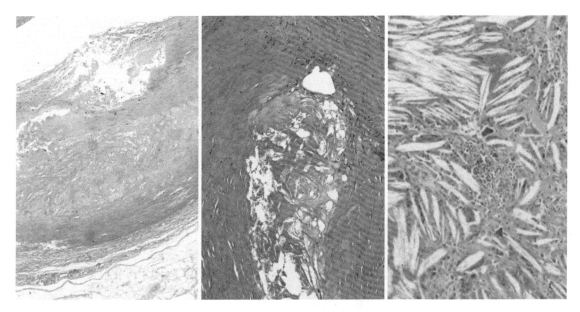

内膜损伤处为大量无定形的坏死崩解物质、细胞外脂质及胆固醇结晶，少量泡沫细胞和淋巴细胞浸润。内膜下胶原纤维玻璃样变性。

In endothelia injury，necrotic core contains numerous unstructured disintegrations，extracellular lipid and cholesterol clefs. Subendothelial collagenous fibers show hyaline degeneration.

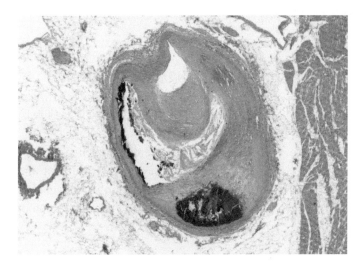

冠状动脉狭窄，内膜局灶性增厚形成纤维帽，胶原纤维玻璃样变，胆固醇结晶和钙盐沉着，其底部和边缘可见肉芽组织，外周有少量泡沫细胞和淋巴细胞浸润。中膜平滑肌萎缩变薄。

Coronary arteries stenosis，focal intima is thickened and forms a fibrous cap. There are collagenous fibers hyaline degeneration，cholesterol clefs and calcification. Graulation tissue is observed at the bottom and edge. Foam cells and lymphocytes infiltrate at periphery. Tunica media smooth muscle is atrophy.

6-2 心肌梗死 Myocardial infarction

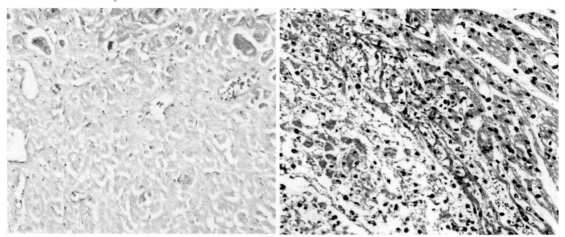

心肌梗死属凝固性坏死，肌原纤维及细胞核溶解消失。坏死心肌细胞核碎裂、胞浆凝固、颗粒样（左）。梗死灶边缘可见充血、出血及中性白细胞浸润。

Myocardial infarction belongs to coagulative necrosis, myofibril and nucleus dissolution and disappearance can be seen. The left inferior part of the photograph show necrotic cardiac muscle cells. The nuclei have fragmented and the cytoplasm is coagulated and granular. The margin of infarcts shows hemorrhage, hyperemia and infiltration of leukocytes.

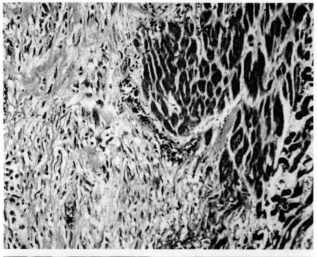

心肌梗死，纤维化（myocardial infarction and fibrosis）
心肌梗死机化阶段示心肌细胞消失，成纤维细胞增生。

Organizing stage of myocardial infarction reveals disappearance of muscle cells and proliferatin of fibroblasts.

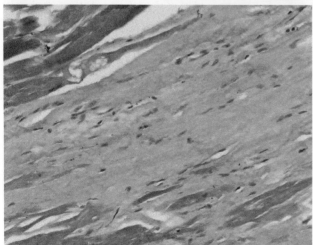

瘢痕形成（scar appears）
在心肌梗死病灶中其机化阶段示成纤维细胞增生，胶原纤维玻璃样变性。

In myocardial infarction forcal, the proliferation of fibroblast and hyaline degeneration of collagenous fibers are observed at organization of myocardial infarction.

6-3　高血压病 Hypertension

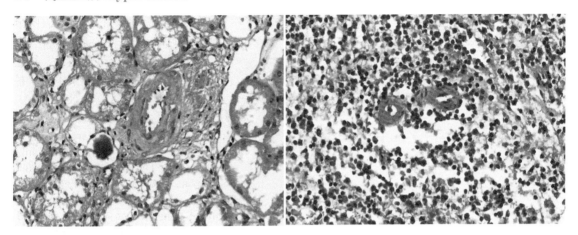

肾小球毛细血管和小动脉壁增厚、均匀红染无结构玻变，管腔狭窄甚至闭塞。

Glomeruli capillary and arteriolar wall are thickened, hyaline degeneration, with a homogenous pink unstructured appearance, cavity shows stenosis or even occlusion.

高血压肾小动脉管壁玻变（左）、脾小动脉玻变（右）。

Arterioles hyaline degeneration, kindney of hypertension（left）, spleen of hypertension（right）.

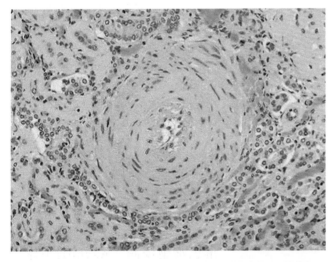

高血压性细小动脉硬化（hyperplastic arteriolosclerosis）

葱皮样血管壁常见于恶性高血压的细小动脉硬化中。

The arteriole has an "onion skin" appearance typical of malignant hyperplastic arteriolosclerosis.

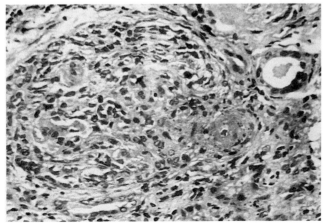

纤维素样坏死性小动脉（fibrinoid necrotizing arteriolitis）

多见于恶性高血压的肾脏小动脉。

Particularly in the kidney arteriole with malignant hypertension.

6-4 风湿性心脏病 Rheumatic heart disease

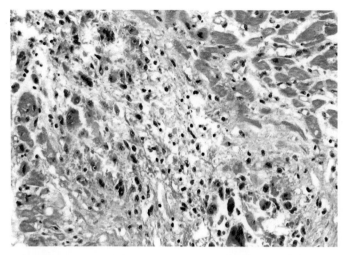

Aschoff细胞体积大，卵圆形或不规则，胞浆丰富，嗜碱性，颗粒状。核大，圆形或椭圆形，核膜厚、清晰，染色质集中于中央，核的横切面似枭眼状（枭眼细胞），纵切面呈毛虫状（毛虫细胞）。

Aschoff cells are large, oval or irregular, and have granular basophilic cytoplasm. The nucleus is big, round or oval, and the nuclear membrane is thick, clear, chromatin accumulating in the centre. Cross section shows owl-eyed shape, vertical section shows caterpillar nucleus.

风湿性心内膜炎（rheumatic endocarditis）

心瓣膜上赘生物由血小板和纤维素构成，病变瓣膜伴小灶状的纤维素样坏死。其周围可出现少量的Aschoff细胞。

Cardiac valve vegetations are composed of platelets and fibrin, the valve is accompanied with focal fibrinoid necrosis, with few Aschoff cells around.

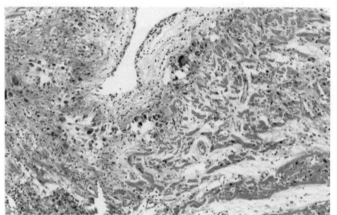

风湿性心肌炎（rheumatic myocarditis）

病变心肌间质水肿，在间质血管附近可见Aschoff小体和少量淋巴细胞浸润。Aschoff小体呈卵圆形或梭形结节，中央为纤维素样坏死，胶原纤维肿胀崩解。Aschoff细胞围绕坏死周围。

Myocardial stroma shows edema, Aschoff body around the stromal vessels and some lymphocytes infiltration. The Aschoff body is an oval or spindle nodule, central areas show fibrinoid necrosis, collagen fibers swelling and disintegration. Aschoff cells are around the necrotic areas.

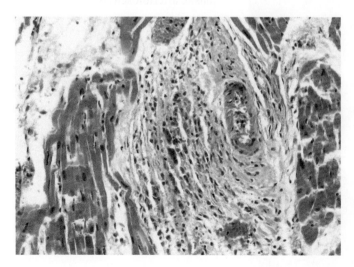

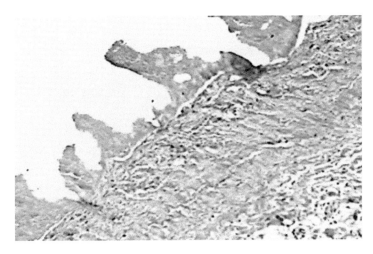

风湿性心外膜炎（rheumatic pericarditis）

镜下为纤维素性或浆液纤维素性炎。可导致心包腔局部纤维素性粘连或完全闭锁（肉眼绒毛心）。

It is a fibrinous or serofibrinous inflammation，which may lead to fibrous adhesions with partial or complete obliterations of the pericardial cavity（corvillosum grossly）.

6-5　感染性心内膜炎 Infective endocarditis

亚急性细菌性心内膜炎（subacute bacterial endocarditis，SBE）

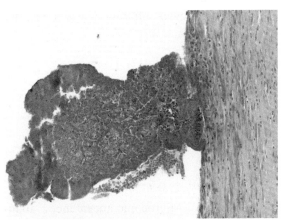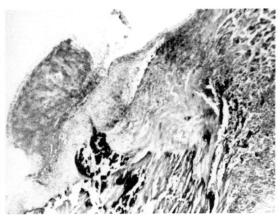

病变瓣膜上见赘生物。赘生物由血小板、纤维蛋白、细菌菌落、坏死组织、中性粒细胞组成，赘生物底部见风湿病背景及少量淋巴细胞和单核细胞浸润（左）。已发生钙化和纤维化的瓣膜表面见小赘生物（右）。

Vegetation is seen in the injured valve. The vegetation is composed of platelets，fibrin，bacterial colonies，tissue necrosis and neutrophil cells. At the bottom of the vegetation rheumatism background，lymphocytes and monocytes infiltrations are seen（left）. Small vegetation is noted on the valvular surface occurred in calcified and fibrotic valve（right）.

6-6 病毒性心肌炎 Viral myocarditis

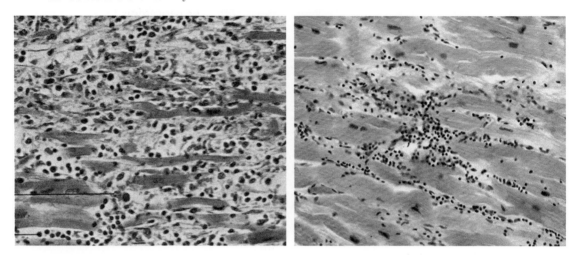

其特征为心肌间质中单核细胞和淋巴细胞浸润，伴灶性坏死。

The interstitial mononuclear inflammatory cells and lymphocytes infiltration shown here are characteristic with focus necrosis.

6-7 心脏黏液瘤 Cardiac myxoma

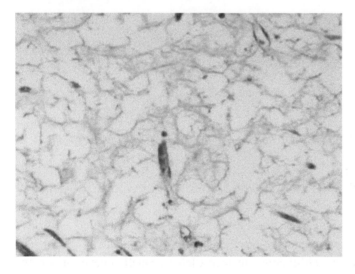

镜下大量无定型的细胞外基质中弥散分布黏液瘤细胞。

Microcopic appearance, abundant amorphous extracellular matrix, in which are scattered myxoma cells.

第七章 口腔及头面部疾病
Chapter 7 The Oral Cavity and Head Facial Diseases

7-1 口腔黏膜白斑 Leukoplakia，oral cavity

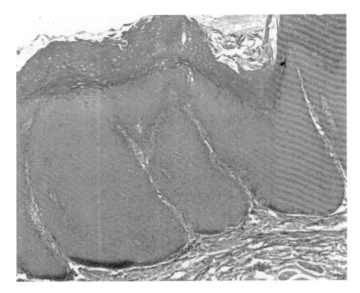

上皮全层增厚，主要为棘细胞层增生，表层呈过度不全角化，钉突整齐增粗，基底膜清晰，固有层少量炎症细胞。

The whole layer of epithelial is thickening, mainly acanthosis, surface hyperkeratosis, clear basement membrane and epithial foot flattening, a small amount of inflammatory cells in the lamina propria.

7-2 口腔扁平苔藓 Lichen planus，oral cavity

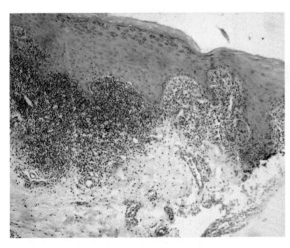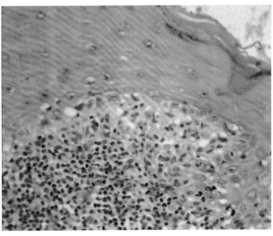

低倍见上皮不全角化或无角化，棘层增生，锯齿状钉突及固有层内有密集的淋巴细胞浸润带（左）；高倍示基底细胞液化，变性，以及黏膜固有层内圆形或卵圆形的胶样小体（右）。

Low magnification showed epithelia parakeratosis or unkeratosis, acanthosis, serrated spikes and dense lymphocytic infiltration in lamina propria.（left）

At high magnification showed liquifaction, degeneration of basal layer, round or oval colloid bodies in lamina propria.（right）

7-3 慢性盘状红斑狼疮 Chronic discoid lupus erythematosus

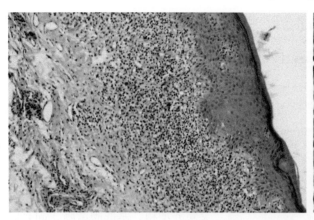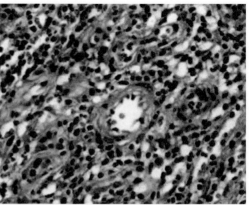

左：上皮表面过度角化及角质栓塞；上皮棘层萎缩变薄；钉突增生，不规则伸长；基底细胞液化变性，基底膜不清晰；固有层见淋巴细浸润，血管周可呈现袖套状。

右：毛细血管扩张、较多中性粒细胞、淋巴细胞、浆细胞浸润。

Left：The epithelial surface has hyperkeratosis and keratosis embolism；acanthocytes atrophy；epithelial ridge hyperplasia，irregular elongation；liquifaction degeneration of basal cells，and basement membrane is not clear；lymphocyte infiltration can be seen in lamina propria，even formed sleeve shape.

Right：Capillary telangiectasia，infiltration of many neutrophils，lymphocytes and plasma cells.

7-4 牙源性上皮囊肿 Odontogenic epithelial cyst

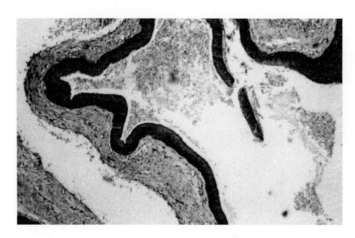

含牙囊肿（dentigerous cyst）

纤维性结缔组织囊壁内衬较薄的复层鳞状上皮，无角化，无上皮钉突，伴感染时上皮增生，见大量炎细胞浸润。

The cystic wall with fibrous connective tissue is lining with thin, stratified squamous epithelium, without keratosis, without epithelial ridge hyperplasia. When accompaning infection, it may stimulate the epithelial proliferation and a large number of inflammatory cells infiltration.

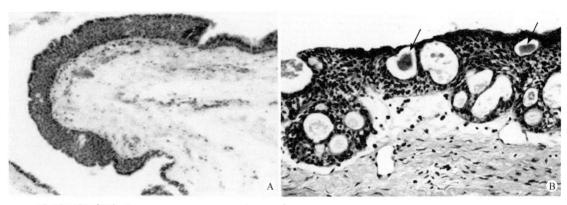

腺牙源性囊肿（glandular odontogenic cyst）

A：低倍示纤维结缔组织囊壁，衬里部分为复层鳞状上皮，并呈乳头状突向囊腔，其表层细胞嗜酸性立方或柱状，另部分无明显特征；B：高倍示衬里内隐窝或囊性小腔，内含黏液（箭头所示）。

A：Low magnification showed the cystic wall is one partial with fibrous connective tissue lining stratified squamous epithelium, and papillary growth protruding into the cystic cavity, the surface cells with eosinophilic cuboidal or columnar, the other part without obvious characteristics；B：High magnification shown in the crypt or cystic cavity contain mucus（↑）.

7-5 根尖周囊肿 Radicular cyst

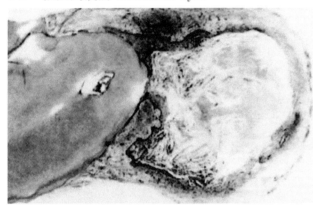

囊肿内壁衬以无角化的复层鳞状上皮，在其衬里上皮内可见大量弓形线状或环状的均质嗜伊红小体，此为透明小体（Rushton body）。

The cystic wall is lined with a non keratinized stratified squamous epithelium containing numerous arcuate, linear or ring-shaped homogeneous eosinophilic bodies, which is Rushton body.

7-6 血管性龈瘤 Vascular epulis

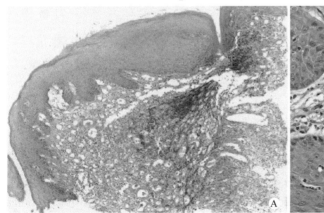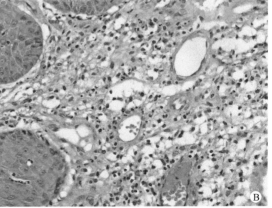

牙龈黏膜下方见炎性肉芽组织，由大量的薄壁血管和纤维组织构成，伴不同程度的炎症细胞浸润。

It can be seen that inflammatory granulation tissue under gingival mucosa, which composed of a large number of thin wall blood vessels and fibrous tissue, with varying degrees of inflammatory cells infiltration.

7-7　颗粒细胞瘤 Granular cell tumor

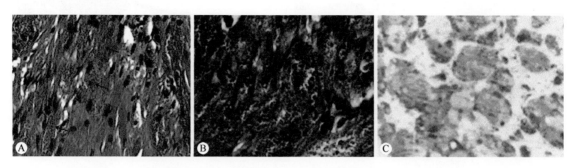

A：瘤细胞较大，圆形或多边形，界限不清，合胞体样，胞浆内含有大量均匀分布的嗜酸性颗粒（箭头所示）。B：肿瘤细胞内颗粒呈PAS阳性。C：颗粒细胞S-100蛋白弥漫性强阳性。

A：tumor cells is larger，round or polygon，unclear boundary，synplasmiod，the cytoplasm contains a large number of uniform distribution of eosinophilic granules（↑）. B：granules in tumor cells are positive for PAS. C：tumor cells are diffusely positive for S-100 protein.

7-8　成釉细胞瘤 Ameloblastoma

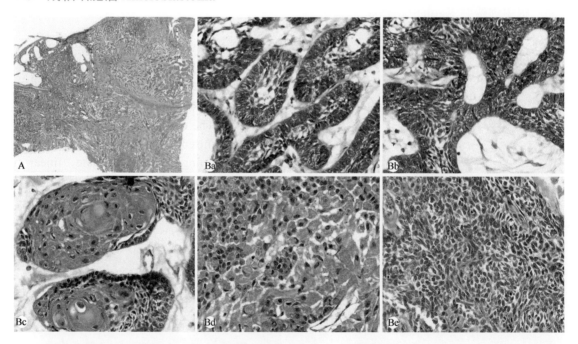

实性/多囊型成釉细胞瘤丛状为主型伴多种结构。

A为低倍视野（×40），示肿瘤细胞巢的多种排列方式混合存在。B为A图各局部的高倍视野，abcde分别为滤泡状结构区、丛状区、棘皮瘤区、颗粒细胞样结构区及基底细胞样结构区。

Solid / polycystic ameloblastoma is mainly clustered with many kinds of structures。

A：low magnification field（×40），showing tumor cell nests with multiple growth patterns. B：high magnification visual field of A，and abcde is follicular，plexiform，acanthosis，granular cells and basal cells like structure areas，respectively.

7-9　成釉细胞癌 Amelocarcinoma

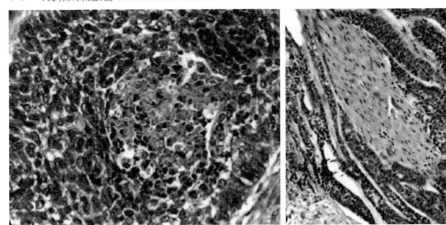

肿瘤实质排列似成釉细胞瘤结构，但见癌细胞多形、核深染及核分裂，癌巢中央见粉刺样坏死灶（左）。癌细胞包绕并浸润一中等大小的外周神经束（右）。

The parenchyma of the tumor is arranged in the shape of ameloblastoma, but the tumor cells are pleomorphic, dark stained and mitosis. Comedo necrosis exists in the central of cancer nests（left）; The cancer cells surround and infiltrate to a medium-sized peripheral nerve（right）.

7-10　牙源性钙化上皮瘤 Calcifying epithelial odontogenic tumor

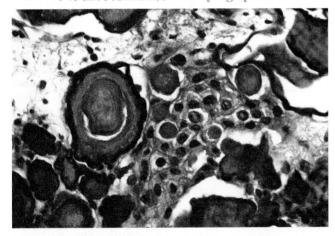

多边形嗜酸性上皮细胞，境界清楚，核大小不等，可见多核，但几乎无核分裂。间质极少。上皮团中出现淀粉样小体，伴发钙盐沉着构成砂粒体。

Polygonal eosinophilic epithelial cells with clear boundaries, unequal size of nuclear and polynuclei are seen, but almost without nuclear division. Interstitial is few. Amyloid granules appear in the epithelial masses, accompanied by calcium deposits, which constitute the so-called psammoma.

7-11　牙骨质纤维瘤 Cementifying fibroma

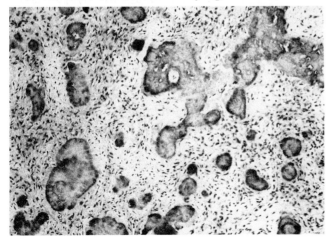

纤维瘤的背景中散在分布的不规则岛状牙骨质成分。

The irregular island cementum components scattered in the background of fibroma.

7-12 多形性腺瘤 Pleomorphic adenoma

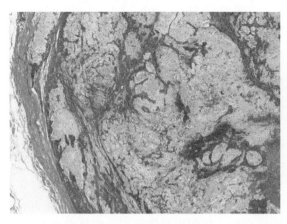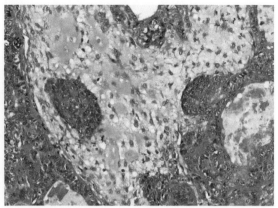

肿瘤由上皮和黏液软骨样基质组成。肿瘤上皮排列成片状、条索状，或导管样，或散在分布。导管样结构由腔面细胞和一些腔外的肌上皮细胞构成，导管腔内常含嗜伊红的分泌物。排成实性的肌上皮细胞团块中心可见鳞状细胞团（鳞化）。软骨样基质与黏液样组织相互移行，其中散在的上皮细胞周边有空晕似软骨细胞。

Tumor is composed of epithelium（epithelial and myoepithelial cells）and mucus-chondroid matrix. Tumor epithelial arranged in sheet，cords，or duct-like structures，or scattered distribution. The duct-like structures are composed of luminal cells and several abluminal layer of myoepithelial cells，the ducts often contain eosinophilic secretory material. Squamous cells mass（squamous metaplasia）can be seen in the center of myoepithelial cells mass. Chondroid matrix is continuing with myxoid matrix，presents scattered epithelial cells surrounded by halos like cartilage cells.

7-13 腺淋巴瘤（Warthin 瘤）Adenolymphoma（Warthin Tumour）

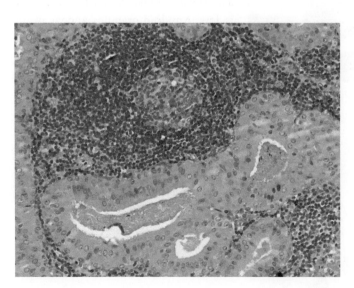

肿瘤由上皮和淋巴样组织组成。肿瘤上皮两层细胞排列成不规则的腺管及囊腔，腔面层为高柱状细胞栅栏状排列；基底层为立方形细胞。肿瘤间质中含密集的淋巴细胞，并有淋巴滤泡形成，也有肥大细胞和S-100蛋白阳性的树突细胞。

Tumor is composed of epithelial and lymphoid tissue. The two layer epithelium arranged to irregular glandular duct and cystic cavities.The cells of cavity surface are tall and columnar，palisadin arrangement. The basal layers are disorder flattened or cuboidal cells. The stroma contains intensive lymphocytes with lymphoid follicle formation，mast cells and S-100 positive dendritic cells.

7-14 嗜酸性腺瘤 Oxyphilic adenoma

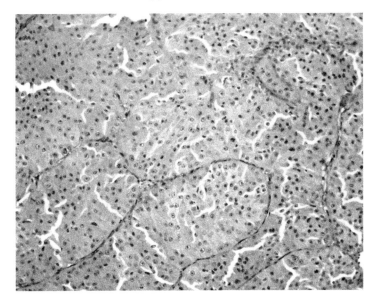

瘤细胞呈嗜酸性胞浆，核小居中。

The tumor cells were eosinophilic cytoplasm with small central nuclei.

7-15 黏液表皮样癌 Mucoepidermoid carcinoma

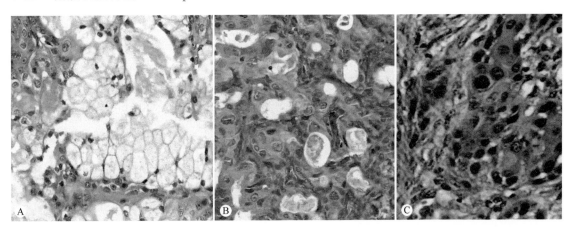

由表皮样细胞、中间细胞及黏液细胞构成。A：高分化型：黏液细胞占肿瘤细胞 50% 以上，并常形成腺腔及囊样腔隙；表皮样细胞成熟；中间细胞较少。B：中分化型：表皮样细胞、中间细胞与黏液细胞数量大致相等混合而成；瘤细胞有轻度异形性，偶见核分裂。C：低分化者：肿瘤主要以表皮样细胞和中间细胞构成；黏液细胞不足 10%；瘤细胞异型性明显，核分裂像多见。

It is composed of epidermoid cells, intermediate cells and mucus cells. A：Well differentiated：mucous cells account for over 50% of tumor cells, and often form lacuna lumens and cyst. Epidermoid cells are mature, and intermediate cells are less. B：Moderately differentiated：mixed with roughly equal number of epidermoid cells, intermediate cells and mucous cells. Tumor cells have mild atypia and occasionally mitosis. C：Low differentiationed：mainly composed of epidermoid cells and intermediate cells, mucous cells are less than 10% of the tumor cells, with obvious atypia and more nuclear mitosis.

7-16 腺样囊性癌 Adenoid cystic carcinoma

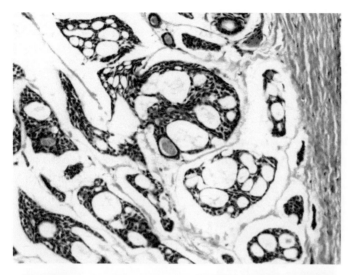

主要由导管细胞和变异的肌上皮细胞这两类细胞构成。瘤细胞似基底细胞，大小一致，圆形、卵圆形，核深染。按瘤细胞排列结构不同，该肿瘤可分成三型：腺样（筛状）型、小管型、实性或基底样型。

It consists of two main cell types: ductal epithelval cells and modified myoepithelial cellss. Tumor cells are similar to basal cells, same size, round or ovoid, nuclear hyperchromatism. According to the different cell structures, the tumor can be divided into three types: adenoid（cribriform）type, small tube type, and solid or basaloid type.

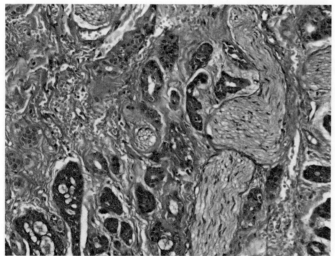

小管型腺样囊性癌伴神经浸润。

The figure showed a small tube type ACC with infiltrating nerve.

7-17 基底细胞腺瘤 Basal cell adenoma

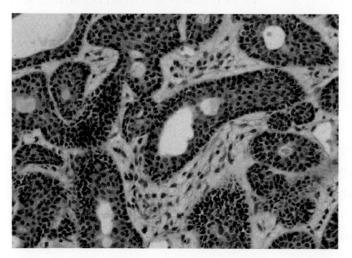

肿瘤由形态一致的立方或柱状基底样细胞构成，胞浆少，核圆形或卵圆形深染，可见核仁。

The tumor is composed of morphologically consistent cuboidal or columnar basaloid cells, with less cytoplasm, round or oval nuclei, and dark staining nucleoli.

7-18　肌上皮瘤 Myoepithelioma

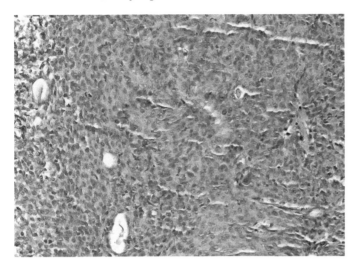

肿瘤性肌上皮细胞呈梭形细胞、上皮样细胞、浆细胞样细胞或透明变细胞，束状排列。

Neoplastic myoepithelial cells are long spindle, or epithelioid cells, or plasmacytoid cells, or hyaline degeneration cells, beam pattern.

7-19　上皮肌上皮癌 Epithelial-myoepithelial carcinoma

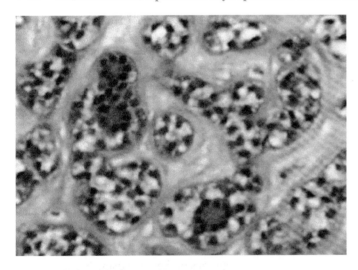

双层细胞常围成管样结构，内层为单层立方或矮柱状；外层为单或多层多角形细胞，细胞大，胞质透明状。

Double layer cells usually surrounded to form the tubular structures, the inner layer is single layer cubic or dwarf columnar, and the outer layer is single or multilayers polygonal cells. The cells are large with clear cytoplasm.

7-20　腺泡细胞癌 Acinic cell carcinoma

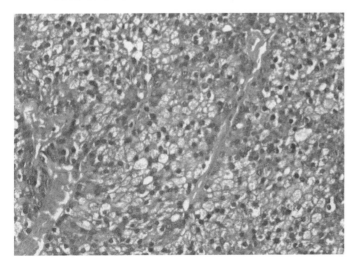

肿瘤细胞相似于正常腮腺的浆液细胞大圆细胞伴嗜碱性细颗粒状物（酶原颗粒），透明胞质，核居中或偏位，核仁不明显，核分裂像罕见。

The tumor cells are resemble normal serous cells of salivary gland. Large round cells with basophilic fine granules（zymogen granules）clear cytoplasm, and nuclei centered or biased, the nucleoli are not prominent, and the mitosis is rare.

7-21　鼻息肉 Nasal polyp

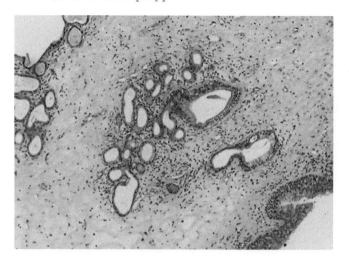

可见大量炎症细胞，黏液浆液腺增生，间质水肿。

It can be seen that a large number of inflammatory cells，the proliferation of mucus or serous glands，interstitial edema.

7-22　鼻血管瘤 Nasal hemangioma

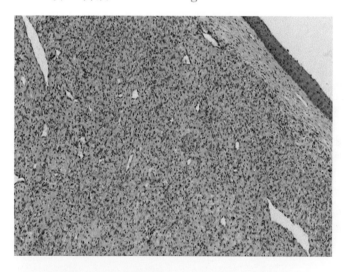

鼻腔毛细血管瘤（capillary hemangioma）

鼻腔血管瘤以毛细血管瘤最多，其次是海绵状、静脉性血管瘤、血管内皮细胞瘤、血管瘤病。毛细血管瘤由管径一致的、较小的小动脉构成。

Capillary hemangioma is the most common type of nasal hemangioma followed by the cavernous hemangioma，vein hemangioma，vascular endothelial hemangioma，angiomatosis. Capillary hemangioma is composed of smaller arteries of the same diameter.

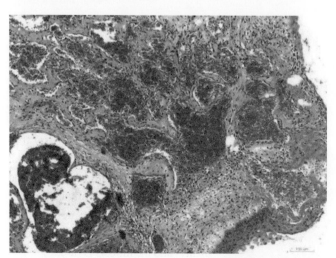

海绵状血管瘤（cavernous hemangioma）

由囊性扩张的薄壁血管构成，在扩张的血管内，有时可有血栓形成，或机化，或钙化而形成静脉石。

It is composed by cyst-dilated thin-walled blood vessels. In the dilated blood vessels，sometimes thrombosis，or organization，or calcification forms phlebolith.

7-23 鼻咽纤维瘤 Nasopharyngeal fibroma

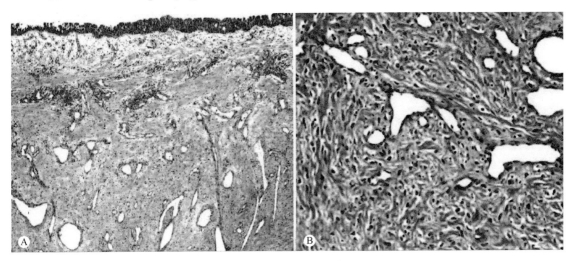

A：完整的呼吸道上皮覆盖于富含血管的瘤体表面，肿瘤内有大小不等的血管，血管由含胶原的细胞性成纤维间质所包绕；B：密集的瘢痕瘤样胶原包绕薄壁血管，可见星状成纤维细胞。

A：The tumor surface with rich blood vessels is coveraged with the complete respiratory epithelial，unequal blood vessels is surrounded by fibroblasts or collagen in the tumor；B：Dense keloid collagen wrapped around thin-walled vessels，with visible stellate fibroblasts.

7-24 鼻咽癌 Nasopharyngeal carcinoma

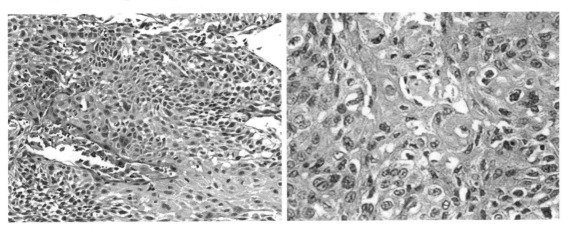

角化型鳞状细胞癌（keratinizing squamous cell carcinoma）
肿瘤细胞相互衔接呈片状、巢状排列，肿瘤细胞有明显的细胞间桥和鳞状细胞分化，后者包括细胞外角化、细胞内胞浆粉染。
The tumor cells are opposed to one another in a "mosaic tile" in sheets and nests with histologic evidence of intercellular bridges and squamous differentiation in the form of extracellular keratin or intracellular pink cytoplasm.

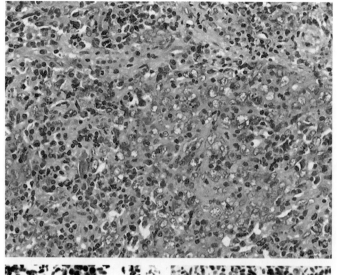

非角化性分化型癌（nonkerati-nizing differentiated carcinoma）

肿瘤细胞被纤维结缔组织分隔，呈巢状排列，其中可见散在淋巴细胞。肿瘤细胞胞浆粉染，无明显角化和细胞间桥。

The tumor is arranged in nests, separated by fibrous connective tissue, and admixed. with numerous small lymphocytes. The neoplastic cells have pink cytoplasm and unde-tecble keratinization and intercellular bridges.

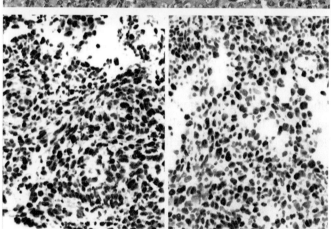

原位杂交结果显示EB病毒阳性，免疫组化结果显示鳞状细胞癌标记P40阳性。

Hybridization *in situ* is positive for EBV. Immunohistochemistry is positive for P40, a marker of squmous cell carcinoma.

7-25 低分化鼻咽癌（淋巴上皮癌）Lower differentiation nasopharyngeal carcinoma（Lymphoepithelioma）

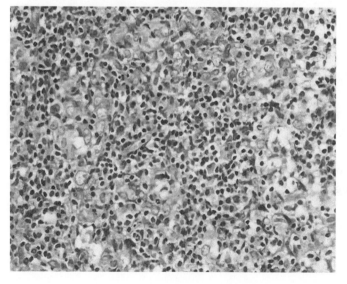

属于低分化鳞癌的一种类型，癌细胞胞质丰富，境界不清合体状。细胞核大，圆形或卵圆形，空泡状，有大而明显的核仁，又称泡状核细胞癌。瘤细胞排列密集甚至重叠。间有淋巴细胞浸润。所以称为"淋巴上皮癌"。

One of the poorly differentiated squamous cell carcinoma. Outline of cancer cell is not clear but confused with plenty cytoplasm. Nucleus is large, round or oval, vesicular, with large and prominent nucleoli（vesicular nucleus cell carcinoma）. Tumor cells are arranged densely even overlap with lymphocytic infiltration so that called as lymphoepithelioma.

7-26 颈部淋巴结鼻咽癌转移 Nasopharyngeal carcinoma metastasis，neck lymph node

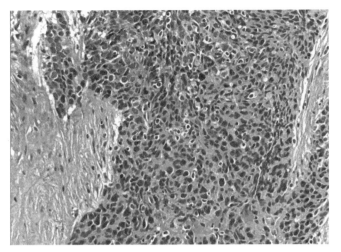

淋巴结被膜增厚，被膜下可见转移的鼻咽癌细胞癌细胞胞浆粉染，无明显角化和细胞间桥。

The capsule of lymph node is thickened. The nest of nasopharyngeal cancer cells visible under the capsule. The cancer cells have rich cytoplasm with pink staining and inconspicuous keratinization and intercellular bridges.

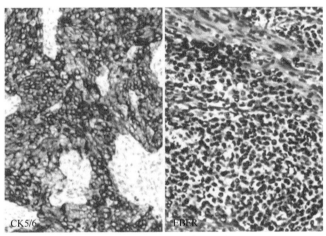

CK5/6   EBER

免疫组化结果显示鳞状细胞癌特异性标记CK5/6阳性，鼻咽癌常用标记EBER阳性.

Immunohistochemistry is positive for CK5/6, a specific marker of squamous cell carcinoma and EBER usually used in nasopharyngeal carcinoma.

7-27 鼻嗅神经母细胞瘤 Olfactory neuroblastoma，nasal

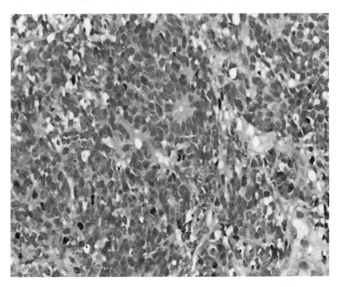

肿瘤被纤维血管间隔分隔成小叶状。一个大的假菊形团显示其中央的神经原纤维基质。

The tumor lobule is divided by the fibrovascular septum. A large pseudorosettes mass shows its central neurons fiber matrix.

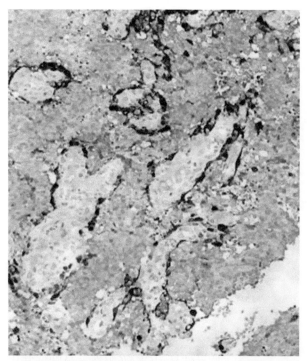

免疫染色显示癌巢S-100蛋白阳性的支持细胞围绕肿瘤癌巢的特征性形态。

Immunostaining revealed the characteristic morphology of S-100 protein positive supporting cells surround the tumor nests.

7-28 外耳道鳞状细胞乳头状瘤 Squamous cell papilloma, external auditory canal

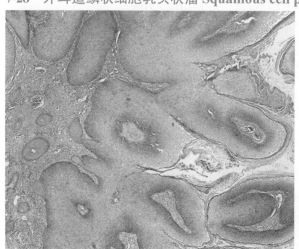

被覆鳞状上皮及间质增生，并向表面呈乳头状突起，表层细胞呈角化过度及角化不全，透明细胞层常明显可见，细胞大而圆，多呈空泡状。

Squamous epithelium and interstitial hyperplasia, and papillary projections to the surface. The surface cells are hyperkeratosis and hypokeratosis, and transparent cell layer is often visible, large and round cells, mostly in a vacuolar shape.

7-29 耵聍腺腺瘤 Ceruminoma

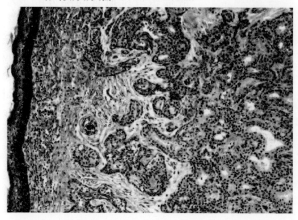

鳞状上皮下肿瘤界限清楚但无包膜，注意腺样及小囊性结构。

Under squamous epithelium, tumor is with well-defined margins but no envelope, noting glandular and small cystiod structures.

7-30 耵聍腺癌 Adenocarcinonma，ceruminous glands

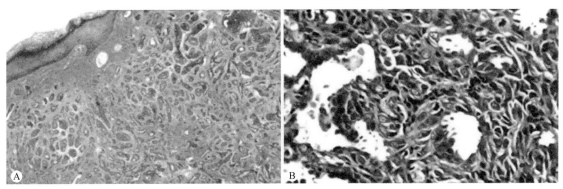

　　A. 完整的表面上皮下可见致密纤维中"双相性"分化的肿瘤浸润。B. 显示中央腺体的顶浆分泌，同时在"浸润性"生长方式中可见显著的不典型细胞。

　　A. Biphasic differentiated tumor with dense fiber invasion is seen under the intact surface epithelum； B. shows apocrine secretion of the central gland，while significant atypical cells are seen in the "invasive" mode of growth.

7-31 副神经节瘤 Paraganglioma

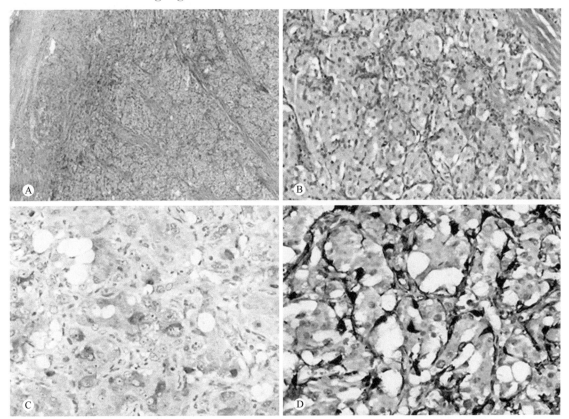

　　A，B：肿瘤由主细胞和支持细胞构成纤细的纤维血管间质分隔成境界清楚的巢状或腺泡状结构。肿瘤细胞含有细颗粒和嗜碱或嗜酸性的胞质；C：瘤细胞CgA阳性；D：支持细胞S-100阳性。

　　A，B：Tumor is composed of chief cells and supporting cells. Well-defined nests or acinaroid structures is divided by a delicate fibrovascular stroma（zellballen）.Tumor cells have a finely granular and basophilic or eosinophilic cytoplasm；C：Tumor cells are positive for CgA；D：Supporting cells are positive for S-100.

7-32 中耳血管球瘤 Glomus tumor，middle ear

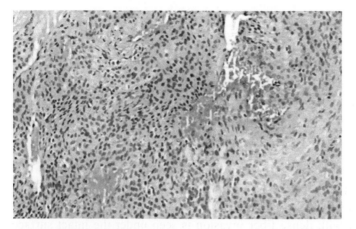

血管周围可见大量上皮样细胞呈巢状或条索状排列。

A large number of perivascular epithelioid cells with nests or cords patterns.

7-33 睑板腺腺癌 Adenocarcinoma，meibomian gland

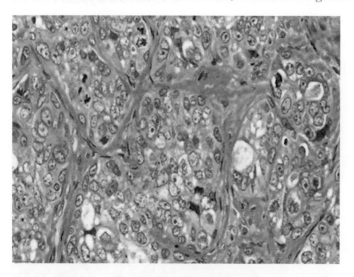

该肿瘤具有皮脂腺癌的特点，由泡沫状或透明状多形性皮脂腺细胞组成小叶状细胞巢，癌细胞脂肪染色阳性。个别癌细胞可浸润皮肤表皮形成Pagetiod现象。也可呈基底细胞型或梭形细胞型。

It is characterized of sebaceous carcinoma. Lobular cell nests composed of foamy or clear pleomorphic sebaceous cells，cancer cells positive staining for fatty. Individual cancer cell can infiltrate the epidermis of skin，forming Pagetiod phenomenon，or basal cell or spindle cell types.

7-34 视网膜母细胞瘤 Retinoblastoma

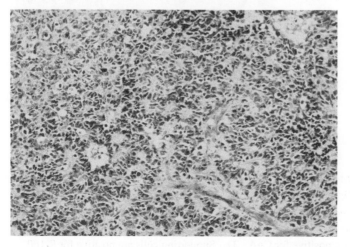

小圆细胞巢，高染色质的核，胞质少，大量瘤细胞形成菊形团。

The tumor is composed of small round cell nests with hyperchromatic nuclei and scantly cytoplasm. Tumor cells arranged cocentrically to many rosettes.

第八章 肺、胸膜和纵隔的疾病
Chapter 8 Diseases of the Lung, Pleural and Mediastinum

8-1 支气管肺隔离症 Bronchopulmonary sequestration

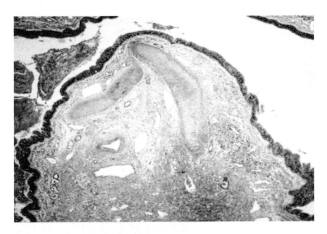

叶外型肺隔离症（extralobar seque-stration）

支气管被覆假复层纤毛柱状上皮，周围是纤维肌性管壁，内含有软骨板。

The bronchial with the coating pseudostratified ciliated columnar epithelium is surrounded by fibromuscular septum, which containing cartilage.

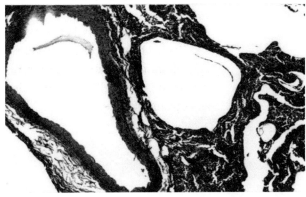

叶内型肺隔离症（intralobar seque-stration）

肺实质内可见硬化和囊性区，有动脉直接进入病变部位。囊性扩张的细支气管伴有肺组织炎症、纤维化。

There is a sclerosing and cystic area in the lung parenchyma, and the arteries enter the lesion directly. Cystic dilatation of the terminal bronchioles accompanied by inflammation and fibrosis of the lung.

8-2 支气管源性囊肿 Bronchogenic cysts

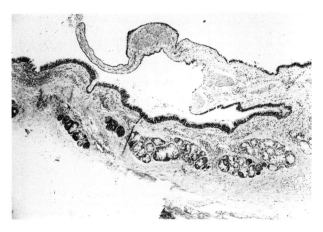

囊壁内衬假复层纤毛上皮细胞，外层为结缔组织、平滑肌纤维、黏液腺、软骨等。

The cystic wall is lined with pseudostratified ciliated columnar epithelium with connective tissue, smooth muscle bundles, mucous glands and cartilage and so on.

8-3 慢性支气管炎 Chronic bronchitis

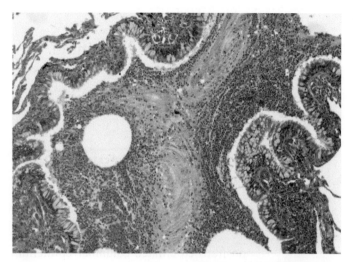

（1）支气管和细支气管的管壁增厚伴平滑肌束增生、肥大，支气管周围肺泡间质软骨变性、萎缩；慢性炎细胞浸润。

The wall of the bronchi and bronchioles are thickened and accompanied by smooth muscle hyperplasia, hypertrophy, cartilage can show degeneration, atrophy between peribronchial alveolar interstitium there is chronic inflammatory cell infiltration.

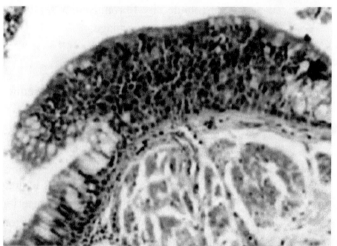

（2）部分支气管纤毛柱状上皮变性、坏死脱落，再生的上皮杯状细胞增多，并发生鳞状上皮化生。

Partial bronchial ciliated columnar epithelium degeneration, necrosis, increased goblet cells in regeneration and squamous metaplasia.

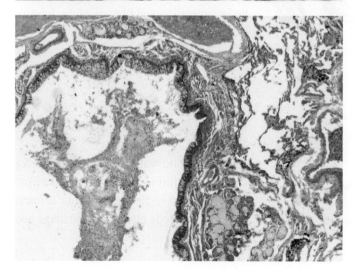

（3）黏膜下腺体增生肥大和浆液性腺上皮发生黏液腺化生。

Under mucosa, the glands occur hypertrophy and hyperplasia and serous epithelial occur mucous metaplasia.

8-4　支气管扩张 Bronchiectasis

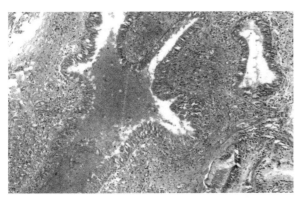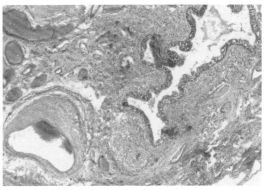

　　支气管扩张，管壁增厚，黏膜上皮增生伴鳞化，可有糜烂及小溃疡形成。黏膜下血管扩张充血，淋巴细胞、浆细胞或中性粒细胞浸润，管壁腺体、平滑肌、弹力纤维和软骨不同程度损伤，代之以肉芽组织或纤维组织。邻近肺组织常发生纤维化或肺气肿。

The bronchus shows dilation，the wall is thickened obviously，and the mucosal epithelial cells show proliferation with squamous metaplasia，erosion and small ulcers may form. Vessels under mucous show dilation and hyperemia，with inflammation of lymphocyte，plasma cell or even neutrophils. Glands，smooth muscle，elastic fibers and cartilage in the wall show various degrees of destruction，replaced by granulation tissue or fibrous tissue. Adjacent lung tissues often show fibrosis or emphysema.

8-5　肺气肿 Emphysema

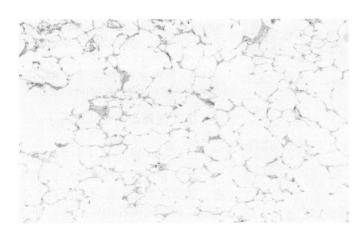

　　肺泡扩张，间隔变窄，肺泡间孔扩大，部分肺泡间隔断裂，扩张的肺泡可融合成大囊腔，肺毛细血管床明显减少。间质内肺小动脉内膜纤维性增厚。

　　Alveolar dilates，septum narrows，alveolar hole dilates，and some alveolar septums rupture，the dilated alveolar can be confluent to a large cavity，pulmonary capillary is significantly reduced. Pulmonary arteriloe tunica intima in stroma shows fibrous thickened.

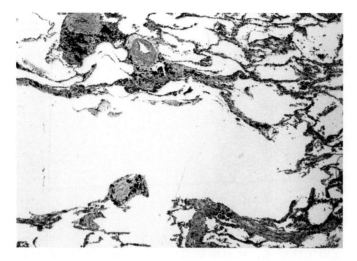

肺气肿和肺大泡（emphysema and bulla）

肺泡间隔破坏、纤维化。

The alveolar septa rupture and fibrosis.

8-6 肺炎 Pneumonia

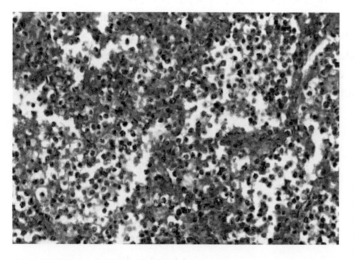

大叶性肺炎（lobar pneumonia）

大叶性肺炎灰肝期，扩张的肺泡腔内充满纤维素互相连接成网，并经肺泡间孔到达相邻肺泡，在纤维素网中有大量中性粒细胞和少量的巨噬细胞，少量红细胞，肺泡壁毛细血管受压。

Lobar pneumonia, gray hepatization. The alveolar spaces are distended and there is consolidation by a chumping of fribin, passing through the Gohn's pores, with a large amount of neutrophils, but fewer macrophages and red blood cells in the fibrin network. The alveolar wall capillary is oppressed.

小叶性肺炎（lobular pneumonia）

以细支气管为中心，管腔及其周围肺泡腔内出现较多的中性粒细胞、少量红细胞及脱落的肺泡上皮细胞。病灶周围肺泡壁毛细血管充血，可有浆液渗出，部分肺泡过度扩张。肺泡结构尚存。

Bronchioles are in the center of lesions, many neutrophils, fewer red blood cells and shedding alveolar epithelial cells are observed in the bronchiolar cavities and alveolar spaces around. Alveolar wall capillary shows hyperemia with serous exudates, some alveolar overexpansion. Alveolar structure is preserved.

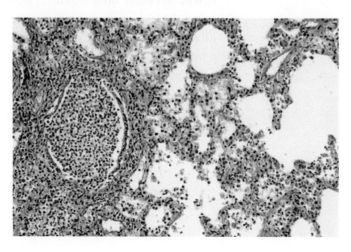

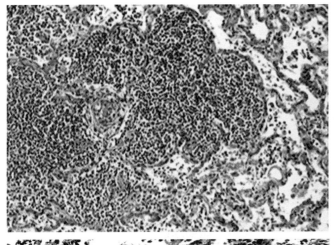

小叶性融合性肺炎（confluent lobular pneumonia）

在以细支气管为中心的小叶性肺炎病变的基础上，病灶相互融合形成大片融合性改变，以中性粒细胞渗出为主。

On the basis of lobular pneumonia（bronchioles at the center of lesions）, the lesion merge to form large fusion changes, mainly with neutrophils exudation.

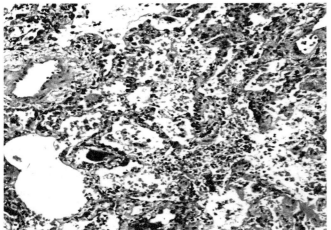

病毒性肺炎（麻疹病毒）[viral pneumonia（measles virus）]

可见巨细胞和间质炎症。肺泡中充满渗出物和新鲜出血。

Giant cells and interstitial inflammatin are seen. The alveolar spaces are filled with excudate and fresh hemorrage.

巨细胞病毒性肺炎［cytomegalovirus（CMV）pneumonitis］

为少见的一种间质性肺炎，表现为肺泡间隔明显增宽，血管扩张、充血，间质水肿及多核巨细胞（其中可见巨细胞病毒包涵体）与其他炎症细胞，包括淋巴细胞、单核细胞浸润，肺泡腔内一般无渗出物或仅有少量浆液。

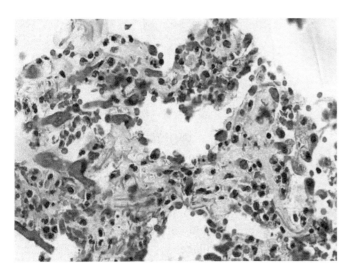

One rare form of interstitial pneumonia, shows significantly widened alveolar septa, vascular dilation, hyperemia, interstitial edema and polynuclear giant cells with CMV inclusions, and other inflammatory cells, including lymphocytes, mononuclear cell infiltration, alveolar spaces generally shows no exudation or only a small amount of serous exudation.

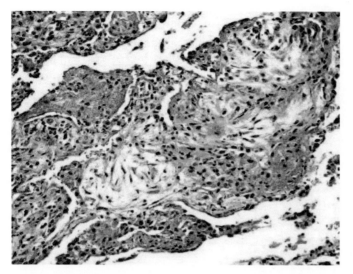

机化性肺炎（organized pneumonia）

肺泡腔内增生的纤维母细胞/肌纤维母细胞灶通过肺泡间孔从一个肺泡到邻近的肺泡形成蝴蝶样的结构。

In the alveoli the fibroblasts/myofibroblasts proliferated from alveolar to adjacent alveoli through alveolar pores to form a butterfly like structure.

8-7　肺肉质变（机化）Carnification（Organization），lung

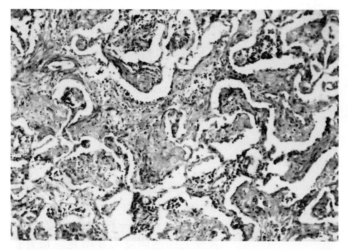

光镜下渗出的纤维蛋白被肉芽组织取代而机化——肺肉质变。

Microscopically, the fibrinous exudate is organized by granulation tissue, which is pulmonary carnification.

8-8　硅肺 Silicosis

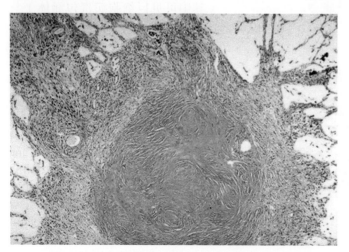

肺中硅结节（silicotic nodule in lung）

结节由间隔排列的粉染胶原纤维束组成。

A silicotic nodule is composed mainly of bundles of interlacing pink collagen.

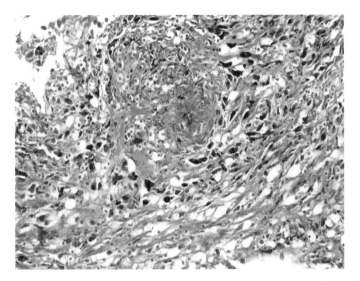

硅结节形成的初始阶段是由吞噬硅尘的巨噬细胞聚集组成的细胞性结节，以后纤维化。由粉染胶原纤维束呈同心圆状排列。结节中央也可见到异常小血管（管壁增厚、管腔狭窄）。

The initial stage of the silicon nodules formation is due to the silica dust phagocyted by macrophage cell. Then later becomes fibrotic nodules. Concentric arrangement of the eosinophilic collagen fibers，abnormal small blood vessel can also be seen in the nodules center（wall thickened，the cavity stenosis）.

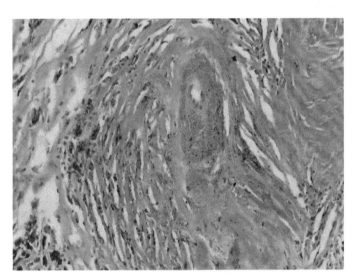

肺组织中见大小不等的硅结节，结节内可见玻变的胶原纤维呈同心圆或旋涡状排列；硅结节周围可见碳末沉积及巨噬细胞浸润；结节中央也可见到异常小血管。相邻的硅结节可以融合形成大的结节状病灶。

Silicon nodules of varying sizes are shown in the lung tissue，the hyaline collagen fibers are concentric or spiral-shaped arranged in the nodules；coal dust deposition and macrophage infiltration can be seen around silicon nodules；abnormal small blood vessels can also be seen in the center. Adjacent silicon nodules can fuse to form large nodular lesions.

8-9　肺石棉沉着病 Asbestosis，lung

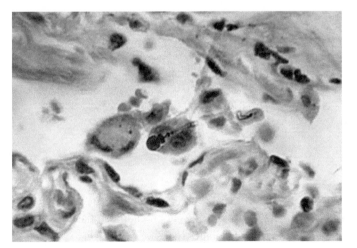

石棉小体（asbestos body）

图中见巨噬细胞吞入了石棉小体，但不能将其消化分解。这在其致病性中起主要作用。

Asbestos bodies are engulfed by macrophages，macrophages are unable to dispose of them. Failure of macrophages to dispose of asbestos fibers plays a major role in their pathogenicity.

8-10 肺透明膜病 Hyaline membrane disease，lung

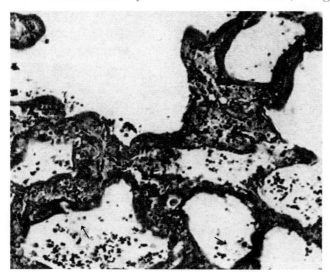

有些肺泡萎陷，有些扩张，许多肺泡壁衬有粉红色透明膜（箭头所示）。

Some alveoli are collapsed，other are ditended. Many alvedar walls are lined by bright pink hyaline membrane（arrows）.

8-11 支气管乳头状瘤 Bronchial papilloma

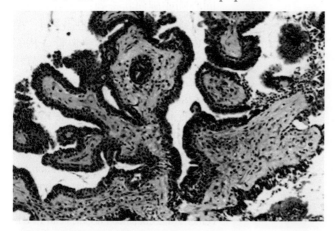

瘤组织呈乳头状结构，由上皮组织构成，以纤维血管为轴心。

The tumor tissue is papillary and consists of epithelial tissue with fibrovascular axis.

8-12 肺错构瘤 Hamartoma，lung

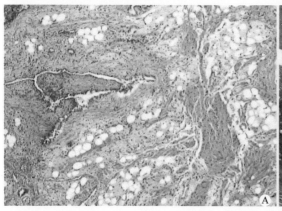
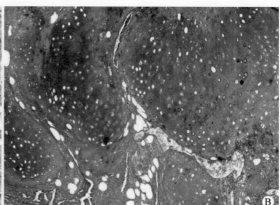

A：瘤组织主要为纤维、平滑肌和脂肪组织。B：肿瘤组织可由分化成熟的软骨组织构成。

A：The tumor tissues composed of mature fibers，smooth muscle and adipose tissue. B：The tumor tissue can be composed of differentiated and mature cartilage tissue.

8-13 炎性肌纤维母细胞瘤 Inflammatory myofibroblastic tumor

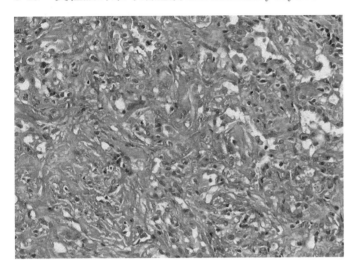

炎性肌纤维母细胞肿瘤是炎性假瘤的一个亚群，由胶原、炎细胞和在细胞学上常显示肌纤维母细胞分化的、温和的梭形细胞不等量混合而成。

It is a subgroup of inflammatory pseudotumor, it mixed with collagen, inflammatory cells, and well spindle cells from cytologically myofibroblasts differentiated.

8-14 支气管鳞化上皮和肺泡上皮不典型增生 Epithelial squamous metaplasia and dysplasia, bronchial and lung

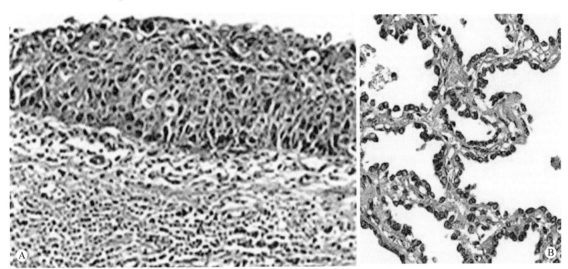

A：支气管鳞化上皮不典型增生和上皮内瘤变该分级类似宫颈上皮。

A：The grades of bronchial epithelial squamous metaplasia and dysplasia and intraepithelial lesion are similar to those of cervical epithelium.

B：肺泡由均匀一致核的柱状上皮内衬，细胞密度不高，无明显的不典型性，几乎没有病理性核分裂，病灶常小于5mm，呈多灶性。免疫组化显示CEA阴性或弱阳性，Ki67显示较低的增生活性。

B：The alveoli are lined by a uniform nuclear, brush like epithelium. The density of the cells is not high, and there is no significant atypical, almost no pathological mitosis. The lesions are usually less than 5mm and multifocal. Immunohistochemistry showed CEA negative or weakly positive, and Ki67 lower proliferative activity.

8-15 肺鳞癌 Squamous cell carcinoma，lung

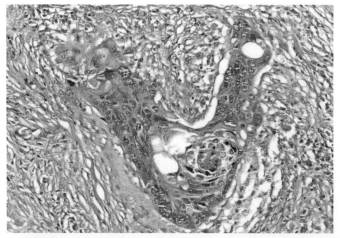

起源于鳞化的支气管上皮，多为中央型肺癌。肿瘤细胞胞浆丰富，红染；核大，深染，核仁明显，呈实性巢状分布。高分化时，角化和细胞间桥明显。

The tumor originates from bronchial epithelium of squamous metaplasia. Tumor cells are rich of cytoplasm with eosinophilic staining and atypically hyperchromatic nuclei with prominent nucleoli，and consist of sheets or nests. Keratin pearl formation and/or intercellular bridge are prominent in well-differentiated tumors.

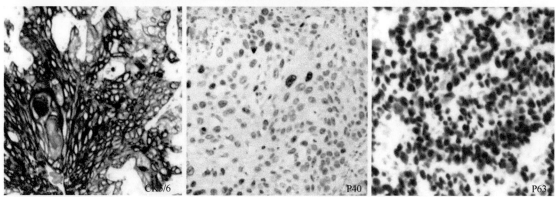

免疫组化结果显示鳞状细胞癌标记CK5/6和P40分别胞质和核阳性。P63核阳性。

Immunohistochemical result shows the marker of squamous cell carcinoma，CK5/6 is positive with cytoplasm and membranous staining pattern，P40 and P63 is positive with nuclear staining pattern.

8-16 肺腺癌 Adenocarcinoma，lung

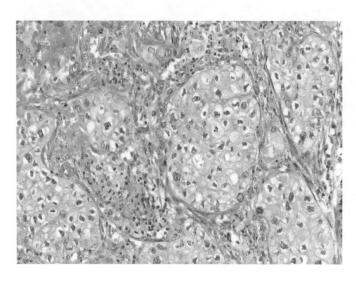

分化好的癌细胞呈腺样分化的特征，表现为癌细胞排列成管状、腺泡状，或乳头状，或有黏液分泌。分化差者，上述分化特征不明显，呈实性，可见细胞内黏液，或仅见小灶性腺样结构，腺癌的间质常有明显的促纤维结缔组织形成反应。

Well-differentiated cancer cells have features of adenoidal differentiation，the cancer cells differentiating into tubular，acinar，or papillary structures，or with mucus secretion. Poorly differentiated cells show solid，or only small focal gland-like structures. Adenocarcinoma stroma often shows significant desmorplastic reaction.

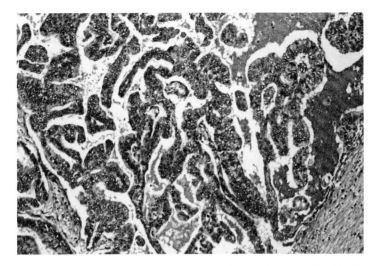

腺癌（adenocarcinoma）

切片显示腺体形成肿瘤，呈乳头样生长。

Glandiod structure with papillary grows pattern.

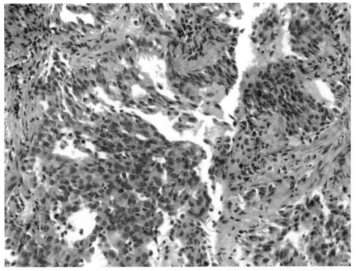

实体性腺癌（solid adenocarcinoma）

肿瘤细胞较大、多角形，实性片状排列，不形成腺泡、乳头、微乳头、贴壁等结构。

Large and polygonal tumor cells consist of sheets or solid, without acinar, papillary, micropapillary adherent and other structures.

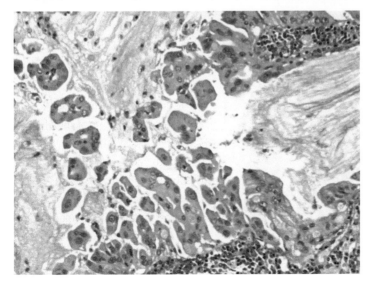

黏液腺癌（mucinous adenocarcinoma）

肿瘤中含有大量的黏液肿瘤细胞漂浮在黏液中。肿瘤细胞似杯状细胞或柱状细胞形态。

Tumor contains amount of mucin. Tumor cells resemble goblet cells or columnar cells, floating in mucin.

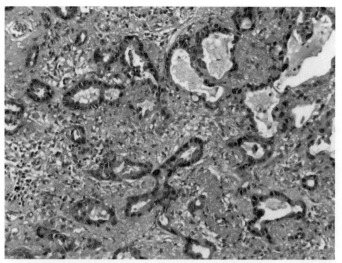

腺泡型腺癌（acinar adenocarcinoma）

肿瘤细胞在纤维间质中形成不规则圆形-椭圆形腺体结构，肿瘤细胞核大、深染，肿瘤细胞或腺腔内含有黏液。

Tumor cells form irregularly round to oval-shaped glands with malignant cytology exhibiting hyperchromatic nuclei in fibrous stroma. Neoplastic cells or glandular spaces contain mucin.

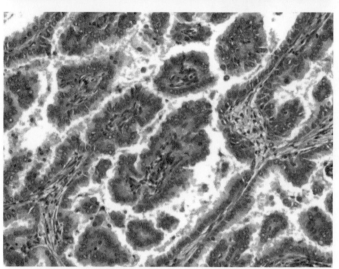

乳头型腺癌（papillary adenocarcinoma）

肿瘤细胞具有以纤维血管为轴心的乳头结构，原有的肺泡结构被复杂的二级、三级乳头状结构所取代。

Malignant cuboidal to columnar tumor cells grows on the surface of fibrovascular cores. The secondary and teritary papillary structures replace the underlying lung tissue.

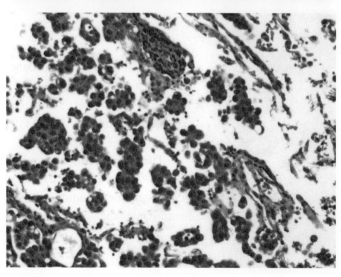

微乳头型腺癌（micropapillary adenocarcinoma）

肿瘤细胞排列成乳头状，乳头无纤维血管轴心，有时乳头似癌巢漂浮在肺泡腔内。

Tumor cells grows in papillary tufts lacking fibrovascular cores. Sometimes papillary tufts resemble cancer nest float within alveolar spaces.

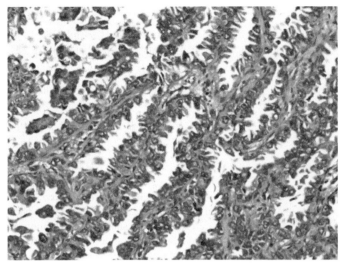

贴壁型腺癌（lepidic adenocarcinoma）

肿瘤细胞沿着尚存的肺泡结构生长，间质增宽伴有硬化，肿瘤细胞核大、深染，异型性明显，并有间质浸润。

Tumor cells grow along the pre-exsiting alveolar structure, accompanied by septal widening with sclerosis. Tumor cells are atypically hyperchromatic nuclei and prominent nucleoli with stromal invasion.

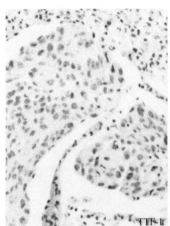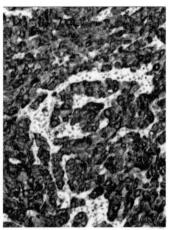

免疫组化结果显示TTF-1和CK7阳性。

Immunohistochemical results show TTF-1 and CK7 positive with nuclear and cytoplasm staining pattern respectively.

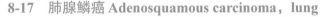

8-17 肺腺鳞癌 Adenosquamous carcinoma，lung

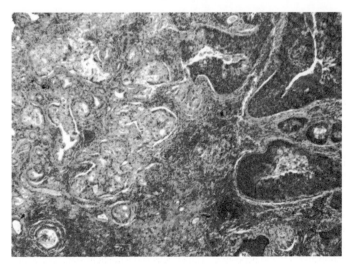

肿瘤由两种细胞成分组成，一种为排列成不规则腺样结构的上皮细胞（左侧），另一种为排列成巢状的具有鳞样分化的上皮细胞（右侧）。

The tumor is composed of two kinds of cell components, one kind of epithelial cells are arranged in irregular glandular structures（left）and the other kind of epithelial cells are arranged in nests with squamous differentiation（right）.

8-18 肉瘤样癌 Sarcomatoid carcinoma

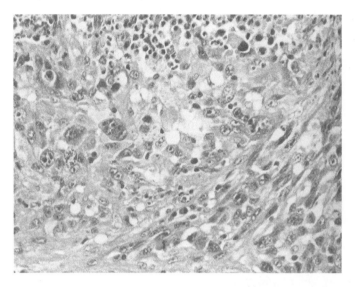

这是一组分化差的含梭形和（或）巨细胞分化的非小细胞癌，缺乏腺样或鳞状分化。目前有5种亚型代表其形态学谱系：多形性细胞癌、梭形细胞癌、巨细胞癌、肉瘤样癌、肺母细胞瘤。肺母细胞瘤除了癌的成分外还含有异源性肉瘤样成分，如恶性骨、软骨、甚至骨骼肌。

It is a group of poorly differentiated and （or）non small cell cancers that have a lack of adenoid or squamous differentiation. There are currently five subtypes representing the morphological pedigree：pleomorphic cell carcinoma, spindle cell carcinoma, giant cell carcinoma, carcinosarcoma, pulmonary blastoma, the latter, in addition to the components of carcinoma, contains heterogenous sarcomas compositions, such as malignant bone, cartilage and even skeletal muscle.

8-19 肺神经内分泌肿瘤 Neuroendocrine tumor，lung

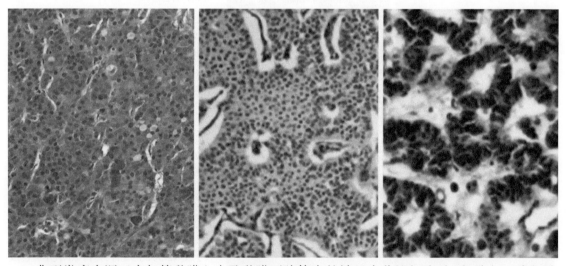

典型类癌来源于支气管黏膜上皮及黏膜下腺体中的神经内分泌细胞（K细胞）。癌细胞通常排列成实性片块、条索、小梁状、带状、栅栏状、器官样结构，亦可呈腺样或菊形团样结构及真假乳头状排列。癌间质富于毛细血管，透明变性，偶见钙化、骨化及淀粉样物质沉着。肿瘤细胞中等大小形状一致。细胞核圆形或卵圆形，位于中央，染色质细而分布均匀（盐粉状）。无明显核仁，分裂像罕见或无。一般无坏死。有时可见血管侵袭现象。免疫组化CgA、Syn、NSE等阳性。

Typical carcinoid originates from the bronchial epithelium and neuroendocrine cells （K cells）in submucosal glands. Tumor cells arranged in solid pieces, cord, trabecular, ribbon, fence-like, organ-like structure, also showing adenoid or rosettes-like structure and genuine papillary arrangement. Interstitial associated with rich capillaries, hyaline degeneration, occasionally calcification, ossification and amyloid deposition. Tumor cells show medium size, cell shape is consistent. Round or egg-shaped nucleus garden, located in the centre, thin and evenly distributed chromatin （salt powder）. No prominent nucleoli, mitotic figures are rare or absent；Generally no necrosis. Sometimes there is visible vascular invasion phenomenon. Immunohistochemical markers CgA, Syn, NSE and so are positive.

8-20　肺小细胞癌（燕麦细胞癌）Small cell carcinoma（Oat cell caecinoma），lung

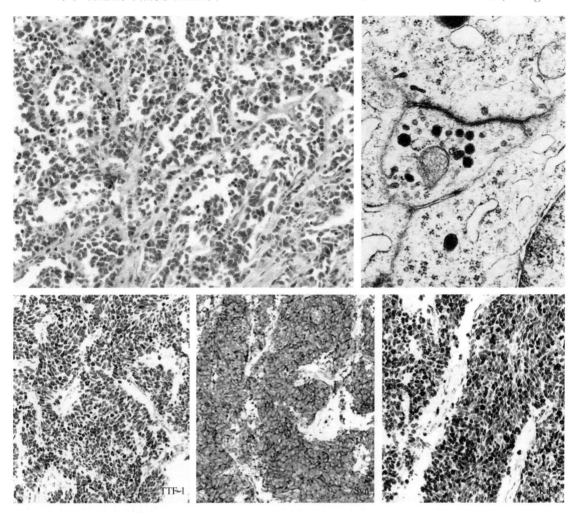

　　属于神经内分泌癌，癌细胞小，圆形、卵圆形或梭形似燕麦，伴有深染的核，相对少胞浆，成巢或成簇排列，没有鳞状上皮或腺样的结构。有时也可围绕小血管形成假菊形团结构。坏死常见且广泛。肺小细胞癌电镜下有神经内分泌颗粒。免疫组化TTF-1和Ki67呈核染色强阳性。Syn为胞质和胞膜阳性。

　　The tumor belongs to neuroendocrine cancer，cancer cell is small，round，oval or spindle-like oats，deeply stained nuclei with relatively little cytoplasm arranged in nests or clusters，no squamous or adenoid structure. Sometimes it can be around small blood vessels forming a pseudorosettes structure. Necrosis is common and widespread.There are neuroendocrine granules under electron microscopy.

　　TTF-1 and Ki67 are positive with nuclear staining pattern. Syn is positive with cytoplasm and membranous staining pattern.

8-21 肺大细胞癌 Large cell carcinoma，lung

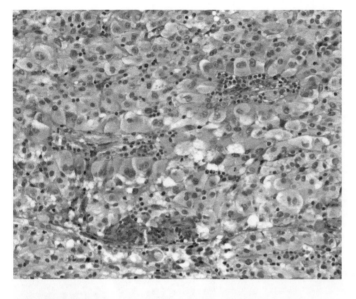

癌组织常呈实性团块或片状，或弥漫分布。癌细胞体积大，多角形，胞质丰富，通常均质淡染，也可呈颗粒状或胞质透明。核呈圆形、卵圆形或不规则形，胞核空泡状，核仁明显，无鳞样和腺样分化。异型明显，核分裂像多见。

Cancer tissue often shows solid clumps or flakes，or diffuse. Cancer cells are large with abundant cytoplasm，usually homogeneous lightly stained，also cytoplasmic granular or clear. Nuclei are round，oval or irregularly shaped，vesicular nuclei and prominent nucleoli，not accompanied by squamous and glandular differentiation，obvious atypia，mitotic figures common seen.

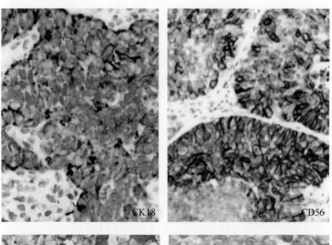
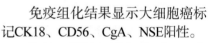

免疫组化结果显示大细胞癌标记CK18、CD56、CgA、NSE阳性。

Immunohistochemical result shows the marker of large cell carcinoma，CK18、CD56、CgA and NSE are positive with cytoplasm and membranous staining pattern.

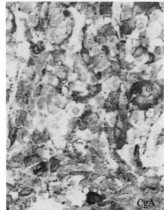
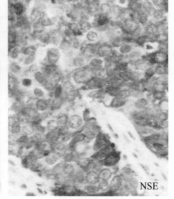

8-22 肺癌的其他类型 Other types of lung cancer

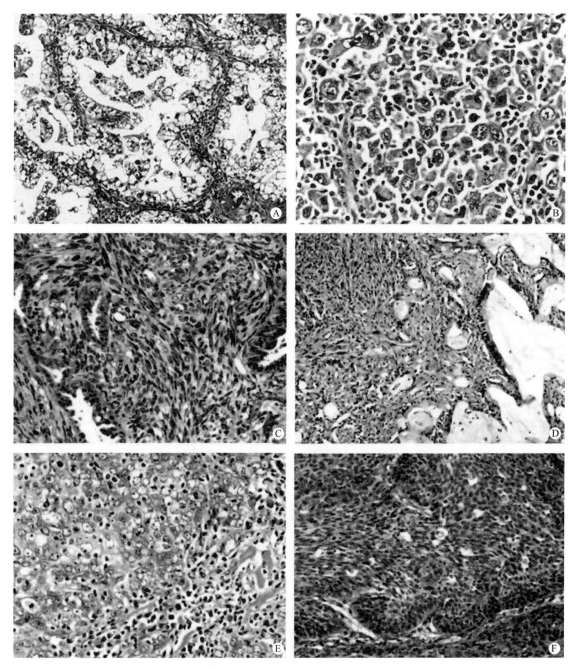

　　A：透明细胞癌。B：巨细胞癌。C：梭形细胞癌。D：多形性癌，见黏液腺癌及梭形细胞癌成分。E：淋巴上皮癌。F：基底细胞癌。

　　A：Clear cells carcinoma；B：Giant cell carcinoma；C：spindle cell carcinoma；D：pleomorphic carcinoma，（main mucinous adenocarcinoma and spindle cell carcinoma componants）；E：lymphatic epithelial carcinoma；F：basal cell carcinoma.

8-23 肺复合性小细胞 Compositive small cell carcinoma，lung

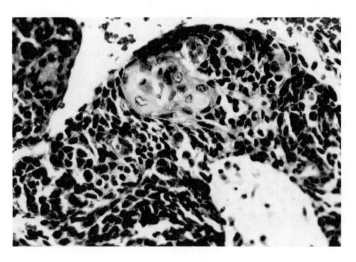

小细胞癌与任何其他非小细胞癌成分复合组成的癌，大细胞成分应不少于10%。免疫组织化学检测：大多数病例CD56、CgA、Syn阳性。少数神经内分泌标记阴性。约90%TTF-1阳性。

Small cell carcinoma and any other non-small cell carcinoma component compose of cancer，large cell composition should be at least＞10%. Immunohistochemistry： most cases were CD56，CgA，and Syn positive. A small number of neuroendocrine markers were negative. About 90% TTF-1 is positive.

8-24 细支气管肺泡癌 Bronchiolo alveolar carcinoma

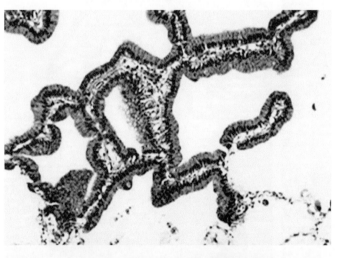

杯状细胞细型支气管肺泡癌（goblet cell，BAC）

黏液性BAC（化生的黏液细胞，20%～25%），属低级别，由高柱状或柱状、或杯状细胞组成，癌细胞沿着细支气管壁生长，无间质侵袭。

Mucinous BAC（metaplastic mucus cells，20%～25%），low grade，composed of tall columnar or columnar，or goblet cells，grows along the bronchioles wall，without invasion.

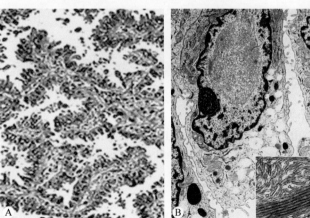

非黏液型Clara细胞型细支气管肺泡癌（A），电镜下癌细胞中具有胞浆突起，含致密颗粒和微绒毛（B）。

Non mucinous clara cell type BAC（A），under electron microscopy，cytoplasmic protrusions with dense granules and microvilli（B）.

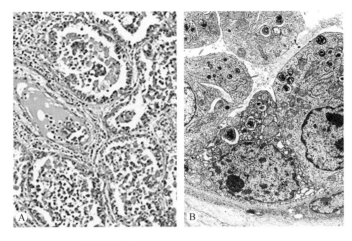

非黏液型Ⅱ型肺泡细胞型细支气管肺泡癌（A），电镜下癌细胞中含板层小体（B）。

Non mucinous type Ⅱ pneumocytes BAC（A），with lamellar bodies（B）in the cancer cells under electron microscopy.

8-25　肺硬化性血管瘤 Pulmonary sclerosing hemangioma（PSH）

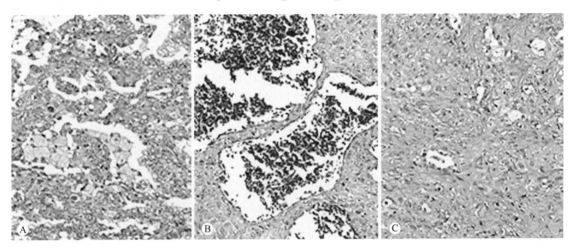

肿瘤由圆形间质细胞和表面立方型上皮样细胞组成。三个特点：①索状或乳头结构：立方型Ⅱ型肺泡上皮索状或乳头状生长，乳头柄中含有圆形间质细胞（A）。②出血区：较大的出血腔内衬Ⅱ型肺泡细胞、灶性出血、含铁血黄素沉着、胆固醇结晶（B）。③硬化区，在乳头柄或索状区有致密的透明变性的胶原灶周围出血或钙化（C）。肿瘤细胞HMB45（+），vimentin（+），EMA（+），Syn（+）。

Tow cell types occur，round stromal cells and surface cuboidal epithelialioid cells，three characteristics：①Solid and papillary pattern：cuboidal epithelialioid cells are growing in the solid and papillary patterns，the stalk of papillary contains round stromal cells（A）.②Heamorrhagic patterns，tumor forms large blood filled spaces lined by typeⅡ pneumocytes or foci of heamorrhage，or heamosiderin deposition，or cholesterol clefts（B）.③Sclerotic pattern dense foci of hyaline collagen at the periphery of heamorrhage areas or calcification，within papillary stalks or within solid areas（C）. Tumor cells HMB45（+），vimentin（+），EMA（+），Syn（+）.

8-26　肺透明细胞肿瘤 Clear cell tumour，lung

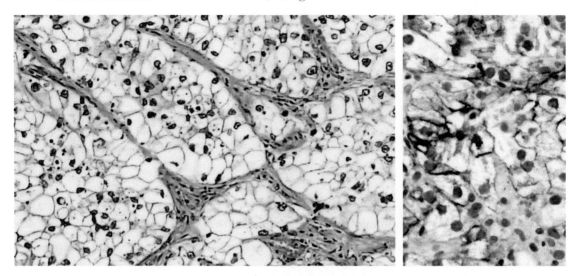

　　可能是起源于血管周细胞的良性肿瘤，由含有大量糖原和富含透明或嗜酸性胞浆的肿瘤细胞构成。HMB45，vimentin，EMA 和Syn阳性（右图. vimentin阳性）。

　　A benign neoplasm that may originate from perivascular epithelioid cells，composed of tumor cells containing large amounts of glycogen and rich in hyaline or eosinophilic cytoplasm. Tumor cell is positive for HMB45，vimentin，EMA and Syn.（Right picture：tumor cell is positive for vimentin）.

8-27　胸膜间皮瘤 Pleural mesothelioma

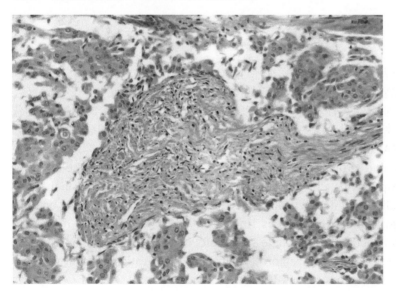

　　瘤组织由梭形的成纤维细胞样瘤细胞和上皮性瘤细胞组成，可形成鱼骨样、乳头状、腺管状或实体结构。（双向性间皮瘤）

　　Tumor tissues are composed of spindle fibroblast-like tumor cells and epithelial tumor cells，can be fishbone，papillary，glandular or entity structures.（biphasic mesothelioma）.

8-28 弥漫性恶性间皮瘤 Diffuse malignant mesothelioma

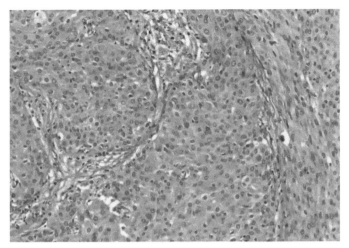

组织学构象复杂，肿瘤细胞具有恶性特征。按肿瘤主要细胞成分的不同，分为腺管乳头状型或上皮样型、由梭形细胞和胶原纤维构成者称肉瘤样型；上述两种成分混合构成者称为混合型（或双向型）。

Histological conformation is complex, has the characteristic of malignant tumor cells. Due to different major tumor cell components, it can be divided into tubular or papillary type, epithelioid type, sarcomatoid type composed of spindle cells and collagen fibers; these two ingredients are mixed to form mixed type（or biphasic）.

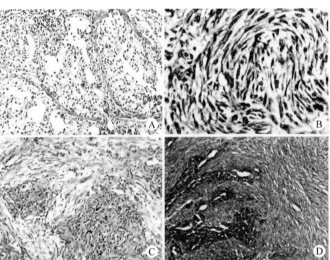

A：上皮样间皮瘤；B：肉瘤样间皮瘤；C：促纤维组织增生性间皮瘤；D：双相型间皮瘤。

A：epithelial type；B：sarcoma like；C：desmoplasia；D：biphasic mesothelioma.

8-29 胸膜肺母细胞瘤 Pleural pulmonary blastoma

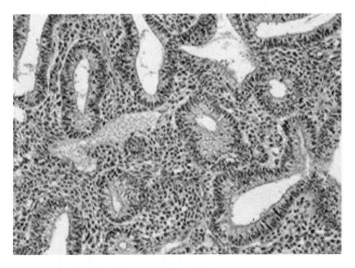

幼稚始基细胞，原始胚胎性小卵圆细胞或鳞状上皮实性桑椹样，菊形团。上皮成分呈密集分支腺管。

Immature basal cell, primitive embryonic small round cells or squamous epithelium, solid mulberry-like, rosseles mass. Epithelial components are dense branched glands.

8-30 胸腺瘤 Thymoma

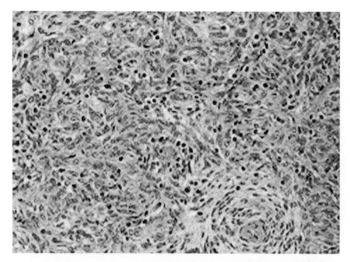

A型胸腺瘤（梭形细胞性胸腺瘤）

Type A thymoma （spindle cell thymoma）

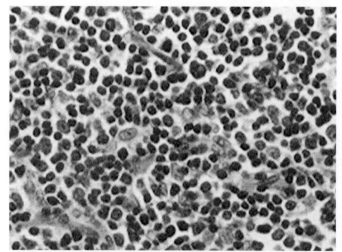

B1型胸腺瘤（淋巴细胞性胸腺瘤）

Type B1 thymoma （lymphocytic thymoma）

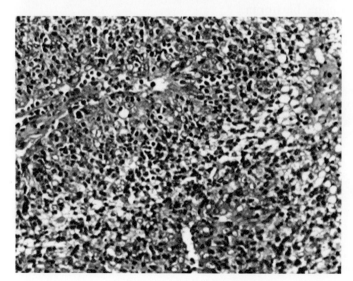

B2型胸腺瘤（皮质型胸腺瘤）

Type B2 （cortical thymoma）

瘤细胞类似正常胸腺皮质上皮细胞。细胞排列成松散网状结构，围绕血管周围间隙或沿着间隔呈栅栏状排列。有小灶性表皮样细胞（但是髓质岛消失或不明显），偶见典型的胸腺小体。

The tumor cells are similar to normal thymic cortical epithelial cells. The cells are arranged in a loosely meshed structure around a perivascular space or along a spaced fence. There is focal epidermaloid cells （but not obvious or disappeared medulla islands）, typical thymic body is occasionally seen.

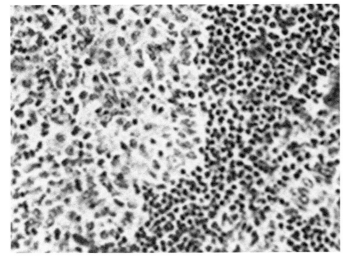

B3型胸腺瘤（上皮细胞型胸腺瘤）

TypeB3（epithelial thymoma）

较厚的纤维性间隔分割成小叶状，上皮性肿瘤细胞常伴有核折叠或核沟，可见酷似胸腺小体的角化灶。

Thicker fibrous segments divided into small lobes, tumor epithelial cells often accompanied by nuclear folds or nuclear sulci, keratinized foci resembling the thymus corpuscle can be seen.

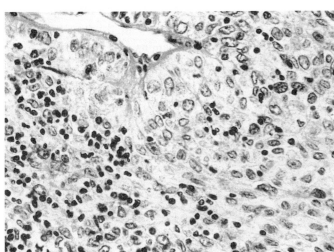

AB型胸腺瘤（混合型）淋巴上皮型胸腺瘤

Type AB（lymphoepithelial thymoma or mixed thymoma）

胸腺上皮样细胞与淋巴细胞数量大致相等。

The number of thymus epithelioid cells is approximately equal to that of lymphocytes.

第九章　消化系统疾病
Chapter 9　Disease of Digestive System

9-1　反流性食管炎 Reflux esophagitis

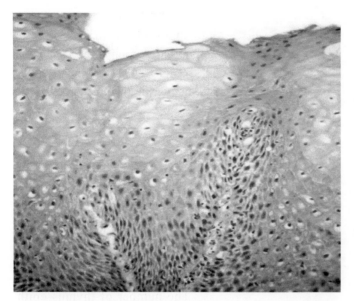

①基底细胞增生（超过黏膜厚度的1/5）；②固有膜乳头延长（达黏膜的上1/3）；③黏膜内炎细胞浸润；④固有膜乳头内血管扩张。

①Basal cell hyperplasia（exceeding mucosal thickness 1/5）；②The lamina propria extends（to the upper mucosal 1/3）；③Infiltration of inflammatory cells in mucous membrane；④Vascular dilatation in papillary of lamina propria.

9-2　胃异位胰腺 Ectopic pancreas，stomach

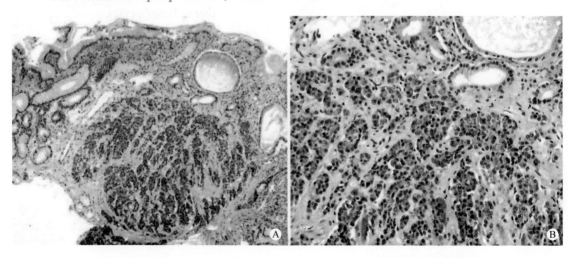

胃中出现正常胰腺组织有腺泡、导管等小叶结构，约1/3的病例可见胰岛。

Normal pancreatic tissue in stomach has acinus, duct and other lobular structures, and pancreatic islets can be seen in about 1/3 of cases.

9-3 胃炎 Gastritis

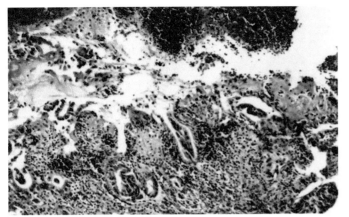

急性糜烂性胃炎（acute erosive gastritis）

胃黏膜上有多灶性小出血糜烂病灶。

Multifocal small hemorrhagic erosions are noted in the gastric mucosa.

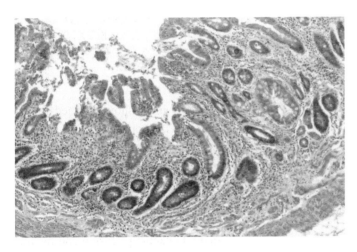

慢性萎缩性胃炎（chronic atrophic gastritis）

①胃黏膜固有腺体不同程度萎缩或消失。②肠上皮化生或假幽门腺化生。③固有层内有淋巴细胞、浆细胞弥漫浸润，可形成淋巴滤泡。④黏膜肌层相对增厚。

①Gastric mucosal lamina propria glands show different degrees of atrophy or disappearance. ②Intestinal metaplasia or pyloric gland metaplasia. ③Diffuse infiltration of the lamina propria containing lymphocytes and plasma cells, may form lymphoid follicles. ④Mucosal muscular is thickened relatively.

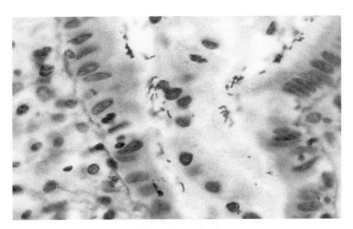

幽门螺杆菌

（helicobacter pylori）

Steiner银染显示胃黏膜上皮腔面的黏液层中大量染成黑色的螺旋形病原体。

A Steiner silver stain demonstrates the numerous darkly stained helicobacter organisms along the luminal surface of the gastric epithelial cells.

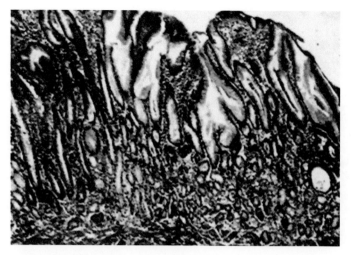

慢性肥厚性胃炎（chronic hypertrophic gastritis）

黏膜上皮增生，结缔组织增生，伴慢性炎症细胞浸润。

Mucosal epithelial hyperplasia, connective tissue proliferation, accompanied by chronic inflammatory cells infiltration.

9-4　胃溃疡 Gastric ulcer

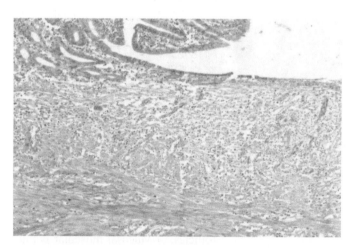

溃疡呈斜漏斗状。溃疡底向上分为四层：①炎性渗出层；②坏死层；③肉芽组织层；④瘢痕层，其中细胞成分较少，胶原纤维增粗融合后发生玻璃样变。

The ulcer show inclined-funnel shape. The bottom can be divided into four layers from the inside out：①zone of active inflammation exudate；②necrotic layer；③granulation tissue；④scar tissue base cellular component is fewer, collagen fibers thickening, fusion and hyaline degeneration later.

9-5　阑尾炎 Appendicitis

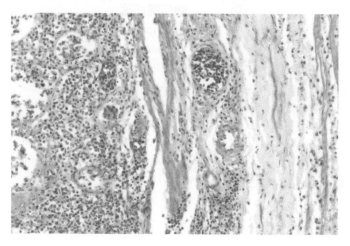

阑尾蜂窝织炎（phlegmonous appendicitis）

阑尾各层血管充血，组织水肿，可见大量中性粒细胞弥漫浸润。阑尾腔内充满脓性渗出物。

All layers of appendix show hyperemia, edema, with diffuse infiltration of a large number of neutrophils. Appendix grandular lumen filled with purulent exudates.

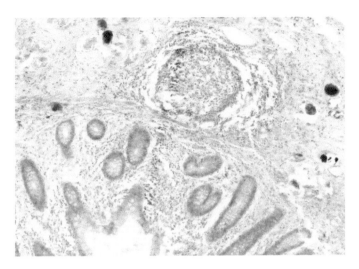

亚急性阑尾炎（subacute appendicitis）

阑尾各层炎细胞浸润，特别是肌层内有嗜酸性粒细胞和淋巴细胞浸润。此例可在黏膜下层见到钙化的血吸虫卵。

All layers of appendix show inflammatory cell infiltration, especially with eosinophils and lymphocytes in the muscle layer. Schistosome eggs calcification can be seen in the submucosa in this case.

9-6 结肠克罗恩病 Crohn's disease，colon

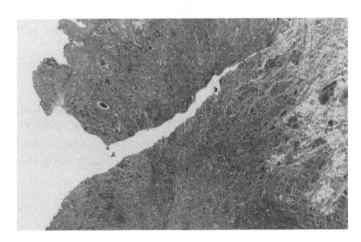

病变组织显示裂隙状溃疡表面被覆坏死组织，其下肠壁各层可见大量淋巴细胞、巨噬细胞与浆细胞浸润（穿壁性炎症），以及淋巴组织增生并有淋巴滤泡形成。肠黏膜下层增厚、水肿，炎症反应。

Pathological tissue shows necrotic tissue along the fissuring ulcer surface. Layers of intestinal wall show a lot of lymphocytes, macrophages and plasma cells（transmural inflammation）, and lymphoid hyperplasia and lymphoid follicles.Intestinal submucosa is thickened, edema and inflammation.

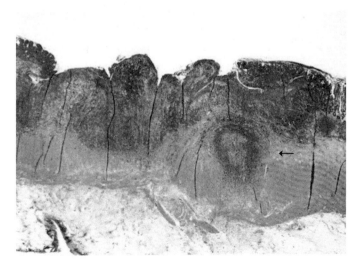

慢性炎症纤维化和非干酪样坏死肉芽肿（箭头所示）。

Chronic inflammation and fibrosis with a noncaseating granuloma（arrow）.

9-7 慢性溃疡性结肠炎 Chronic ulcerative colitis

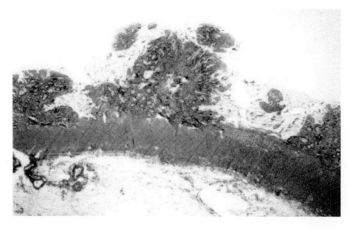

较深而直接的溃疡周围残存黏膜明显炎症呈息肉状。

Pronounced inflammatory changes of surviving mucosa appear polypoid as the ulcerations are deep and immediate.

9-8 食管上皮内瘤变 Esophageal intraepithelial neoplasia

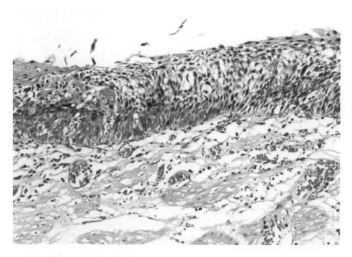

鳞状上皮原位癌（Tis/m1）

（esophageal squamous cell carcinoma in situ）

食管被覆鳞状上皮全层异型增生，失去正常成熟极性，细胞大小不一，核浆比增大，细胞核深染。

All layers of esophageal squamous epithelium display dysplasia, loss of normal mature polarity, cell size varies, karyoplasmic ratio increased, hyperchromatic nuclei.

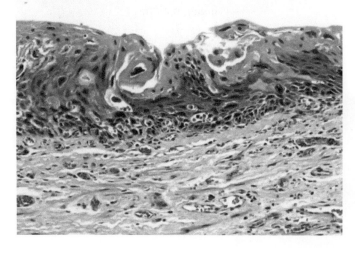

鳞状上皮中-重度异型增生（高级别上皮内瘤变）

[esophageal moderate-severe dysplasia（intraepithelial neoplasia, hight grade）]

鳞状上皮异型增生，但基底膜完整，未见间质浸润。

The squamous epithelium dysplasia, but the basement membrane was intact without interstitial invasion.

9-9　食管鳞状上皮癌 Esophageal squamous cell carcinoma

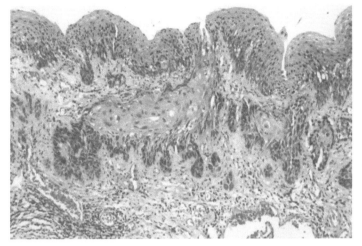

分化性鳞状细胞癌呈钉突样浸润黏膜固有层（T1a/m2），有成熟角化现象，癌细胞多角形，核大深染，异型性大。

The differentiated squamous cell carcinoma showed nail like infiltrating the lamina propria, with mature keratinization, and the tumor cells are polygonal, large nuclei, deep staining, and dysplasia.

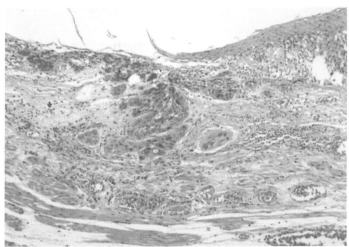

鳞癌细胞巢侵犯固有膜到黏膜肌层（T1a/m3）。视野右侧上皮浅层可见正常上皮残留。

The cancer nests infiltrate the lamina propria to the mucous membrane muscle, the normal epithelial remnant is seen in the right view.

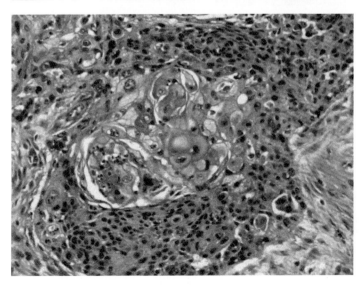

食管鳞状细胞癌Ⅰ级（well differentiated squamous cell carcinoma of the esophagus）

肿瘤细胞片状排列，核分裂低。形成角化珠。

Keratinization, which Component shows tumor cells are arranged in sheets and mitotic counts are lower with keratinized pearl formation.

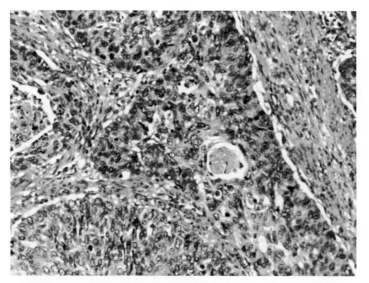

食管鳞状细胞癌Ⅱ级（moderately differentiated squamous cell carcinoma of the esophagus）

肿瘤细胞具有鳞状细胞分化，一般没有角化珠形成。肿瘤细胞片状排列。

The tumor has squamous-cell differentiation. Generally, keratinized pearl is absent. Tumor cells are arranged in sheets.

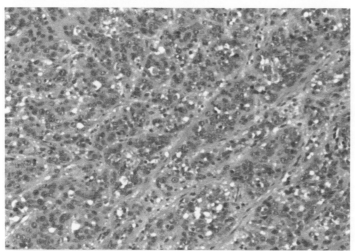

食管鳞状细胞癌Ⅲ级（poorly differentiated squamous cell carcinoma of the oesophagus）

肿瘤主要由基底样细胞形成大小不等的癌巢构成。核分裂相高。

This consists predominantly of basaloid cells forming unegual size nests. The mitosis figures are more.

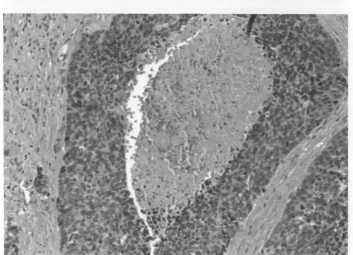

食管基底样鳞状细胞癌（basaloid squamous cell carcinoma of the esophagus）

一种少见的鳞状细胞癌特殊亚型。肿瘤由基底样细胞构成，排列成实性或筛状小叶样伴粉刺样坏死。

It is a rare type of squamous cell carcinoma. It consists of basaloid cells with oval to round nuclei arranged in solid or cribriform lobules with comedo necrosis.

9-10 食管腺癌 Adenocarcinoma，esophagus

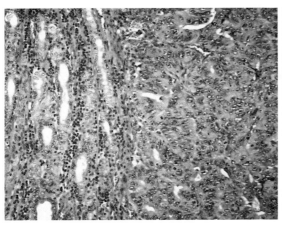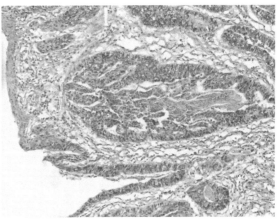

①肿瘤来源于食管黏膜下腺体，或Barrett食管；②肿瘤必须在贲门柱状上皮与食管鳞状上皮交界线以上；③分化差时必须用特殊染色证明确实分泌黏液；④应同腺棘癌与腺鳞癌鉴别。腺癌主要由柱状或立方细胞组成，多分泌黏液，常形成管状结构。

①Tumor originates from esophageal submucosa glands，mainly Barrett esophagus；②Tumor must locate above the junction of cardia columnar epithelium and esophageal squamous；③In poor differentiation，special staining proveits mucus secreting；④Tumor should be distinguished with adenoacanthoma or adenosquamous carcinoma. Gland is mainly composed of columnar or cubic cells with much mucus secretion and tubular structure.

9-11 食管癌肉瘤 Carcinosarcoma，esophagus

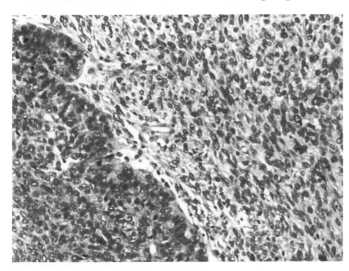

肿瘤细胞有两种成分构成：一种是左边呈巢状分布的鳞状细胞癌成分。癌细胞核大、深染，核浆比增高，核分裂多见；另一种是右边呈束状、编织状排列的梭形细胞成分；二者不相互混杂。

The tumor is composed of two components：on the left is squamous cell carcinoma in nests with enlarged，hyperchromatic nuclei，increased nuclei-cytoplasm ratio and visible mitotic activity. On the right are spindle cells in an interlacing arrangement. The two components are not intermingled with each other.

9-12 胃腺瘤 Adenoma，stomach

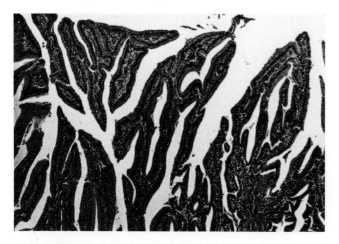

腺瘤上皮呈轻度不典型增生，形成指状或分支状乳头状。上皮内有散在的神经内分泌细胞。

The adenomatous epithelium is slight atypical，forms a finger or branched papillary patterns. There are scattered neuroendocrine cells in the epithelium.

9-13 胃息肉 Polyps，stomach

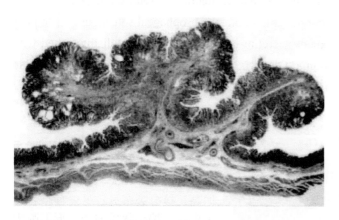

增生性息肉（hyperplastic polyps）

息肉表面腺窝皮增生构成大型腺管，中心部为增生的幽门腺或胃体腺，夹杂血管纤维平滑肌组织，深部腺体常呈囊性扩张。有些增生性息肉中可见由表面上皮内褶的锯齿状形态。

The large glandular duct composed of hyperplastic and enlarged crypt epithelium on the surface of the polyp, the central part of which is a hyperplastic pyloric gland or stomach gland. It is filled with vascular fibrous smooth muscle tissue，and the glands in the deep part often present cystic dilatation. Some hyperplastic polyps are visible from the surface epithelium into a serrated fold.

胃底腺息肉（fundic gland polyp）

息肉内有被覆胃底腺上皮即含有壁细胞和主细胞的囊肿，表面腺窝短或缺如。

In polyp，glandular epithelium covering the fundus of the stomach contains parietal cells and chief cells，and the surface glands are short or absent.

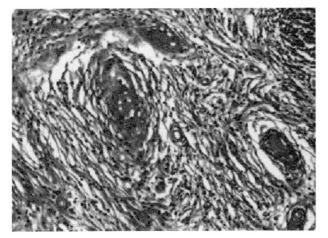

炎性纤维性息肉（inflammatory fibroid polyp）

息肉由许多小血管和成纤维细胞呈漩涡状生长。

Polyps is composed of many small blood vessels and fibroblasts with whirlpool growth.

9-14 胃上皮内瘤变 Gastric intraepithelial neoplasia

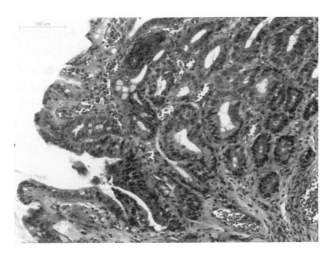

胃（角）高级别上皮内瘤变［Gastric（angle mucosal glands）high grade intraepithelial neoplasia］

腺管拥挤，细胞失去正常成熟趋势，核多数呈杆状，增生复层，核染色质增多，病理性核分裂。见核仁，未见固有膜浸润。

The glandular tubes arrange crowded. The cells lost the normal mature tendency. Most of the nuclei were rod-shaped，multilayer hyperplasia with increasing chromatin and mitosis. The nucleolus is seen. But no the lamina propria infiltration is seen.

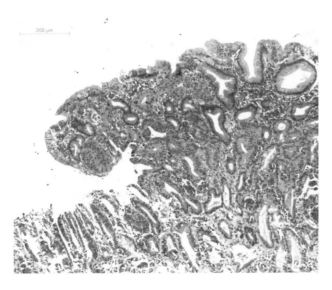

（胃角）高分化-中分化管状腺癌（Tub1>Tub2），浸润固有膜及黏膜肌（T1a/m）；未见血管/淋巴管浸润。

Gastric（angle）highly-moderately differentiated tubular adenocarcinoma（Tub1>Tub2），invasion of lamina propria and mucous membrane muscle（T1a/m）. No vascular / lymphatic infiltration.

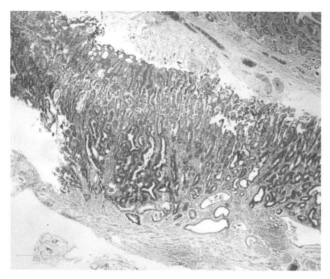

黏膜表面腺管密集拥挤，固有膜深部腺体大小形状不规则，异型深染的腺体失去正常成熟趋势。

The surface mucosa glands were irregular shapes and densely packed with- out normal maturation tendency.

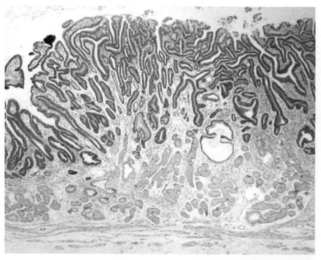

（胃窦）管状腺癌，高-中分化（Tub1>Tub2），浸润固有膜（T1a/m）

［（Gastric antrum） tubular adenocarcinoma with high-moderately differentiation（Tub1>Tub2）, infiltrating lamina propria（T1a/m）］

未见血管/淋巴管浸润，水平切缘及基底切缘均未见癌累及。

No vascular/lymphatic invasion was observed. No tumor involvement was found in both horizontal and basal margins.

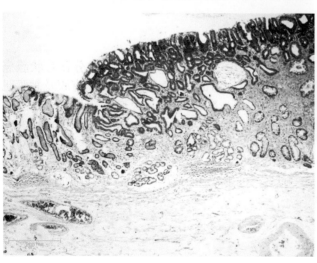

（胃窦）腺体高级别上皮内瘤变/高分化管状腺癌（Tub1），浸润固有膜（T1a/m）。伴神经内分泌细胞不典型增生，未见血管/淋巴管浸润。

Gastric antrum high grade intraepithelial neoplasia/highly differentiated tubular adenocarcinoma （Tub1）with invasion of the lamina propria （T1a/m）. and neuroendocrine cell dysplasia. No vascular/lymphatic invasion was found.

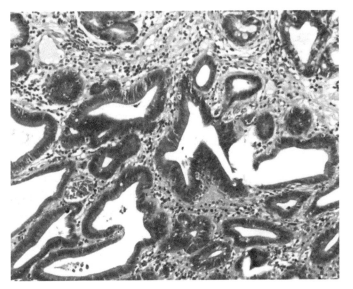

上图局部放大［image amplification（400*）］

异型深染的腺管失去正常成熟趋势，极向紊乱，大小形状不规则，分枝、出芽、成角或向外形成子腺体浸润固有膜。

The irregularly glands lose normal maturation tendency and polarity, with irregular in size and shape, branching, budding, angular, or external glands infiltrating the lamina propria.

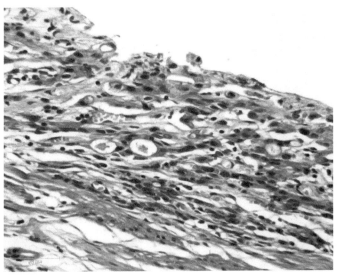

胃（体）低分化腺癌（Por2）呈梁索状浸润黏膜下层（SM1/T1b1）；未见血管/淋巴管浸润。

Lower differentiated adenocarcinoma（Por2）with trabecular pattern infiltrate submucosa（SM1/T1b1）；No vascular/lymphatic invasion was found.

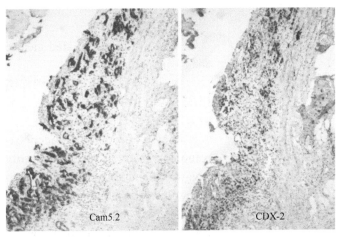

免疫组化：Cam5.2（左）和CDX-2（右）阳性清楚显示黏膜下浸润。

Immunohistochemistry：Cam-5.2（left）and CDX-2（right）poitive clearly showed submucosal invasion.

9-15 胃癌 Gastric carcinoma

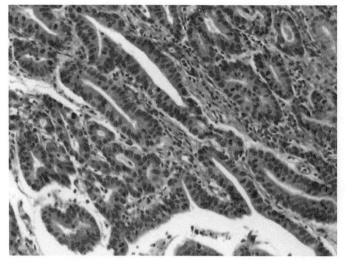

胃腺癌Ⅰ级（well differentiated gastric adenocarcinoma）

由完好的腺体组成，腺体的大小和形状显示轻度异型，比较规则，癌细胞呈柱状或立方形。

Well-differentiated adenocarcinomas are composed of well-formed glands，which size and shape show slightly different，relatively regular in a columnar or cuboidal.

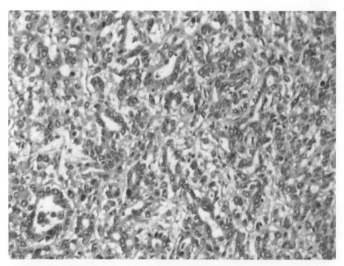

胃腺癌Ⅱ级（moderately differentiated gastric adenocarcinoma）

介于高分化和低分化之间的肿瘤，腺管结构不规则，或形成不完整的腺腔，异型较为显著。

Moderately differentiated adenocarcinomas are composed of neoplasm intermediated between well-and poorly differentiated. The glands are irregular with relatively remarkable atypia.

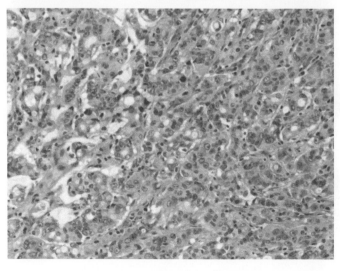

胃腺癌Ⅲ级

（poorly differentiated gastric adenocarcinoma）

由难以辨认的高度不规则腺体组成。腺管样结构不明显，或几乎没有腺管样结构，构像变异很大。

Poorly differentiated adenocarcinomas are comprised of highly irregular glands that are difficulty to recognize. The tubular structure of gland are not obvious or almost absent，variable greatly in morphology.

9-16 胃黏液腺癌 Mucinous adenocarcinoma，stomach

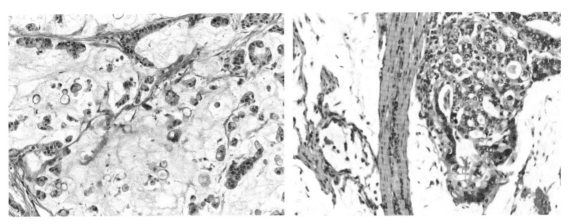

由恶性上皮成分和细胞外黏液池构成。一般情况下，肿瘤中的细胞外黏液成分大于50%。有两种生长方式：①腺体由柱状黏液分泌上皮组成，间质腔隙中存在黏液；②细胞呈链状或不规则串状散在漂浮于黏液湖。

This tumor is composed of malignant epithelium and extracellular mucinous pools. By convention，the tumor shows more than 50% extracellular mucin. Two kinds of growth modes：①the glands are composed of columnar epithelium with mucus secretion，and stromal compartments exist some mucus；②the cells scatter in the chain or irregular cluster patterns and float in the mucinous pools.

9-17 胃印戒细胞癌 Signet ring cell carcinoma，stomach

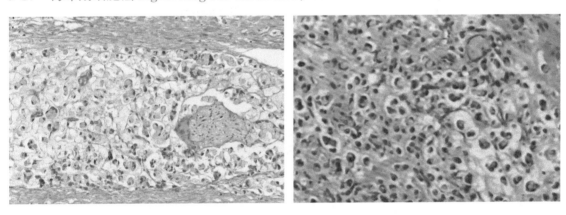

肿瘤细胞中50%以上为印戒细胞，印戒细胞弥漫分布，细胞内充满黏液，黏液将胞核推挤到一侧，形似戒指。胃印戒细胞癌浸润神经纤维。

More than 50% of tumor cells are signet ring cell，signet ring cell diffuse distribution. The cell contains more mucin，mucin pushes the nuclei to the side of the cell，showing ring-like appearence.

Gastric signet ring cell carcinomas invade nerve.

9-18 胃低黏附性癌 Poorly cohesive carcinomas，stomach

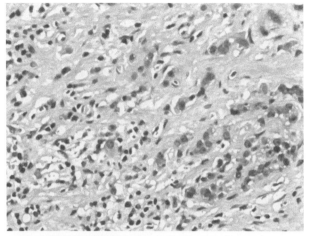

肿瘤细胞呈孤立的或排列成小簇状，可以为印戒细胞、组织细胞样或淋巴细胞样、或浆细胞样，常有深染伊红细胞。

Poorly cohesive carcinomas are composed of neoplastic cells with isolated or arranged in small cluster. These encompass：signet-ring cells，resembling histiocytoid or lymphocytoid，or plasmacytoid cells often with deeply eosinophilic cytoplasm.

9-19 胃混合性癌 Mixed carcinoma，stomach

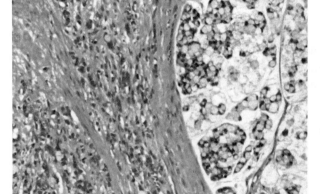

由腺样（梁状/乳头状）和印戒细胞/低黏附性的癌细胞成分混合组成。

The tumor displays a mixture of glandular （tubular/papillary） and signet ring/poorly-cohesive cellular histological components.

9-20 胃神经内分泌肿瘤 Neuroendocrine neoplasm，stomach

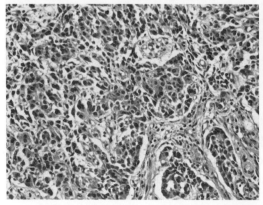 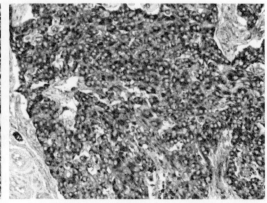

Ⅰ级（grade Ⅰ）：由规则排列的细胞聚集成微小叶状、梁状结构。肿瘤细胞核形态单一，核仁不明显，胞质较丰富且显著嗜伊红，极少有核分裂像。神经内分泌标记物CgA免疫组化阳性，增殖指数Ki67低。

The tumor is characterized by small，microlobular-trabecular aggregates formed by regularly distributed. Tumor cells often aligned cells，with regular，monomorphic nuclei，usually unapparent nucleoli，and rather abundant，fairly eosinophilic cytoplasm. Mitoses are almost absent. Immunohistochemistry is positive for CgA，a neuroendocrine marker and the proliferation index Ki67 is extremely low.

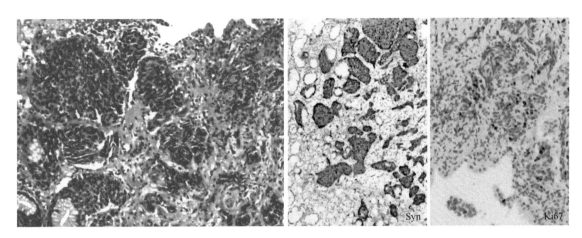

　　Ⅱ级（gradeⅡ）：圆形到梭形及多角形肿瘤细胞实性生长，排列呈大的梁状、密集且不规则分布。肿瘤细胞核小、深染，核仁小。可伴灶性坏死。神经内分泌标记物Syn免疫组化阳性，增殖指数Ki67较低。

　　Round to spindle and polyhedral tumor cells show solid aggregates with large trabeculae, crowding and irregular distribution. Tumor cells are smaller, hyperchromatic nuclei and small nucleoli. There may be small focal necrosis. Immunohistochemistry is positive for syn, a neuroendocrine marker and the proliferation index Ki67 is relatively low.

9-21　胃神经内分泌癌 Neuroendocrine carcinoma，stomach

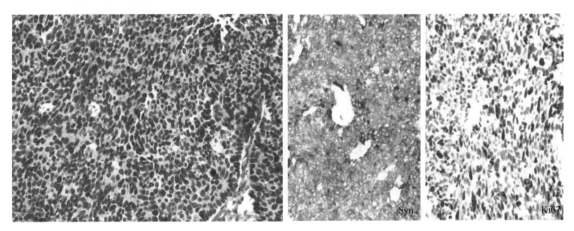

　　肿瘤细胞较原始，呈圆形、多边形及梭形。细胞大小不一，排列紊乱呈巢状结构，伴有坏死。神经内分泌标记物Syn免疫组化阳性，增殖指数Ki67高。

　　Anaplastic round, polyhedral to spindle tumor cells, small to fairly large in size poorly form nests with necrosis. Immunohistochemistry is positive for Syn, a neuroendocrine marker and the proliferation index Ki67 is relatively high.

9-22 胃癌肉瘤 Carcinosarcoma，stomach

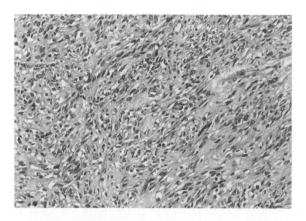

肿瘤细胞有两种成分构成：一种是上皮样细胞，胞浆透亮；另一种是核呈杆状、深染的梭形细胞，二者相互混杂存在。核分裂多见。

The tumor has two components：one is epithelioid cells with clear cytoplasm. The other is spindle cells with rhabditiform，hyperchromatic nuclei. The two components are intermingled with each other. Nuclear mitotic activity is visible.

9-23 左锁骨上淋巴结胃腺癌转移 Gastric adenocarcinoma metastasis，left supraclavicular lymph node

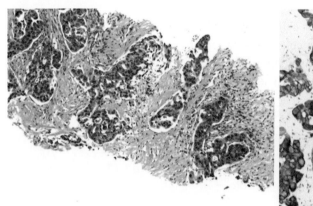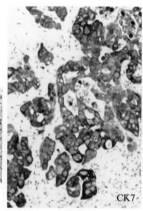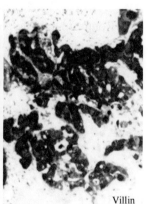

CK7   Villin

淋巴结中肿瘤细胞呈不规则腺管排列，被纤维结缔组织分隔，瘤细胞浆丰富，核大、深染。免疫组化结果显示腺上皮特异性标记CK7和Villin阳性。

In lymph nale，the tumor cells have rich cytoplasm and large，hyperchromatic nuclei arranged in nests and separated by fibrous connective tissue. Immunohistochemistry is positive for CK7 and Villin，as specific markers of glandular epithelia.

9-24 Peutz-Jeghers 息肉 Peutz-Jeghers polyps

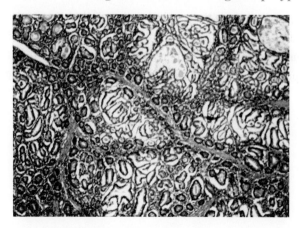

息肉呈小叶状，排列似腺瘤。黏膜肌层的肌纤维增生形成树枝状结构。

Polyps are composed of lobules and arranged like adenomas. The muscle fiber hyperplasia of the muscularis mucosa formed a dendritic structure.

9-25 结直肠腺瘤 Adenoma, colon and rectum

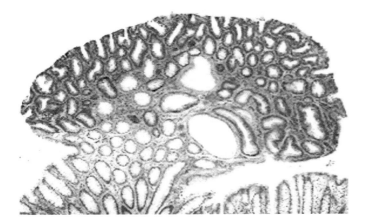

管状腺瘤（tubular adenoma）
由分支小腺管组成，腺管排列紧密。

The consists of branch small glandule tube arranged closely.

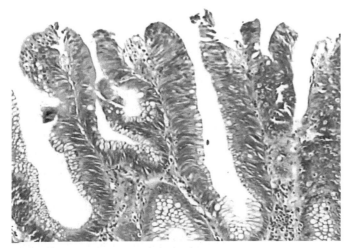

绒毛状腺瘤（villous adenoma）
由指状或分支状乳头组成，乳头中央为固有膜，表面覆盖以柱状上皮。

Composed of finger or branched papillarys, the center of papillary is lamina propria, and the surface is covered with columnar epithelium.

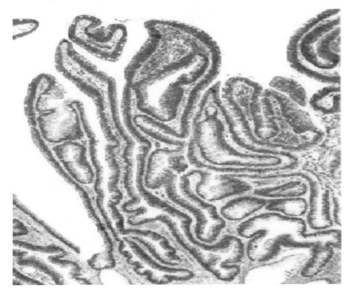

管状绒毛状腺瘤（tubulovillous adenoma）
为管状腺瘤移行至绒毛状腺瘤的过渡类型。管状结构位于深层，绒毛状结构位于表面，两种成分之间有移行。

Transitional type from tubular adenoma to villous adenoma. The tubular structure is located in the deep layer, the villous structure is located in the surface and transition area is between the two components.

9-26　结肠上皮内瘤变 Intraepithelial neoplasia，colon

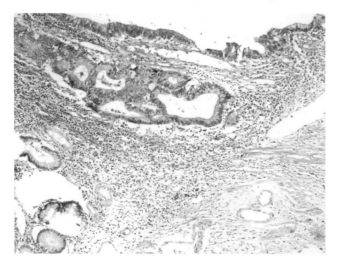

　　管状-绒毛状腺瘤，局部腺体黏膜内癌变，符合高级别上皮内瘤变。

Tubular-villous adenoma，local glands occur canceration accords with high-grade intraepithelial neoplasia.

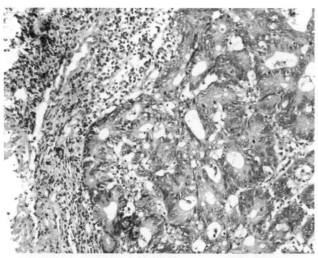

　　腺管密集，细胞排列和极向显著紊乱，共壁和筛状，病理性核分裂。浸润黏膜固有层，但黏膜肌层未受侵犯。

Irregular glanduls densely crowded, the cells arrangement disordered with co-wall and sifler like structures. Nuclear mitosis is active. Irregular glandular epithelial cells infiltrate the mucous lamina propria，but the muscularis mucosae isn't involved.

9-27　结直肠腺癌 Adenocarcinoma，colon and rectum

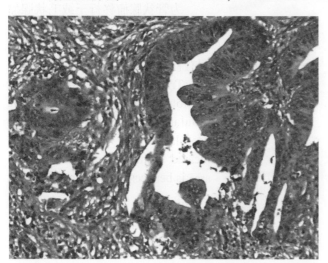

　　肠腺癌Ⅰ级（well differentiated）腺体的大小和形状显示轻度异型，比较规则，癌细胞呈柱状或立方形。

The tumor is composed of columnar or cuboiolal epithelioid cells. The size and shape show slightly atypia，relatively regular.

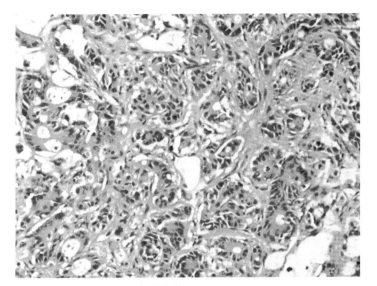

肠腺癌Ⅱ级（moderately differentiated）

这是介于高分化和低分化之间的肿瘤，腺管结构不规则，异型较为显著。

Moderately differentiated adenocarcinomas are composed of neoplasm intermediated between well and poorly differentiated. The glands are irregular with relatively remarkable atypia.

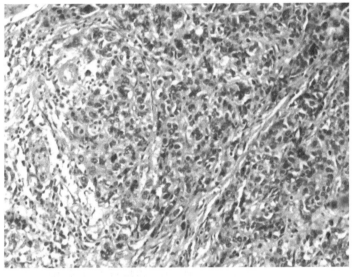

肠腺癌Ⅲ级（poorly differentiated）

由难以辨认的高度不规则腺体组成。腺管样结构不明显，或几乎没有腺管样结构，构像变异很大。

Poorly differentiated adenocarcinomas are comprised highly irregular glands that are difficulty to recognize. The tubular structure of glands are not obvious or almost absent, variable obviously in morphology.

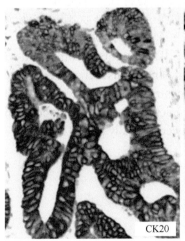
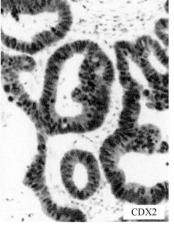

CK20 CDX2

免疫组化结果显示腺上皮标记CK20和CDX2阳性。

Immunohistochemistry shows CK20 and CDX2, that gastrointestinal specific marker, are positive.

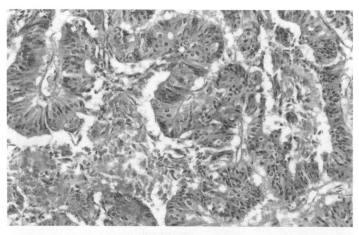

乳头状腺癌（papillary adenocarcinoma）

癌细胞乳头状排列，乳头内间质很少，其中央为纤维血管索。

Cancer cells show papillary arrangement, little stroma in the papillary, its central is fibrovascular cord.

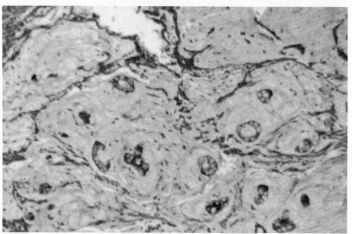

黏液腺癌（mucinous adenocarcinoma）

由恶性上皮成分和细胞外黏液池构成。细胞呈链或不规则串状散在漂浮于黏液湖。

This tumor is composed of malignant epithelium and extracellular mucinous pools. The tumor cells were scattered in the chain or irregular clusters floating mucinous pools.

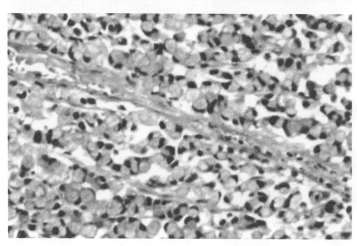

印戒细胞癌（signet ring cell carcinoma）

肿瘤由印戒细胞构成，印戒细胞的特征是细胞中心有一光镜下透明的球状胞浆黏液滴和一个偏心的细胞核。

The tumor is composed of signet ring cells, characterized by a central optically clear, globoid droplet of cytoplasmic mucin with an eccentrically placed nucleus.

9-28 结直肠神经内分泌肿瘤 Neuroendocrine neoplasm，colon and rectum

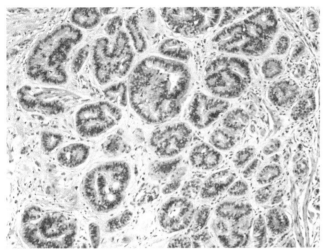

Ⅰ级（grade Ⅰ）

由规则排列的细胞聚集成梁状结构。肿瘤细胞核形态单一，核仁不明显，胞质较丰富且显著嗜伊红，极少有核分裂像。

The tumor is characterized by trabecular aggregates with regularly distributed. Tumor cells are often aligned cells，with regular，monomorphic nuclei，usually unapparent nucleoli，and rather abundant，fairly eosinophilic cytoplasm. Mitoses are almost absent.

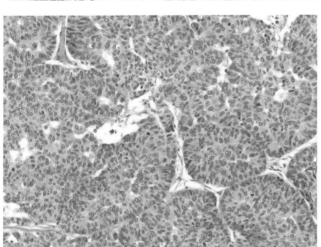

Ⅱ级（grade Ⅱ）

圆形到梭形及多角形肿瘤细胞实性聚集，排列呈大的梁状、密集且不规则分布。肿瘤细胞核小、深染，核仁小。可出现灶性坏死。

Round to spindle and polyhedral tumor cells show solid，aggregates with large trabeculae，crowding and irre gular distribution. The tumor cells are smaller，hyperchromatic nuclei and small nucleoli，often present faci necrosis.

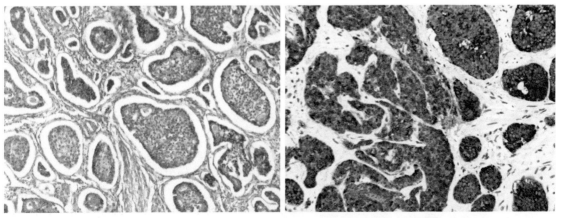

癌细胞呈腺样排列或呈器官状结构，癌细胞形态相对较一致。免疫组化显示神经内分泌标志Syn阳性。增殖指数Ki67极其低。

Tumor cells are adenoid arranged or show organ-like structure. Tumor cells morphology are relatively consistent. Immunohistochemistry is positive for Syn（synaptophysin），a neuroendocrine marker and the proliferation index Ki67 is extremely low.

9-29　结直肠神经内分泌癌 Neuroendocrine carcinoma，colon and rectum

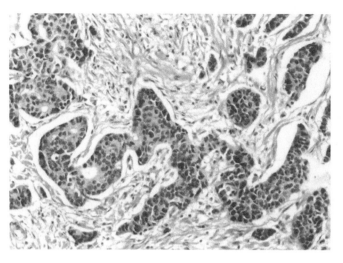

间变性肿瘤细胞呈圆形、多边形及梭形。细胞体积有的较小，有的相对很大，排列成紊乱的巢状结构。核呈盐粉状，核分裂不多，癌间质血管丰富，可有淀粉样变或玻变。

Anaplastic tumor cells show round, polyhedral to spindle，small to fairly large in size，is arrangement disordered nests structures.

Relatively consistent cells，nucleus salt powder，mitotic figures are fewer. Blood vessels in cancer stroma are plenty，may show amyloidosis or hyaline degeneration.

9-30　直肠腺鳞癌 Adenosquamous crcinoma，rectal

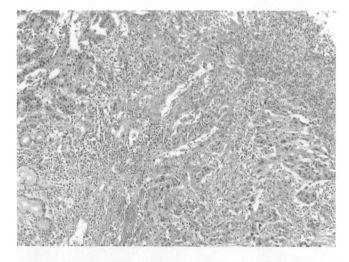

具有腺癌（左上）和鳞癌（右下）结构，伴坏死（右上）。

It is composed of adenocarcinoma（left upper）and squamous cell carcinoma（right down）with necrosis（right upper）.

9-31　胃肠间质瘤 Gastrointestinal stromal tumour（GIST）

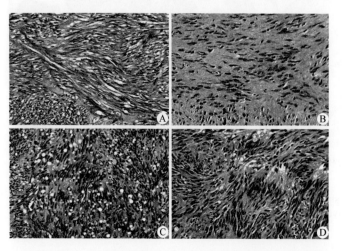

梭形细胞型（spindle cells type）

肿瘤由长梭形细胞组成，呈编织状排列，核略呈梭形，栅状排列，核分裂像极少见。

The tumor is composed of spindle cells with interlacing arrangement, the nuclei are spindle，palisading arrangement and inconspicuous mitotic activity.

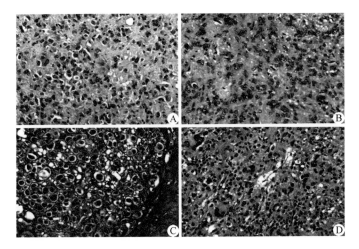

上皮样型（epithelioid type）

肿瘤由上皮样细胞组成，圆形、卵圆形，中等大小，胞质略嗜酸，核圆或卵圆形，单核，无明显异型性，极少核分裂，瘤细胞被纤维血管分隔成巢团状。

The tumor is composed of epithelioid cells that are middle size of round, oval cells with amphophilic cytoplasm and single nucleus without atypia and mitotic activity. The tumor is separated into nests by fibrous vessels.

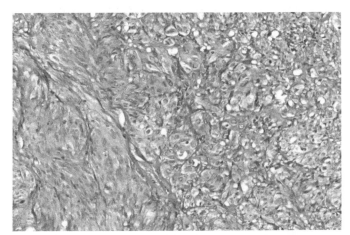

混合型（mixed type）

梭形瘤细胞和多边形上皮样细胞，编织状、栅状排列；分裂像极少见，一般少于2个/10 HPF；基质内含多少不等的胶原，可有玻璃样变和钙化。

Spindle and epithelioid tumor cells show interlacing, palisading-like arrangements; mitosis figures are rare, usually less than 2/10 HPF; containing varying amounts of collagen in matrix, with hyaline degeneration and calcification.

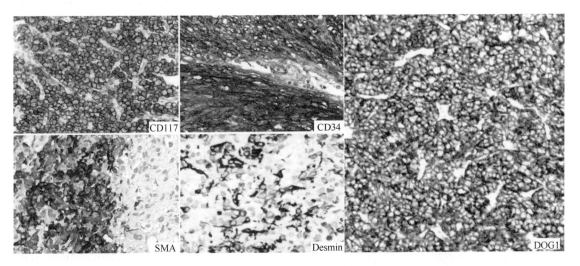

GIST特异性标记物CD117、CD34、SMA、Desmin和DOG1。

Immunohistochemistry is positive for CD117、CD34、SMA and Desmin，DOG1，which are GIST specific markers.

9-32 胃炎性肌纤维母细胞肿瘤 Gastric inflammatory myofibroblastic tumor

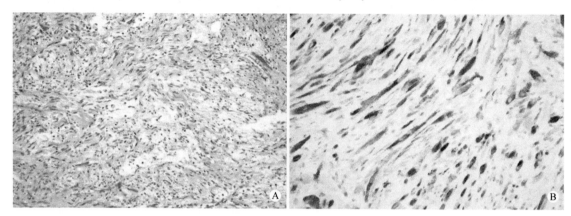

A：肿瘤成分为梭形或上皮样肌纤维母细胞；B：肿瘤细胞可呈ALK免疫标记阳性表达。

A：It is composed of spindle or epithelioid myofibroblastic cells. B：Tumor cells positively expressed ALK marker.

9-33 胃丛状黏液瘤 Gastric plexiform myxoma

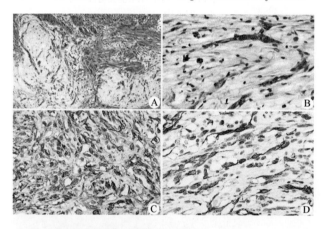

A：肿瘤呈结节状、丛状，累及胃壁肌层；B：肿瘤中较多毛细血管和大量黏液基质，其内细胞相对稀疏，细胞温和呈梭形；C：肿瘤细胞表达SMA；D：肿瘤细胞表达CD10。

A：The tumor was nodular, plexiform, invating to gastric smooth musclar layer；B：More capillaries and mucus matrix, relatively sparse the cells, with mild spindle shaped；C and D：Tumor cells expressed SMA and CD10.

9-34 胃肠道透明细胞肉瘤 Clear cell sarcoma, gastrointestinal tract

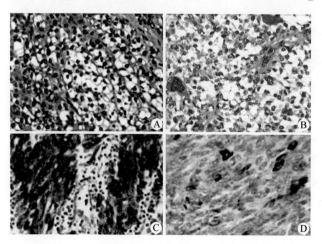

A：肿瘤由片状、圆形到短梭形透明细胞构成；B：肿瘤中常见多核破骨巨细胞样细胞；C：肿瘤细胞表达S100；D：肿瘤细胞表达Syn。

A：The tumor consists of lamellar, round to short spindle clear cells；
B：Multinucleated osteoclastioid giant cells are common in tumor；C and D：Tumor cells express S100 and Syn.

9-35 肝炎 Hepatitis

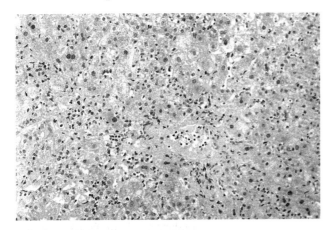

急性病毒性肝炎（acute viral hepatitis）

见小叶中气球样肝细胞杂乱排列，伴灶状坏死。

Note lobular disarray of ballooned hepatocytes with focal necrosis.

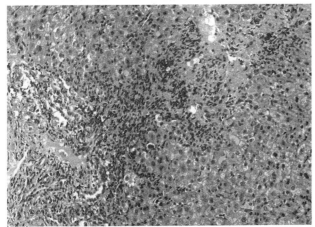

慢性肝炎（chronic hepatitis）

肝细胞变性、坏死形成"碎片状坏死"和"桥接坏死"，其间淋巴细胞浸润，间质纤维化。

Hepatocytes show degeneration and necrosis forming a "piecemeal necrosis" and "bridging necrosis", with lymphocyte infiltration and interstitial fibrosis.

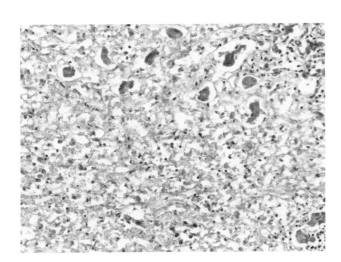

急性重型肝炎（acute severe hepatitis）

肝细胞弥漫性大块坏死，仅门管区周围残留少许变性的肝细胞。网状支架残留，肝窦明显扩张淤血。小叶内及汇管区大量炎细胞浸润，以淋巴细胞、巨噬细胞为主，可有少量中性粒细胞。

Diffuse massive necrosis of hepatocyte, only a few residual degeneration hepatocytes are surrounding the portal area. Mesh scaffolds is residual and liver sinus show obviously dilatation. A large number of inflammatory cells infiltrate in the lobular and portal area, mostly are lymphocytes, macrophages, and a small amount of neutrophils.

9-36 酒精性肝病 Alcoholic liver disease

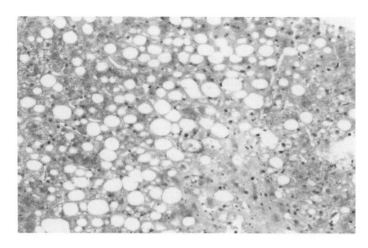

小叶中央区发生肝脂变和中央性纤维化。进展性肝纤维化呈蜘蛛样形态，将肝细胞分隔，严重时累及全小叶。继发炎症中性粒细胞浸润。

Liver fat change and central fibrosis first occurs in the centrilobular area. The progressive fibrosis around the liver parenchyma shows spider-like, separating the liver cells, In severe it involves the entire lobules, secondary alcoholic hepatitis shows neutrophils infiltration.

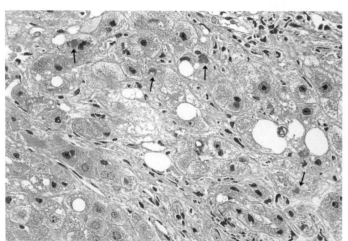

肝细胞水肿，内含Mallory小体（箭头所示），Mallory小体为丝条状、块状亮染的胞浆成分。并可见少量中性粒细胞。

Liver cells are swollen and contain Mallory bodies（arrows）in the form of strands and clumps of brightly stained cytoplasmic material. A few neutrophils are seen.

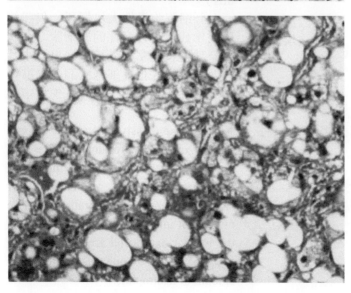

Massontrichrome染色显示小叶中央区肝细胞周围纤维化，胶原纤维呈蓝色。

There is pericellular fibrosis in centrilobular area. Collagen fibers are stained blue in Massontrichrome stain.

9-37　毛玻璃样肝细胞 Ground- glass hepatocytes

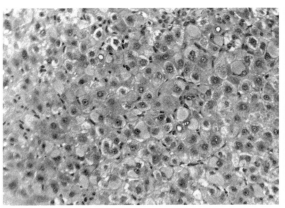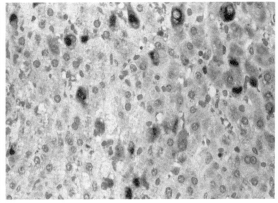

　　毛玻璃样肝细胞内含颗粒样、淡伊红色胞质包涵体，后者由内质网和HBV表面抗原组成。HBsAg免疫组化阳性染色呈棕黄色颗粒。

Ground-glass hepatocytes contain granular，lightly eosinophilic cytoplasmic inclusions，which consist of endoplasmic reciculum and HBV surface antigen can be stained by the immunohistochemical method for HBsAg.

9-38　肝 α1 抗胰蛋白酶缺乏症 Alpha 1 antitrypsin deficiency，liver

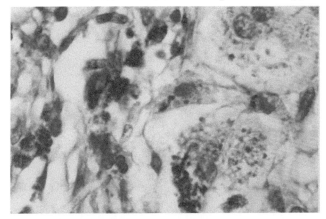

　　PAS染色阳性显示肝细胞质内有大小不等的均质玻璃样小体。

Liver cells contain many magenta haylineloid globules of different size，PAS stain.

9-39　门脉性肝硬化 Portal cirrhosis，liver

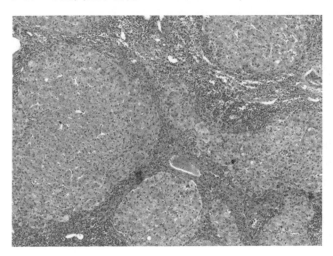

　　肝小叶结构破坏，形成大小较一致的假小叶。假小叶内中央静脉常偏位、缺失或数量增多（两个或两个以上）；肝细胞索排列紊乱，不呈放射状，纤维间隔细而均匀，少量淋巴细胞和单核细胞浸润，并有少量小胆管增生。

Lobular structural damage，forming consistent size pseudolobules. Central vein in pseudolobuli often show deviation，deletions or increase in the number （two or more）；Hepatic cords show arrangement disorder，not radial，fiber septa is thin and uniform，with a small amount of lymphocytes and monocytes and a few small bile duct hyperplasia.

9-40　坏死后性肝硬化 Postnecrotic cirrhosis，liver

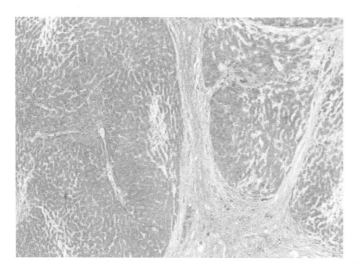

　　肝小叶破坏，假小叶结节较大且大小形态不一，可见残存汇管区的相对集中现象；假小叶内肝细胞变性，坏死更显著。纤维间隔较宽且宽窄不一，其内有较多的炎细胞浸润和小胆管增生。

Lobular shows destruction，pseudolobule nodules are large with varying size and shape，relative concentration of portal area are seen；liver cells within pseudolobules show more significant degeneration and necrosis. Fiber septa is wider and varying width，there are more inflammatory cells infiltration and bile duct hyperplasia.

9-41　肝细胞局灶性结节状增生 Hepatocellular focal nodular hyperplasia

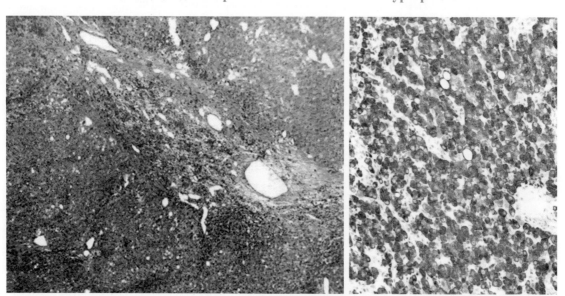

　　良性的肝细胞结节中，肝细胞排列成不厚于2层的肝板，可伴有脂肪变性。纤维间隔中央瘢痕含有一个或多个发育不良的血管和许多小动脉。瘢痕的放射状分支含有多个汇管区样结构，但仅有动脉而无伴行的静脉和胆管。纤维间隔边缘肝组织内见胆小管增生伴炎症细胞浸润。免疫组化显示Ck18阳性表达在增生细胞胞质。

This disease is composed of benign hepatocellular nodules, the liver cells arranged in plates pattern no more than two layers cells with fat change. The central scar in fibrous septum contains one or more dysplastic vessels and many small arteries. The radial branches of scar contain multiple portal areas，but only arteries without accompanying veins and bile ducts. There is ductular proliferation and inflammation at fibroseptal marge. Immunohistochemical Ck18 positive with cytoplasmic expression in proliferating cells.

9-42 肝细胞腺瘤 Hepatocellular adenoma

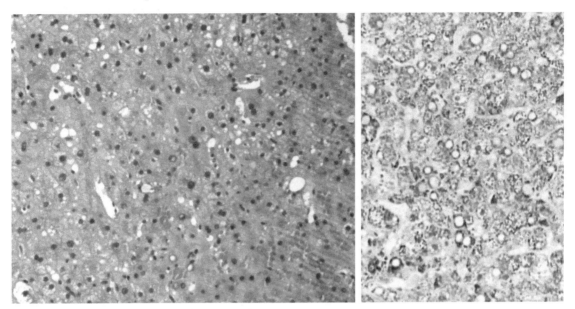

由良性的肝细胞排列成规则的单层或两层的肝板结构。无小胆管，更无门管区结构。肿瘤细胞胞浆丰富，核不典型和核分裂未见。免疫组化显示hepatocyte阳性表达在增生细胞胞质。

The tumor is composed of benign hepatocytes arranged in regular plates of one or two layer cells thick without ductular reaction and portal area. The neoplastic cell is rich cytoplasm without nuclear atypia and mitotic activity. Immunohistochemically positive hepatocyte with cytoplasmic expression in proliferating hepatocytes.

9-43 肝细胞肝癌 Hepatocellular carcinoma

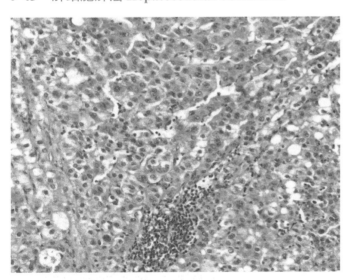

高分化HCC（well differentiated HCC）

癌细胞呈多角形，胞浆丰富，排列呈小梁状；癌组织富含血窦状裂隙；肿瘤间质稀少。部分癌细胞胞浆内可见胆汁颗粒。

Carcinoma cells show well differentiation cancer cells are polygonal with abundant and intensly eosinophilic cytoplasm, trabecular arrangement; cancer stroma shows rare. Some cancer cells contain bile particles.

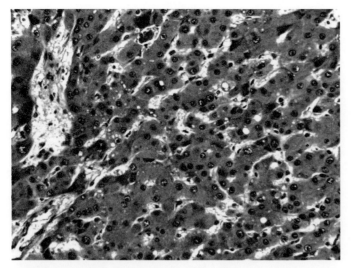

小梁状结构HCC（trabecular pattern HCC）

肿瘤细胞类似肝细胞，呈条索状排列，宽度不一，由被覆单层内皮细胞的血窦样腔隙组成的间质所分隔。

The tumor cells usually resemble hepatocytes and arrange in cords with variable thickness, separated by the stroma that is composed of sinusoid-like blood spaces lined by a single layer of endothelial cells.

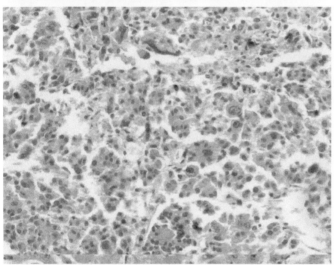

低分化HCC（poorly differentiated HCC）

呈梁状（窦索样）或假腺样排列，细胞嗜伊红的胞浆，大而不规则的异型核。

The tumor cells are arranged in trabecular（sinusoidal）or pseudoglandular patterns. Eosinophilic cytoplasma, larger and more irregular atypical nuclei are seen.

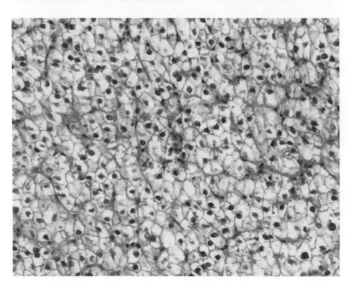

透明细胞亚型（clear cells variants）

透明细胞型作为肝细胞肝癌的一种变异，细胞透明是由于大量的胞浆糖原所致。肿瘤细胞胞浆透亮，核大、深染。

Clear cell pattern as a variant of hepatocellular carcinoma is due to large amounts of cytoplasmic glycogen. Tumour cells have clear cytoplasm with large, hyperchromatic nuclei.

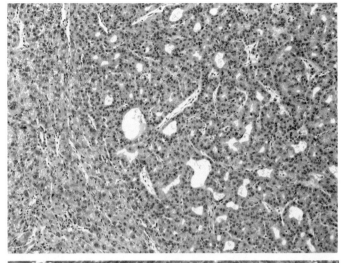

假腺样结构（pseudoglandular pattern）

肿瘤细胞类似肝细胞，呈假腺体排列，这些假腺体常由单层肿瘤细胞所组成。

The tumor cells usually resemble hepatocytes and grow in a gland-like pattern, which is formed mostly by a single layer of tumor cells.

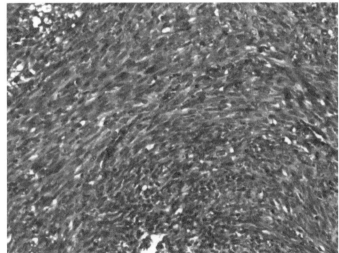

肉瘤样肝细胞肝癌（sarcomatoid hepatocellular carcinoma）

肿瘤由恶性梭形细胞所组成。

The tumor is comprised of malignant spindle cells.

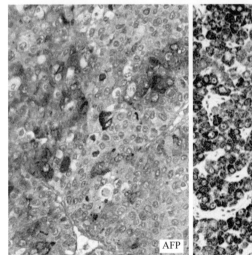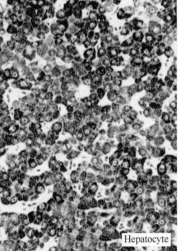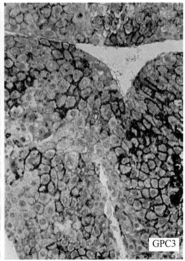

免疫组化显示AFP、Hepatocyte阳性表达在肿瘤细胞胞质，GPC3阳性膜表达。

Immunohistochemistry is positive for AFP, Hepatocyte with cytoplasmic staining pattern, and GPC3 with membrane staining pattern in tumor cells.

9-44　肺肝癌转移 Hepatocellular carcinoma metastasis，lung

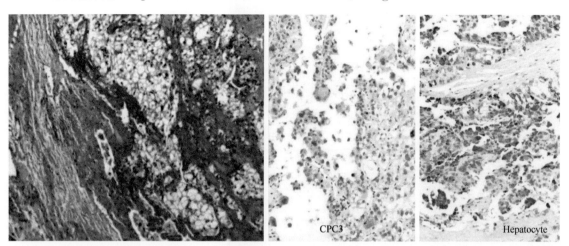

　　肿瘤细胞胞浆透亮或嗜酸性，核大、深染，呈巢状分布。免疫组化结果显示肝细胞特异性标记CPC3和Hepatocyte阳性。

The tumor distributes in nests with clear or eosinophilic cytoplasm and large and hyperchromatic nuclei. Immunohistochemistry shows that liver specific marker，GPC3 and Hepatocyte are positive.

9-45　肝内胆管癌 Intrahepatic cholangiocarcinoma

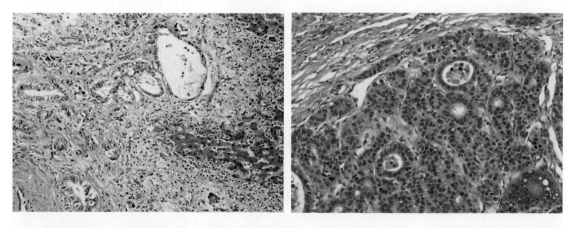

　　癌细胞呈立方形或低柱状，形成腺腔样结构，或呈实性条索状，肿瘤间质丰富，为致密的胶原纤维，促结缔组织反应。

Cancer cells are cuboidal or low columnar，forming glandular-like structures，or in solid cords，the tumor stroma is abundant，with dense collagen fibers with desmoplastic reaction.

9-46 肝母细胞瘤 Hepatoblastoma

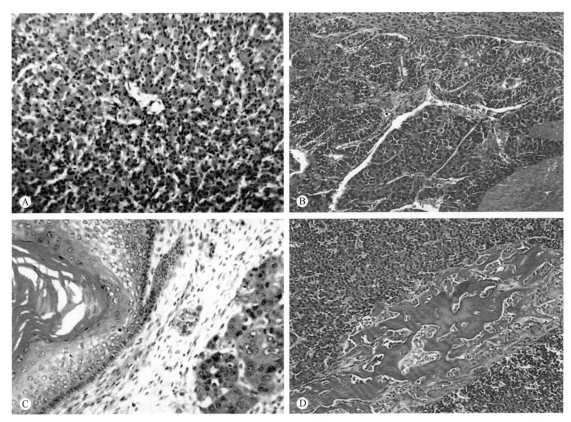

一种具有多种分化方式的恶性胚胎性肿瘤，它由相似于胎儿性上皮性肝细胞、胚胎性细胞，以及分化的间叶成分（包括骨样基质、纤维结缔组织和横纹肌纤维）组成。主要的组织学类型有：单纯胎儿型（A）；混合胎儿型和胚胎型；小细胞未分化型（B）；伴畸胎瘤特征的混合型（C）；混合性上皮和间叶型，伴嗜酸性基质组成的骨样组织（D）。

A kind of multiple differentiation of malignant embryonal tumors, it is composed of similar to fetus epitheliod liver cells, embryo cells and differentiated mesenchymal components (including osteoid matrix, fiber connective tissue and striated muscle fiber). The main types of histology are: simple fetal type (A); Mixed fetal and embryo type; small cell undifferentiated type (B); Mixed type with teratoma characterized (C); Mixed epithelium and mesenchymal type with osteoid tissue with eosinophilic matrix (D).

9-47 肝血管平滑肌脂肪瘤 Angiomyolipoma, liver

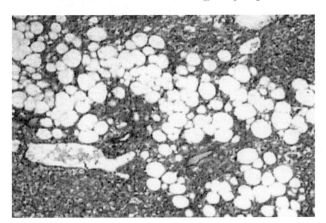

肿瘤由成熟脂肪、扭曲的厚壁玻璃样变的血管和平滑肌构成。

The tumor is composed of mature fat, twisted thick walls and hyaline degeneration blood vessels and smooth muscle.

9-48 肝代谢障碍性疾病 Metabolic disorders，liver

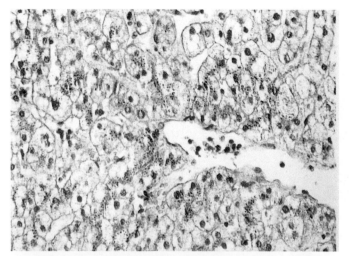

Dubin-Johnson综合征（Dubin-Johnson syndrome）

在中央静脉周围和胆管周围的肝细胞含有大量深褐色色素。

Dark brown pigments accumulate in the liver cells，particularly near centrilobular vein and pericanalicular area.

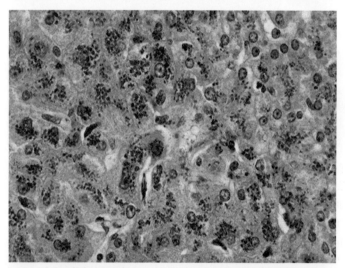

肝含铁血黄素沉积症（liver hemosiderosis）

由于过多的铁在肝脏内聚集，肝细胞和Kupffer 细胞胞浆内充满棕褐色含铁血黄素颗粒。

The hepatocytes and Kupffer cells here are full of brown hemosiderin granules from accumulation of excess iron in the liver.

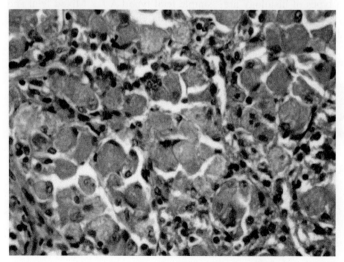

肝糖脂沉积症（戈谢病）[glycolipidosis of liver（Gaucher disease）]

肝细胞体积增大，胞质呈空网状，犹如皱纸。

Liver cell volume increases，the cytoplasm was reticulate，like crepe paper.

9-49 慢性胆囊炎 Chronic cholecystitis

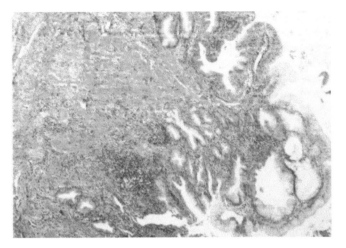

胆囊黏膜萎缩，胆囊壁各层组织中均有淋巴细胞、单核细胞浸润并伴明显纤维化。可见到纤维组织中形成的罗-阿氏窦。

Gallbladder mucosa shows atrophy, whole layers of gallbladder wall show infiltration with lymphocytes, monocytes and significant fibrosis. Romania-A's sinuses formation can be seen in the fibrous tissue.

9-50 胆囊胆固醇沉着症 Cholesterosis，gallbladder

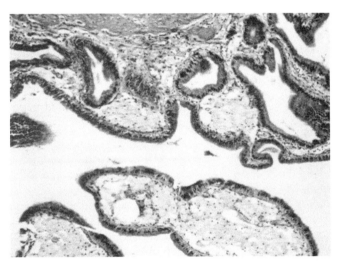

黏膜皱折增大形成绒毛顶端充满含脂质的泡沫样组织细胞。

Enlargement and distention of the mucosal fold into club shape by aggregations of lipid-laden histocytes.

9-51 胆囊腺瘤 Adenoma，gallbladder

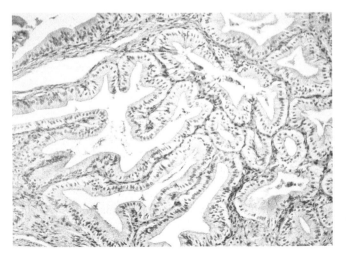

复杂分支的分化好的腺体伴纤维化的间质。

Complex branching prolifiration of well differentiated gland with a fibrotic stroma.

9-52　胆囊癌 Carcinoma，gallbladder

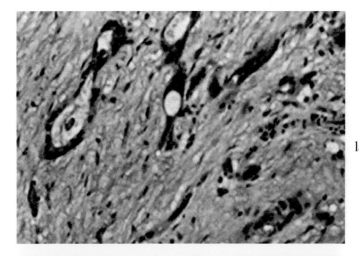

腺癌间质促结缔组织增生反应。
Adnocarcinoma with desmoplastic reaction.

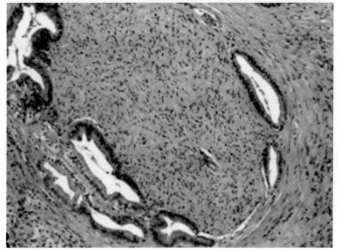

癌神经侵犯。
Carcinoma cells infiltrated nerve fibron.

9-53　胆管癌 Cholangiocarcinoma

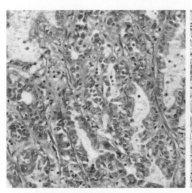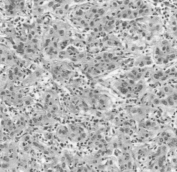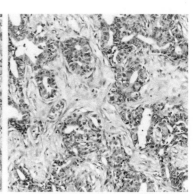

　　肿瘤细胞形成大小不一、形状不一的腺腔结构伴不同分化，或乳头状结构、实性巢状结构。腺体间可有大量纤维间质增生。
　　Most tumor cells form a relatively irregular glandular cavity, with variable differentiation, having tubular structure with variable-sized and shaped lumina, or the structure of solid nests, or papillary structures. Abundant fibrous hyperplasia appear between glands.

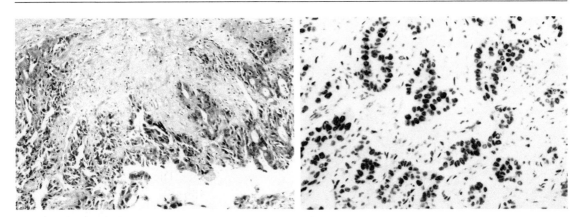

硬化性胆管癌（sclerosing cholangiocarcinoma）

硬化性胆管癌中肿瘤组织分化好并伴广泛纤维化。免疫组化腺上皮标记CK7免疫组化阳性，胆管常用标记CTBP2阳性。

The tumor tissue is well differentiated and has extensive fibrosis. Immunohistochemistry is positive for a glandular epithelium marker CK7 and CTBP2，CTBP2 is common used marker for bile duct.

9-54 胰腺炎 Pancreatitis

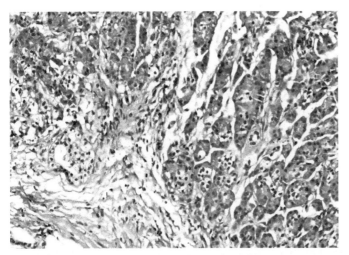

胰腺组织间质充血水肿；中性粒细胞及单核细胞浸润。

Pancreatic tissues show hyperemia and edema；with infilration of neutrophils and monocytes.

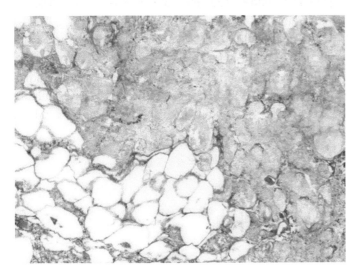

胰腺脂肪坏死（左），胰腺实质坏死（右）。

Fat necrosis（left），and focal pancreatic parenchymal necrosis（right）.

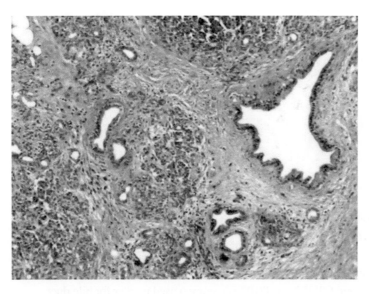

慢性胰腺炎（chronic pancreatitis）

导管上皮增生，间质弥漫性纤维组织增生和淋巴细胞、浆细胞浸润。

The epithelial of duct proliferation with desmoplasia and chronic inflammatory cells infiltration.

9-55 胰腺实性假乳头肿瘤 Solid pseudopapillary neoplasm，pancreas

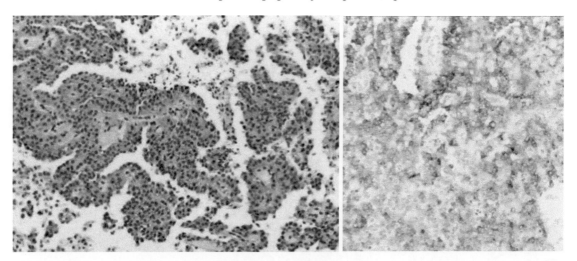

胰腺假乳头状肿瘤又称为胰腺囊实性肿瘤（Solid-Cystic tumor of pancreas）、乳头状和实性上皮性肿瘤（papillary and solid epithelial neoplasm，PSEN）

肿瘤细胞由形态一致的、黏附性差的上皮细胞构成，胞浆嗜酸或空泡状，核圆形或卵圆形，染色质细腻，可见核沟。肿瘤细胞形成实性及假乳头状结构。免疫组化CD10阳性。

The tumor is composed of poorly cohesive monomorphic epithelial cells forming solid and pseudopapillary structures. The neoplastic cells have either eosinophilic or clear vacuolated cytoplasm. The round to oval nuclei of the neoplastic cells have finely dispersed chromatin and the nuclei often have groove. Immunohistochemistry is positive for CD10.

9-56 胰腺浆液性囊腺瘤 Pancreatic serous cystadenoma

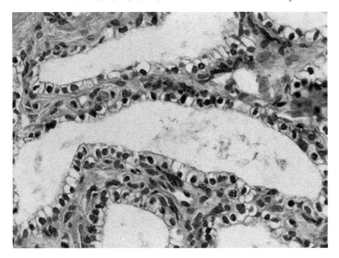

囊肿被覆扁平及立方形的小细胞。胞浆内充满糖原，透明。

The cyst is lined with flattened and cuboidal small cells. The cytoplasm is filled with glycogen and clear.

9-57 黏液性囊性肿瘤 Mucinous cystic neoplasm

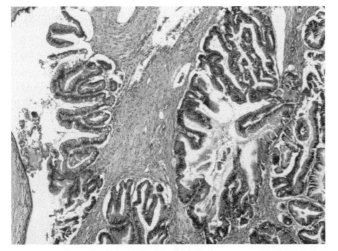

囊壁被覆分泌黏液的高柱状细胞形成乳头。肿瘤细胞可有间质浸润。

Intrcystic growth of tall columnar epithelial cells may form papillary pattern，the tumor cells also infiltrate into stroma.

9-58 导管内乳头状黏液肿瘤 Intraductal papillary mucinous neoplasm（IPMN）

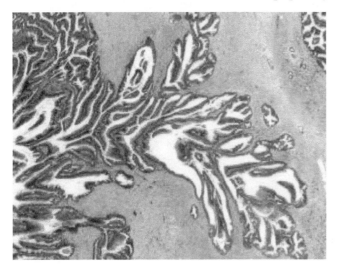

这是一种起源于主胰管或其主要分支的分泌黏液的乳头状肿瘤。根据肿瘤中乳头上皮成分、分泌黏液的程度、囊性导管扩张及是否浸润，将该肿瘤分为良性、交界性、恶性非浸润性和恶性浸润性4类。

This is a kind of secreting mucus papillary tumor originated in the main pancreatic duct or its main branches. According to papillary epithelial components，the degree of secrete mucus, cystic duct expansion and infiltration in tumor, the tumor can be divided into 4 classes：benign，border，malignant without invasive and malignant with invasive.

9-59 胰腺癌 Pancreatic carcinoma

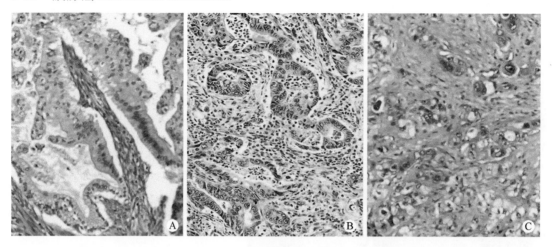

A：Ⅰ级（well differentiated），由完好的腺体组成，腺体的大小和形状显示轻度异型，比较规则，癌细胞呈柱状或立方形。B：Ⅱ级（moderately differentiated）：介于高分化和低分化之间，腺管结构不规则，或形成不完整的腺腔，异型较为显著。C：Ⅲ级（poorly differentiated）：由难以辨认的高度不规则腺体组成。腺管样结构不明显，或几乎没有腺管样结构，构像变异很大。

A：Well-differentiated adenocarcinomas are composed of well-formed glands，which size and shape show slightly different，relatively regular in a columnar or cuboidal form. B：Moderately differentiated adenocarcinomas are composed of neoplasm intermediated between well and poorly differentiated. The glands are irregular or incomplete with relatively remarkable atypia. C：Poorly differentiated adenocarcinomas are comprise of highly irregular glands that are difficulty to recognize. The tubular structure of glands are not obvious or almost absent，variable greatly in morphology.

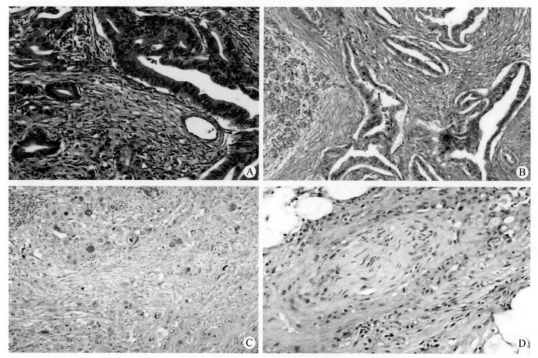

A：高分化；B：中分化；C：低分化；D：胰腺癌神经周围浸润。

A：well differentiated carcinoma；B：moderately differentiated carcinoma；C：poorly differentiated carcinoma；D：perineural invasion carcinoma.

9-60 胰腺腺泡细胞癌 Pancreatic acinar cell carcinoma

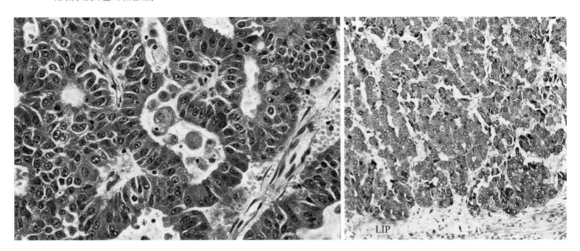

高柱状肿瘤细胞浸润间质，免疫组化LIP阳性

The tall columnar tumor cells infiltrate into stroma. Immunohistochemistry LIP is positive.

9-61 胰母细胞瘤 Pancreatoblastoma

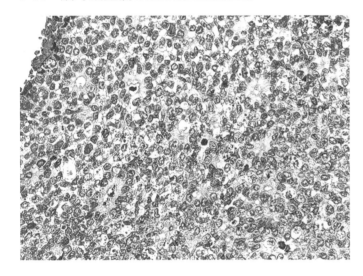

肿瘤细胞密集，实性巢状。间质纤维间隔分割呈"地图样"：以腺泡分化为主，不同程度内分泌及导管分化。有特征性鳞状小体。

The tumor cells arrange dense and solid nests pattern. The interstitial fibrous septa are similar to "map like": major, acinar differentiation, varible endocrine and ductal differentiation. There is characteristic squamous body.

第十章 淋巴造血系统疾病

Chapter 10   Disorders of Hematopoietic and Lymphoid System

10-1   反应性淋巴结增生 Reactive lymphadenopathies

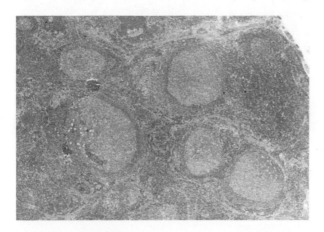

反应性淋巴滤泡增生。Reactive lymphoid follicular hyperplasia.

滤泡中可见数量较多的母化细胞、核分裂像和着色体巨噬细胞。

Lymphoid follicular shows hyperplasia，with a large number of blastic cells，mitotic figures and tingible body macrophages.

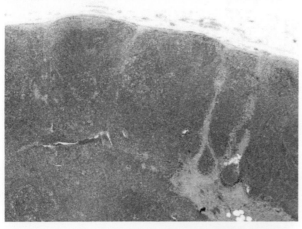

反应性副皮质区增生。Reactive paracortical area hyperplasia.

副皮质区增生、扩大，高内皮小静脉增生显著，大量活化的T免疫母细胞混杂期间。

Para cortex is hyperplastic，expanding，high endothelial venules，with a large number of active T immunoblastic cells.

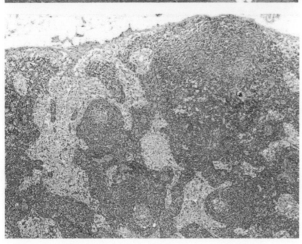

窦组织细胞增生。
Sinus histiocytosis（"sinus catarrh"）.

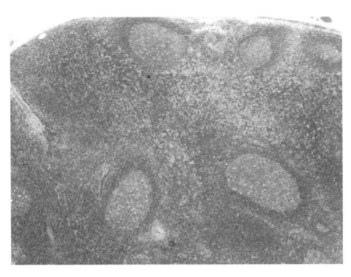

反应性淋巴结增生（混合型）包括：

淋巴滤泡增生、副皮质区增生、窦组织细胞增生。显著的毛细血管后微静脉，以及免疫母细胞、浆细胞和组织细胞增多。

Reactive lymphoid hyperplasia （mixed pattern）including：lymphoid follicular hyperplasia paracortical hyperplasia and sinus histiocytosis. The number of postcapillary venules immunoblasts plasma cells，and histiocytes prominencely increased.

10-2　结节病 Sarcoidosis

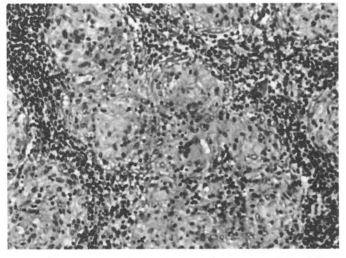

淋巴结中可见主要由上皮样细胞构成的融合性非坏死性肉芽肿。

Numerous confluent nonnecrotizing granulomas mainly composed of epithelioid cells in a lymph node.

10-3　Kimura 病 Kimura disease

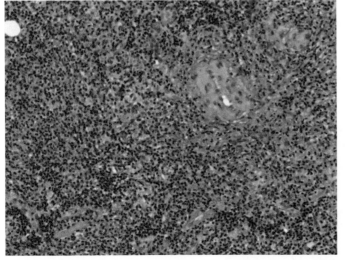

可见大量成熟的嗜酸细胞浸润以及玻璃样变的血管常见于副皮质区。

The lymph nodes show the extensive infiltration of mature eosinophils. Hyalinized degeneration vessels are often seen in the paracortical region.

10-4 血管滤泡性淋巴组织增生 Angiofollicular lymphoid hyperplasia（Castleman disease）

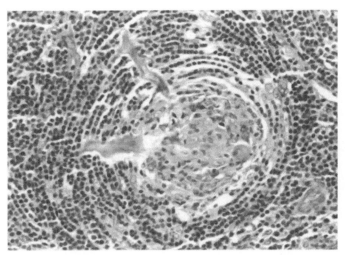

有透明血管型和浆细胞型。

淋巴滤泡内见玻璃样变性的小血管长入，生发中心血管内皮细胞增生，类似胸腺小体。套区增宽，淋巴细胞呈洋葱皮样排列。

It is also known as Castleman disease, hyaline-vascular type and plasma cell type, which typically shows that small vessels with hyaline degeneration grow into lymphoid follicles, hyperplasia of vascular endothelial cells occurs in germinal center, similar to thymus corpuscles and mantle zone broadens with lymphocytes onion peelings arrangement.

10-5 窦组织细胞增生症 Sinus histiocytosis（Rosai-Dorfamn disease）

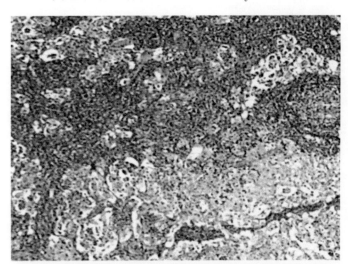

淋巴结包膜增厚，纤维化。

淋巴窦显著扩张，充满特征性组织细胞（明区）。

髓质的索和窦内大量浆细胞（暗区）。

Capsule of lymph node is thicken and fibrosis.

The lymphatic sinus dilated significantly with pale-staining bands of cells（characteristic Rosai-Dorfmanc histiocytes）alternating with dark-staining areas（plasma cells）.

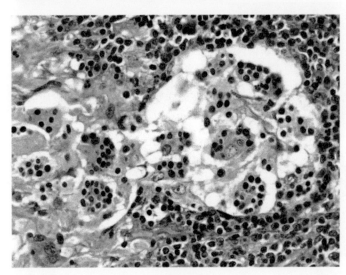

组织细胞体积大，直径为小淋巴细胞核的 6～12 倍，胞浆丰富，可见淋巴细胞被吞噬作用。

Histiocyte is large with rich-cytoplasm, its diameter is 6～12 times that of the small lymphocyte nucleus. Lymphocyte is phagocyted.

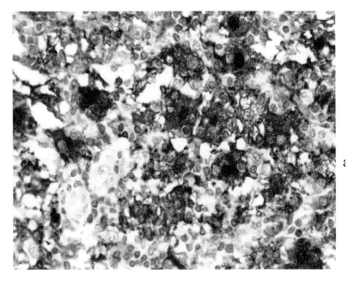

免疫组化染色 S-100 阳性。

S-100 positive for the histiocytes and emperipolesis.

10-6　亚急性淋巴结炎 Subacute lymphadenitis（Kikuchi disease）组织细胞性坏死性淋巴结炎（Histiocytic necrotizing lymphadenitis）

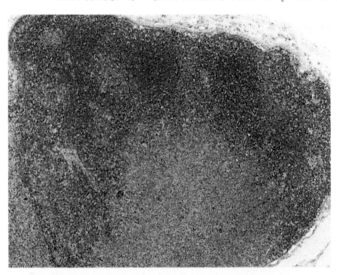

斑片状受累区可融合成不规则地图状嗜伊红凝固性坏死，混有许多组织细胞和核碎屑。

周围为组织细胞，淋巴细胞和免疫母细胞，缺乏中性粒细胞。

The patchy area can be fused into an irregular map eosinophilic necrosis, with many tissue cells and nuclear detritus. The surrounding tissue presents histocytes, lymphocytes and immune cells, lacks neutrophils.

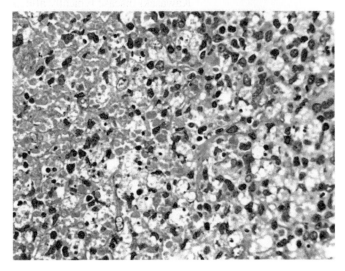

组织细胞胞浆丰富，核呈新月形、扭曲或印戒样，常吞噬细胞碎屑。

Histiocytes have abundant cytoplasm with nucleus crescent-shaped, twisted or insignetic. Histiocytes often phagocyte cell debris.

10-7 传染性单核细胞增生症 Infectious mononucleosis

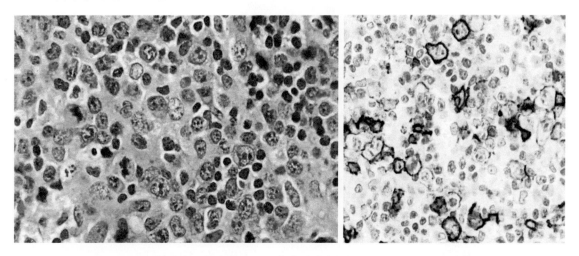

单核细胞样 B 细胞增生伴反应性增生。增生细胞 CD20 阳性，但阳性强度不一（右）。CD30+、LMP1+、EBER+。

Monocyteliod B cell hyperplasia with reactive follicular hyperplasia. Proliferating cell CD20 positive，but the positive expression is vary（right）. CD30，LMP1，EBER is positive，respectively.

10-8 Kawasaki 病 Kawasaki disease

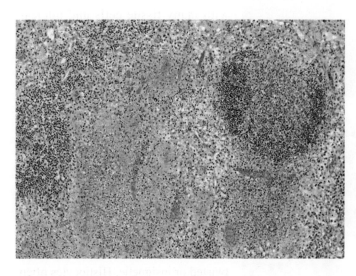

主要累及 5 岁以下儿童，临床上持续高热、皮疹；颈淋巴结肿大和全身血管炎。病理特征为地图样纤维素性坏死、核碎片、不伴细胞增生，可有中性粒细胞浸润。纤维素性血栓。静脉内注射 γ 球蛋白和 / 或高剂量阿司匹林可治愈。

Kawasaki disease typically affects infants and children. Characterized by fever，skin rash，cervical lymphadenopathy and systemic vasculitis Main histologic changes：geographic fibrinoid necrosis in cortex and paracortex without much cell proliferation；There are neutrophils and fibrin thrombi in blood vessels. Early treatment with intravenous immunoglobulin and aspirin reduces the complication.

10-9　化脓性淋巴结炎 Suppurative lymphadenitis

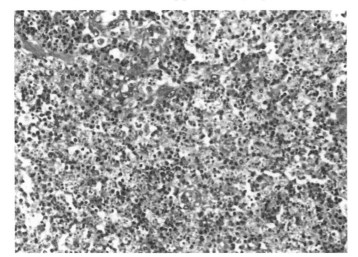

受累淋巴结可见淋巴窦扩张，血管扩张以及多量中性粒细胞浸润，部分病例可有坏死表现。

The involved nodes show sinus dilation，vascular dilation，and accumulation of neutrophils. Necrosis may be seen in some cases.

10-10　淋巴结结核 Tuberculosis，lymph nodes

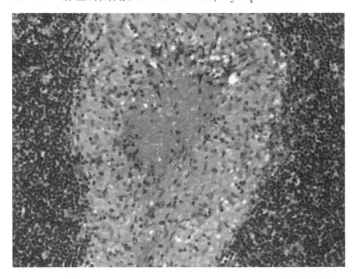

结节中央为干酪样坏死灶，周围为增生的 Langhans 巨细胞、类上皮细胞以及淋巴细胞。

Central caseous necrosis is surrounded by Langhans giant cells，epithelioid cells，and lymphocytes.

10-11　猫抓病 Cat-scratch disease

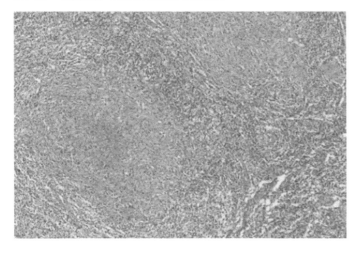

淋巴结中可见大小不等的脓肿形成，脓肿中心可有星芒状坏死，并可见中性粒细胞，组织细胞呈栅状排列在周围。

The lymphnodes present abscesses of various sizes. Stellate necrosis with neutrophils can be seen in the center, surrounded by a palisading of histiocytes.

10-12　霍奇金淋巴瘤中 RS 细胞及其变异 Reed-Sternberg cell and its variants in Hodgkin's lymphoma

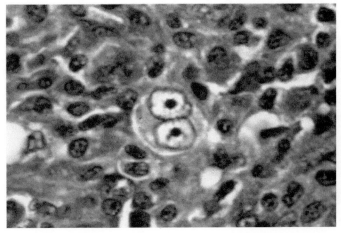

RS 细胞，双核对称，核仁明显。常染色质形成核周空晕，核膜增厚。胞浆丰富，常呈嗜酸性。免疫组化CD30、EBER、EMA 和 Pax5 阳性。

A Reed-Sternberg cell shows a symmetric binucleation with prominent nucleoli. There is prominent parachromatin clearing, leaving a perinucleolar halo with thickened nuclear membrane. The abundant cytoplasm is usually acidophilic.

They are positive for CD30, EBER, EMA and Pax5 in immunohistochemistry.

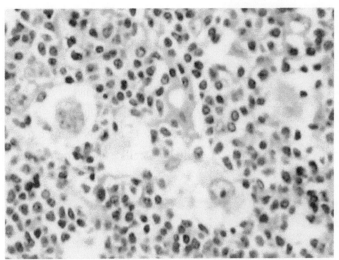

陷窝细胞（lacunar cells）

见于结节硬化型和混合细胞型。

Found in nodular sclerosing subtype and mixed cellularity subtype.

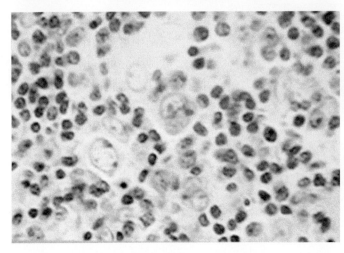

爆米花细胞（popcorn cell）

在淋巴细胞为主型中 RS 细胞变异（爆米花细胞）呈核分叶，染色质细颗粒状，少量透明胞浆和小核仁。

In lymphocyte-rich subtype, RS cells varied（popcorn cell）in nuclei with lobes granules chromatin, and small amounts of clear cytoplasm and small nucleoli.

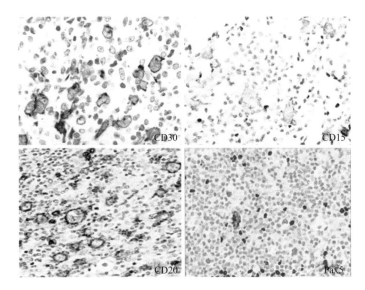

免疫组化染色诊断性 RS 细胞 CD30、CD15、CD20 阳性。陷窝细胞 Pax5 阳性。

Diagnostic Reed-Sternberg cells are CD30、CD15、CD20 positive.

Lacunar cells are positive for Pax5.

10-13　结节性淋巴细胞为主型霍奇金淋巴瘤 Nodular lymphocyte-predominant Hodgkin's lymphoma（NLPHL）

NLPHL 是伴 K 轻链限制的 B 细胞淋巴瘤。淋巴结结构部分或全部被大小不等结节所累及，结节呈斑点状不同于滤泡性淋巴瘤。

在 NLPHL 中缺乏典型 RS 细胞、嗜酸性粒细胞、浆细胞及纤维化；可见较多的 L&H 细胞，该细胞多叶折叠的核伴有小核仁背景富于淋巴细胞，CD20 阳性。

NLPHL is a form of B-cell lymphoma with kappa light chain restriction. The lymph node architecture is partially or totally effaced by nodules which are more irregular in size and have mottled appearance as compared to those seen in follicular lymphoma.

In NLPHL, classic Reed-Sternberg cells, eosinophils, plasma cells, and areas of fibrosis are absent. Instead, numerous L&H cells with multilobed, folded nucleus with small nucleoli are present in a background rich in lymphocytes.

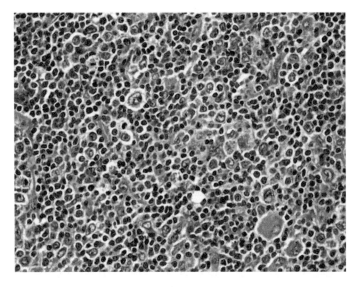

10-14 经典型霍奇金淋巴瘤 Classical Hodgkin's lymphoma

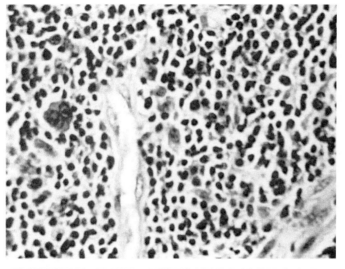

淋巴细胞为主型（lymphocyte-rich subtype）

淋巴结肿大，瘤组织呈结节状或弥漫性生长，其中存在大量淋巴细胞，而其他炎症细胞少见，可找及 L&H 型 RS 细胞。

Lymph nodes swelling, tumor tissues show nodular or diffuse growth with a large number of lymphocytes, and other inflammatory cells are rare to see, L & H type RS cells can be found.

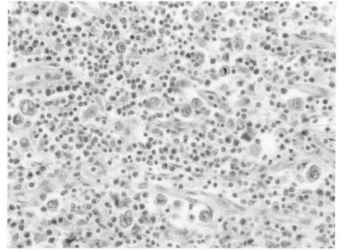

混合细胞型（mixed cellularity subtype）

混合细胞型霍奇金淋巴瘤显示典型的 RS 细胞和一些霍奇金 /RS 细胞，背景中有小淋巴细胞、嗜酸性粒细胞和组织细胞，伴促结缔组织增生。

Mixed cellularity Hodgkin's lymphoma shows a typical RS cells and some Hodgkin / RS cells. There are small lymphocytes, eosinophils and a histiocytes inflammatory background, with desmoplastic figures.

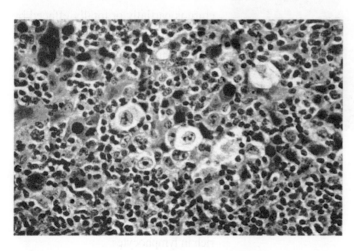

结节硬化型（nodular sclerosing subtype）

①粗大的胶原分隔病变的淋巴结为大小不等的结节。②瘤结节内可见多数陷窝细胞。此外，可见淋巴细胞、组织细胞、嗜酸性粒细胞和浆细胞等多种炎细胞反应。

① Lymph nodes are separated by thick collagen into nodes of varying sizes. ② Most lacunar cells are visible in tumor nodules. In addition, resposing lymphocytes, histiocytes, eosinophils, and plasma cells and other inflammatory cells reactive can be seen.

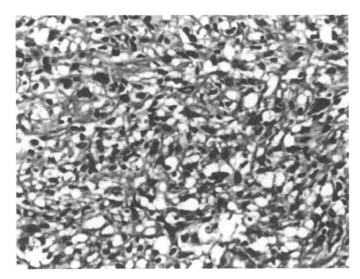

淋巴细胞消减型（lymphocyte depletion type）

致密的纤维性间质中可见较多的非典型细胞，淋巴细胞稀少，瘤细胞 CD30、EBER、Pax5 阳性。

Numerous atypical cells are present in a densely fibrotic stroma. Lymphocytes are scanty. Tumor cells are positive for CD30，EBER and Pax5.

10-15　前体 B 淋巴母细胞性淋巴瘤 Precursor B lymphoblastic lymphoma

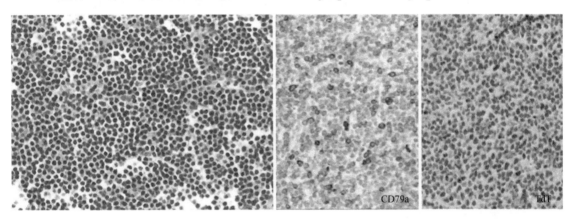

淋巴结结构破坏。瘤细胞弥漫性浸润，相对单一形态的小淋巴细胞增殖，肿瘤细胞胞质少，核圆伴轻微扭曲，染色质细点状，核仁不明显，核分裂象多。其中可见散在分布的大细胞（前淋巴细胞），部分大细胞局部积聚形成所谓的“假滤泡”。可见灶性“星空”现象；免疫组化呈 CD79a、TdT 阳性。

Lymph structural damage. There is a diffuse infiltration and relatively monomorphic small lymphocytes proliferation. The neoplastic cells have scanty cytoplasm and nucleus round with delicate convolutions. The chromatin is finely stippled and nucleoli are inconspicuous. Mitotic activity is extremely high. Large cells（pre-lymphocytes）are scattered，part of the large cells show local accumulation and form “fake follicles”. A focal “starry sky” appearance can be seen in some of the cases. The tumor cells express TdT and CD79a.

10-16　滤泡性淋巴瘤 Follicular lymphoma（FL）

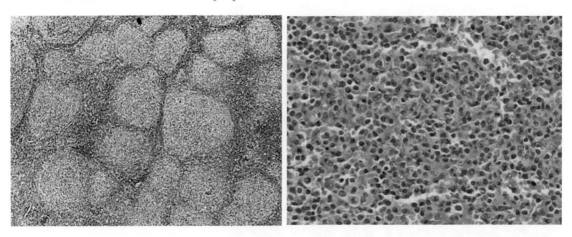

　　属于 B 细胞淋巴瘤，淋巴结正常结构破坏，被密集排列的肿瘤性滤泡所取代。肿瘤性滤泡中包括中心细胞样瘤细胞和中心母细胞样瘤细胞。瘤细胞较大，具有不规则的"裂"核，以显著的锯齿状和线性皱褶为特征。

　　It belongs to B cell lymphoma，lymph node normal structural destroy，replaced by densely packed neoplastic follicles. which include centrocyte-like tumor cells，centroblastic cell-like tumor cells. The cells are large with irregular "cleave" nucleus，with the feature of significantly jagged and linear folds.

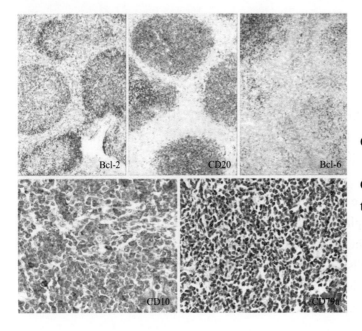

　　滤泡性淋巴瘤免疫组化 Bcl-2、CD20、Bcl-6、CD10、CD79a 阳性。

　　Immunohistochemical Bcl-2，CD20，Bcl-6，CD10，CD79a positive of FL.

10-17 套细胞淋巴瘤 Mantle cell lymphoma（MCL）

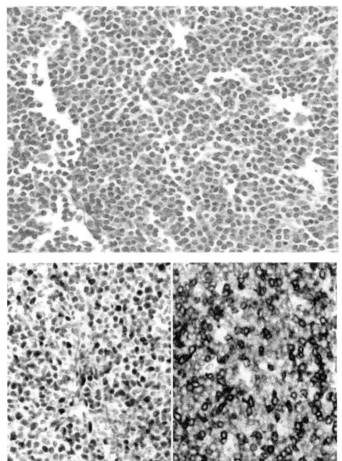

CyclinD1　　CD5

套细胞淋巴瘤往往累及多组淋巴结。淋巴结内瘤组织呈模糊结节状、弥漫或套区生长方式。瘤细胞较正常淋巴细胞稍大，具有不规则核裂或圆形核，核仁不显著。

Mantle cell lymphoma shows a diffuse involvement of lymph node. Tumor tissue in lymph nodes show fuzzy, diffuse or mantle zone growth patterns. The tumor cells are slightly larger than normal lymphocytes and have an irregular cleaved or round nucleus. The nucleoli are inconspicuous.

淋巴结内瘤组织呈模糊的结节状、弥漫或套区增宽的改变，肿瘤细胞较小，核不规则或锯齿状。免疫组化瘤细胞 CyclinD1 核阳性，CD5 阳性表达在肿瘤细胞胞质。

Tumor tissues in lymph node show fuzzy nodular, diffuse or mantle zone enlargement. The neoplastic cells are small, irregular and jagged patterns. The tumor cells express CD5 in cytoplasm and CyclinD1 in nuclei.

10-18 弥漫大 B 细胞淋巴瘤 Diffuse large B cell lymphoma（DLBCL）

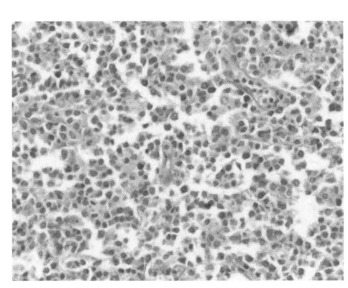

正常的淋巴结结构完全或部分性的被弥漫性的肿瘤组织取代，肿瘤细胞较正常细胞稍大，伴有明显核仁的泡状核，胞质相对丰富，包括具有不规则的"裂"核的中心母细胞样和具 1～2 个居中的显著核仁的免疫母细胞样。

The normal lymph node structure is completely or partially replaced by diffuse tumor tissue. The tumor cells were slightly larger than normal cells, with the vesicular nuclei with obvious nucleoli and relatively abundant cytoplasm, include immunoblastic tumor cells with 1～2 center significantly nucleoli, and centroblastic tumor cells with irregular "cleave" nucleus.

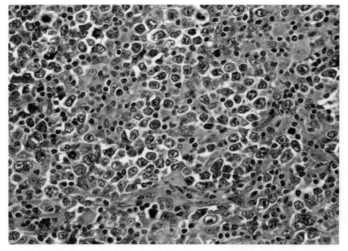

中心母细胞变异是由类似于正常生发中心的细胞组成。有中 - 大的裂和无裂细胞组成。核小，不规则棱角、椭圆 / 圆形，多个小核仁。胞质少，大量核丝分裂和凋亡细胞出现。

Centroblastic variant is composed of cells resemble reactive germinal center. There is an admixture of medium to large size with cleaved or non-cleaved cells. The nuclei are small, irregular and angulated or oval/round with multiple small nucleoli. Cytoplasm is scant and numerous mitotic figures and apoptotic cells are present.

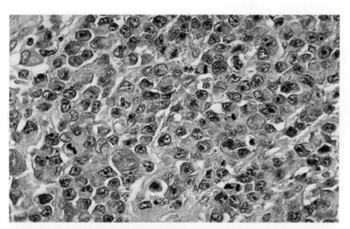

免疫母细胞变异（immunoblastic variant）

有大量的转化细胞，明显单个核仁，适度的胞质。

There are numerous transformed cells with prominent single nucleoli and moderate cytoplasm.

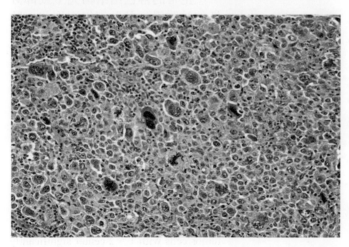

间变细胞变异（anaplastic variant）

肿瘤细胞大、圆、或多边性，异型多核，有类似于 RS 细胞。细胞呈铺路石样排列，可沿淋巴窦生长，貌似癌。

Tumor cells are large, round or multipleated, heteromorphotic multinuclei, which are similar to RS cell. The tumor cells arrange in paving stones, which can grow along the lymphatic sinus and appear to be cancerous.

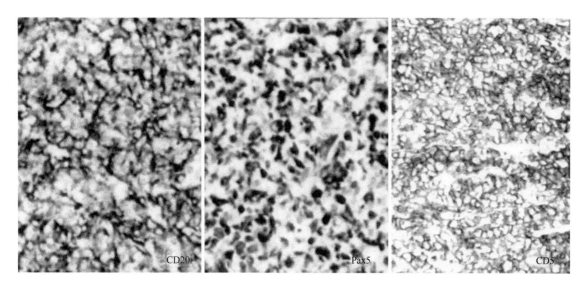

瘤细胞表达 B 细胞标志，如 CD20、Pax5。约 10% 的病例表达 CD5。

The tumor cells express B-lineage markers，such as CD20 and Pax5. CD5 is expressed in 10% of cases.

10-19　ALK 阳性大 B 细胞淋巴瘤 ALK⁺ large B-cell lymphoma

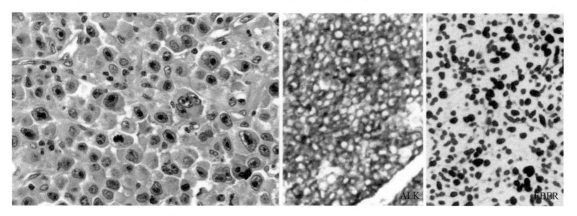

这是 DLBCL 中的少见类型，伴有浆母细胞分化，其肿瘤细胞具有免疫母细胞和浆母细胞形态。瘤细胞表达 ALK 和 EBER。

This is an uncommon form of DLBCL with plasmablastic differentiation. The tumor cells have an immunoblastic or plasmablastic appearance. The tumor cells express ALK and EBER.

10-20　伯基特淋巴瘤 Burkitt's lymphoma（BL）

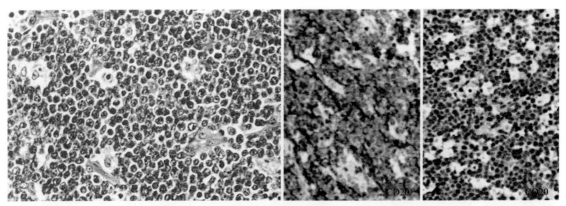

　　形态单一、中等大小的淋巴样肿瘤细胞弥漫性浸润。瘤细胞核圆或卵圆形，染色质分散，有 2～5 个明显的核仁。胞质中等量，嗜碱性。瘤细胞大量核分裂相与细胞凋亡，后者被巨噬细胞所吞噬形成所谓"星空"的图像。瘤细胞 CD20、EBER 阳性。

　　Diffuse infiltration of single-shaped, medium-sized lymphoid tumor cells. Tumor nuclei are round or oval, chromatin dispersion, with 2～5 prominent nucleoli. Moderate amount of basophilic cytoplasm. Tumor cells show more mitotic figures and apoptosis which is engulfed by macrophages present "starry sky pattern". The tumor cells express CD20 and EBER.

10-21　浆细胞瘤 Plasmacytoma

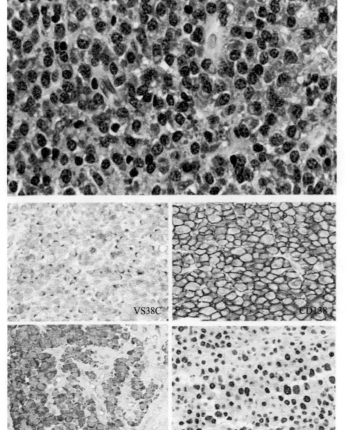

　　肿瘤由分化良好的浆细胞弥漫性增生和浸润，瘤细胞胞质呈嗜碱性，常见核周空晕，核偏于一侧，染色质凝集成车辐状。

　　The tumor is formed by well-differentiated plasma cells, which are proliferation and diffuse infiltration. Cytoplasm of tumor cell is basophilic, perinuclear halos, and nuclei biased side are common, chromatin condensation as wheels shape.

　　免疫组化显示 VS38C、CD138、KAPPA 阳性表达在肿瘤细胞胞质。MUM1 阳性表达在肿瘤细胞核。

　　Immunohistochemical MUM1 positive nuclear expression VS38C, CD138 and KAPPA positive cytoplasmic expression in tumor cells.

10-22 黏膜相关淋巴组织结外边缘区 B 细胞淋巴瘤 Extranodal marginal zone B cell lymphoma of mucosa-associated lymphoid tissue（MALT）

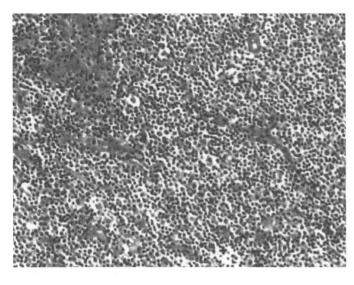

淋巴滤泡边缘区扩张，肿瘤细胞完全是小细胞，包括小圆细胞、单核细胞样 B 细胞、轻微不规则核（中心细胞样）细胞、浆细胞样细胞和浆细胞，偶可见大淋巴细胞。

The marginal zone of lymph follicules expansion. The cell populations are all of small size, including small round lymphocytes, monocytoid B cells with slightly irregular nuclei（centrocyte-like）, plasmacytoid cells, and plasma cells. Large lymphoid cells may occasionally be seen.

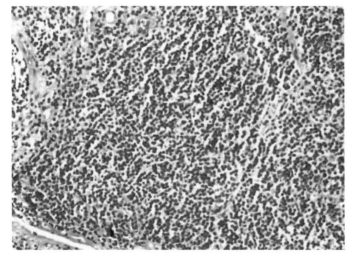

瘤细胞浸润并占据整个淋巴滤泡，被称为滤泡殖入。

Tumor cells infiltrate and occupy the entire lymphoid follicules, known as follicular implantation.

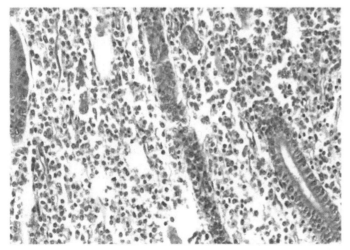

常见 3 个或以上的瘤细胞侵袭破坏腺上皮形成"淋巴上皮病变"。

Commonly three or more tumor cells invade and destroy glandular epithelium form a so-called "lymphatic epithelial lesion".

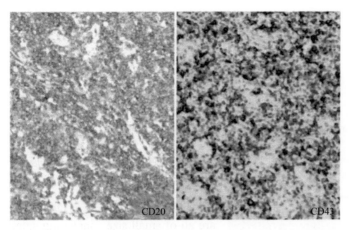

免疫组化瘤细胞 CD20 和 CD43 阳性。

The tumor cells express CD20 and CD43.

10-23　外周 T 细胞淋巴瘤，非特殊型 Peripheral T cell lymphoma，unspecified（U-PTL）

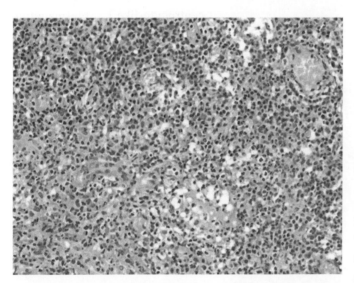

淋巴结结构破坏，呈副皮质区或整个淋巴组织中弥漫浸润，瘤细胞中等细胞和/或大细胞，核不规则，多形，染色深或空泡状，核仁明显。常伴高内皮小静脉增生和数量不等的炎细胞浸润。

The lymphnode structure is destroy The tumor cells diffuse infiltrates to the paracortex or the entire lymph node. The tumor cells are medium-sized or large lymphoidocytes with irregular nuclei, which are hyperchromatic or vesicular with prominent nucleoli. Often accompanied by the proliferation of high endothelial venules and varying amounts of inflammatory cells infiltration.

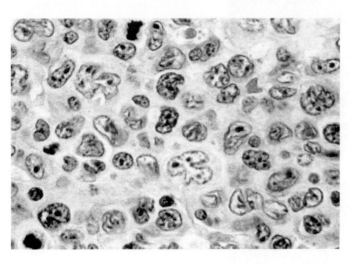

多形性外周 T 细胞淋巴瘤，核显著多形性，分叶状，染色质散在分布，有多个小核仁。

Pleomorphic peripheral T-cell lymphoma marked nuclear pleomorphism and lobulation are seen. Chromatin is dispersed and there are multiple small nucleoli.

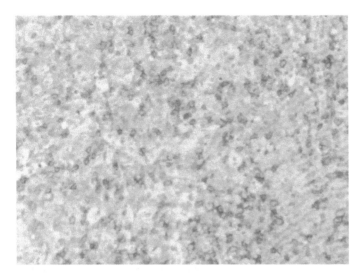

T 细胞标记 CD4 免疫组化阳性。

The cells are positive for CD4, a marker of T cells, used by immunohistochemistry.

10-24　前体 T 淋巴母细胞性淋巴瘤 Precursor T lymphoblastic lymphoma

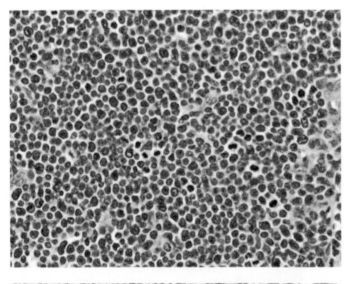

肿瘤细胞胞质少，核圆形，有轻微扭曲，染色质细点状，核仁不明显，核分裂象多，可见灶性"星空"现象。

The neoplastic cells have scanty cytoplasm and a nucleus round with slight delicate convolutions. The chromatin is finely stippled, nucleoli are inconspicuous. Mitotic activity is extremely high. A focal "starry sky" appearance can be seen in some of the cases.

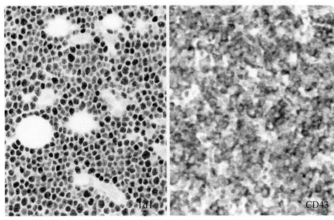

免疫组化呈 TdT 阳性表达在肿瘤细胞核，CD43 阳性表达在肿瘤细胞胞质。

The tumor cells express TdT in nuclear and CD43 in cytoplasmic of tumor cells.

10-25 结外鼻型 NK/T 细胞淋巴瘤 Extranodal NK/T cell lymphoma，nasal type

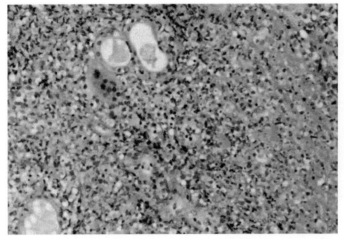

肿瘤常有明显的地图状凝固性坏死，为瘤细胞侵袭和破坏血管的结果。肿瘤由细胞形态由相对单一的中等大的淋巴样细胞组成，核形不规则、胞质淡染，弥漫浸润。并有数量不等的炎细胞混杂其中。

There is commonly prominent Map-like coagulation necrosis in the tumor, as the result of tumor cells invasion and destruction of blood vessels.

The tumor cells are relatively monomorphic medium-sized lymphoid cells with round irregular nuclei and pale-staining cytoplasm and diffuse infiltrates. Amounts of inflammatory ixed with them.

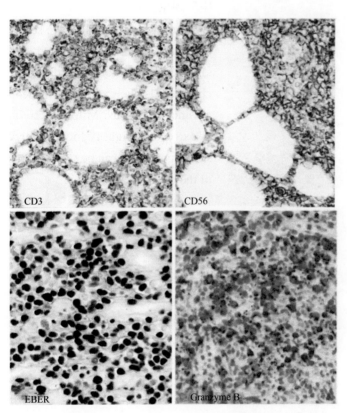

CD3　CD56

EBER　Granzyme B

免疫组化结果显示 CD3，CD56 和 Granzyme B 阳性；原位杂交显示 EBER 阳性。

The cells are positive for CD3, CD56 and Granzyme B detected by immunohistochemistry. EBER is positive detected by in situ hybridization.

10-26　ALK 阴性的间变性大细胞淋巴瘤 Anaplastic large cell lymphoma，ALK-negative

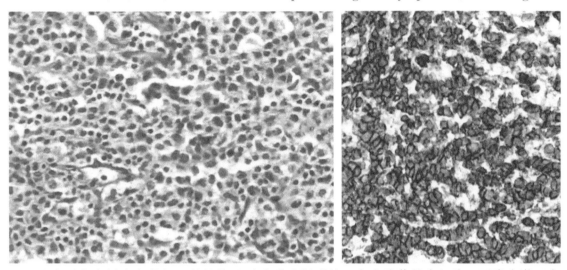

　　肿瘤形态多样存在数量不等的核呈马蹄形或肾形的、富含胞浆的大细胞，通常在淋巴窦内，这种细胞也被称为标志细胞（间变性细胞 CD15/CD30 阳性），属于 B 细胞来源。这种细胞应与转移癌细胞和 Reed-Sternberg 细胞鉴别。免疫组化结果显示 CD30 阳性、ALK 阴性。

　　Tumor morphology varies，large cells with horseshoe-shape or kidney-shape nucleus and abundant cytoplasm，usually in lymphatic sinuses，such cells are also referred to as a flag cell（anaplastic cells CD15/CD30 positive），belonging to B cells. Such cells should be identified with metastatic cancer cells and Reed-Sternberg cells. Anaplastic cells are positive for CD30 and negative for ALK detected by immunohistochemistry.

10-27　血管免疫母细胞性 T 细胞淋巴瘤 Angioimmunoblastic T cell lymphoma

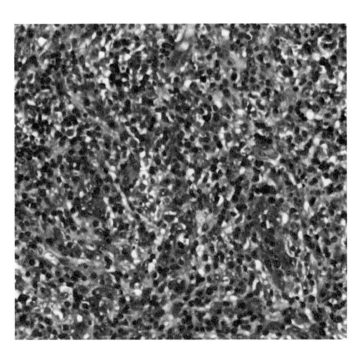

　　淋巴结结构部分破坏，小至中等大的肿瘤性 T 细胞成团或成片生长。瘤细胞具有丰富而透明的胞浆，胞质淡染，细胞异型性轻微，围绕显著增生的高内皮小静脉。肿瘤中可见增生的滤泡树突细胞团（CD21 显示），及较多小淋巴细胞、浆细胞、组织细胞及嗜酸性粒细胞等浸润。原位杂交显示 EBER 阴性。

　　The tumor T cells are small to me-dium-sized and grow in mass or piece patterns，with partial destruction of lymph node structure. Tumor cells appear abundant and clear pale-staining cytoplasm and minimal atypia，surro-unding the proliferated high endothelial venules. Hyperplasia of follicular dendral cell mass（CD21 positive）and the infiltration of small lymphocytes and a variety of inflammatory cells can be seen in tumor. EBER is negative detected by in situ hybridization.

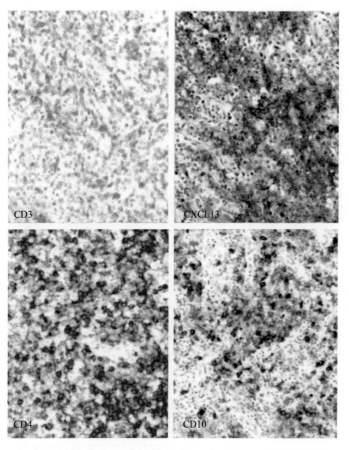

免疫组化结果显示 CD3、CXCL13、CD4、CD10 阳性，

The cells are positive for CD3, CD4, CD10 and CXCL13 detected by immunohistochemistry.

10-28　滤泡树突状细胞肉瘤 Follicular dendritic cell sarcoma

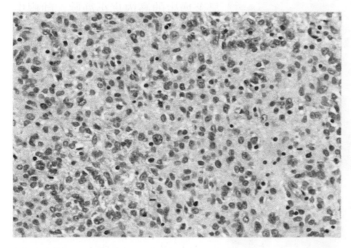

肿瘤细胞呈梭形或卵圆形，束状排列。核卵圆形或梭形，核仁小。肿瘤细胞中常夹杂着小淋巴细胞。

The tumor is composed of spindle or oval cells with spindle or oval nuclei and small nucleoli，growing in fascicles. The tumor is usually infiltrated by small lymphocytes.

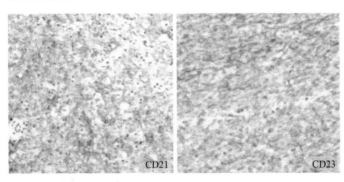

免疫组化结果显示滤泡树突细胞标记CD21, CD23阳性。

The tumor cells are positive for CD21 and CD23, two follicular dendritic markers, detected by immunohistochemistry.

10-29 肠病型 T 细胞淋巴瘤 Enteropathy-type T cell lymphoma

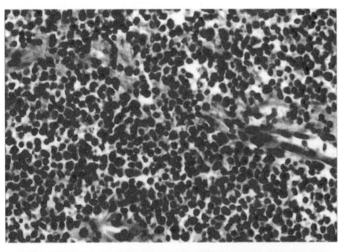

来源于肠上皮内 T 淋巴细胞的肿瘤, 肿瘤细胞由形态相对单一的中等或大的淋巴样细胞组成, 核圆形、空泡状, 核仁明显, 胞质淡染, 可见炎细胞浸润。

The tumor cells originated from intraepithelial Tlymphocytes, which are relatively monomorphic medium-sized to large lymphoidcytes with round vesicular nuclei, prominent nucleoli and pale-staining cytoplasm. The inflammatory cells are visible in the tumor.

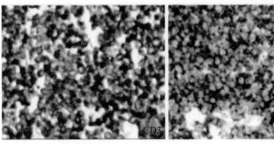

免疫组化结果显示 CD3 和 CD56 阳性, 原位杂交显示 EBER 阴性。

The cells are positive for CD3 and CD56 detected by immunohistochemistry. EBER is negative detected by in situ hybridization.

10-30 皮肤菌样霉菌病 Mycosis fungoides（MF）, skin

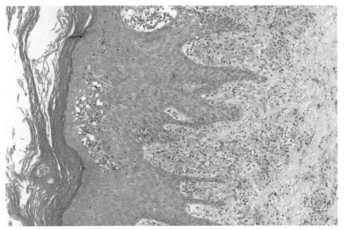

肿瘤性 T 细胞常呈现辅助 T 细胞表型（CD4 阳性）, 在真皮内呈带状浸润, 可侵犯表皮并在其内簇状浸润, 形成所谓的 Pautrier 微脓肿。瘤细胞大于正常淋巴细胞, 核显著不规则呈脑回状改变。

Neoplastic T cells often show helper T cell phenotype（CD4-positive）, zonal infiltration in the dermis, tufted infiltration in the epidermis, forming the so-called Pautrier micro-abscesses. Tumor cells are larger than normal cells, nuclei show significant irregular gyrus pattern.

10-31 粒细胞肉瘤 Granulocytic sarcoma

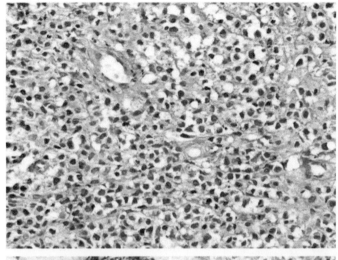

单一性幼稚粒细胞（原始粒细胞或部分分化型早幼粒细胞）弥漫性增生与浸润。

Immature granulocytes（original type or partly differentiated type promyelocytic cells）show unity diffuse hyperplasia and infiltration.

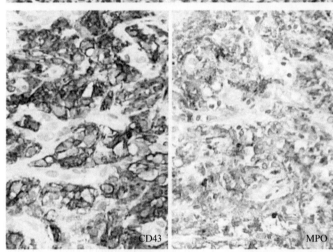

CD43　　　　MPO

免疫组化显示 CD43 和 MPO 阳性表达在肿瘤细胞胞质 / 膜。

Immunohistochemical CD43 and MPO positive cytoplasmic/membranous expression of tumor cells.

10-32 朗格汉斯组织细胞增生症 Langerhans cell histiocytosis

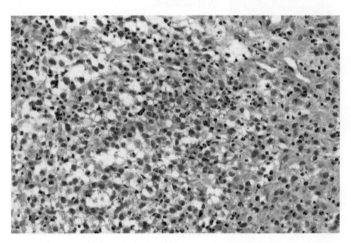

肿瘤性朗格汉斯细胞胞浆丰富、缺乏突起，形态上类似于组织细胞，核呈空泡状，核膜薄，核仁明显，存在特征的核沟或折叠。瘤组织中常混杂各种炎症细胞，其中嗜酸性粒细胞可成片存在。

Neoplastic Langerhans cells show abundant cytoplasm, but the lack of dendritic protrusions, morphologically, is more similar to histiocyte, nuclear vacuolization, nuclear membrane thin, prominent nucleoli, the characteristic of nuclear grooves or folded. Tumor tissueis often mixed with various inflammatory cells, among which eosinophils can be found in sheet existence.

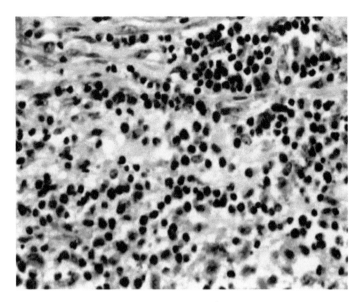

嗜酸性肉芽肿（eosinophilic granuloma）

朗格汉斯细胞、嗜酸性粒细胞、淋巴细胞及浆细胞组成肉芽肿结构。

Granuloma structure is composed of Langerhans cells, eosinophils, lymphocytes and plasma cells.

第十一章 免疫性疾病
Chapter 11 Diseases of Immunity

11-1 红斑狼疮 Lupus erythematosus

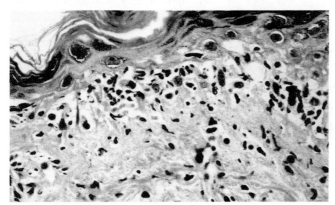

红斑狼疮（lupus erythematosus）

表皮基底层液化，表皮与真皮交界处水肿。

There are liquefactive degeneration of the basal layer in the epidermis and edema at dermal and epidermis junction.

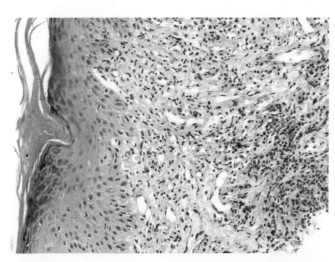

慢性盘状红斑狼疮（chronic discoid lupus erythematosus）

多发生于女性，皮损表现为界限清楚的红斑发展到角化亢进，到萎缩性斑块。多见于面颈和头皮。组织学特点为毛囊显著角化亢进，表皮萎缩，伴基底层液化变性，血管周围明显淋巴细胞浸润。

Most cases occur in women, lesions show well-defined erythema developing to follicular keratosis hyperactivity, to atrophic plaques, common in the face, neck and scalp. Histological features are significant follicular keratosis hyperactivity, skin atrophy, associated with basal liquefaction degeneration, perivascular lymphocytic infiltration is significant.

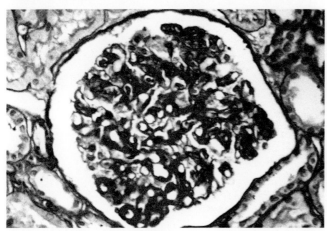

狼疮性肾炎（lupus nephritis）

PAS 染色中肾小球呈数个"线圈"病变。

The glomerulus shows several "wire-loop" lesions in PAS stain.

11-2 硬皮病 Scleroderma

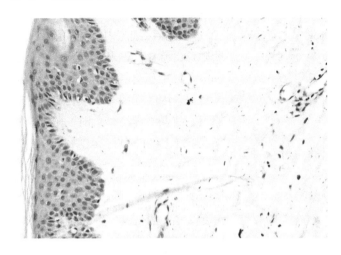

毛细血管与小动脉管壁周围淋巴细胞浸润，部分管腔闭塞或血管透明变性增厚。皮肤进行性纤维化，随之水肿，发生胶原纤维变性。真皮弥漫硬化，皮肤附件丧失，表皮萎缩。

Lymphocytic infiltration surrounding the capillaries and small arteries wall, some cavities occlusion, or vascular hyaline degeneration and thickening. Skin fibrosis, followed by edema and degeneration of collagen fibers. The dermis shows diffuse sclerosis, skin appendages loss and skin atrophy.

11-3 血管炎 Vasculitis

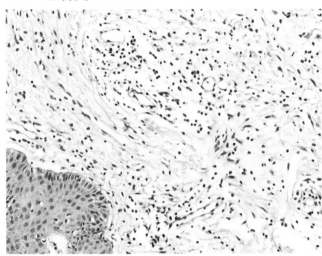

受累血管以真皮乳头部毛细血管、真皮深层的小动脉、小静脉为主，红细胞外漏是主要特点，炎症细胞以中性粒细胞、淋巴细胞为主，也可形成肉芽肿为主，血管壁常为纤维素性坏死。

Vasculitis involved vessels mainly include dermal papilla capillaries, deep dermal arterioles and venules, with the main feature of red blood cells leaking. Main inflammatory cells are neutrophils and lymphocytes, but also granulomatous become main types, blood vessel walls often show fibrinoid necrosis。

11-4 肺隐球菌病 Cryptococcosis, lung

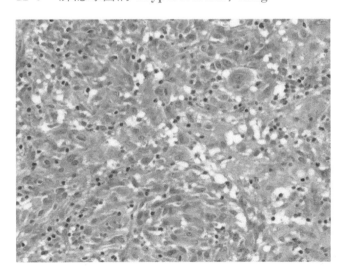

隐球菌组织学改变常表现为肉芽肿性炎症反应。肉芽肿中大量的组织细胞、多核巨细胞、上皮样细胞聚集，伴慢性炎症纤维化为背景。在苏木素-伊红常规染色切片中。隐球菌菌体呈圆形，淡蓝或灰色，在菌体周形成透明的空隙。

Cryptococcus histological changes usually show granulomatous inflammation. Granulomas show in a large number of histocytes, multinucleated giant cells, epithelioid histiocytes gathered fibrosis with chronic inflammation as the background. In HE stained sections, cryptococcus is round, light blue or gray, with a transparent gap is formed in the cell periphery.

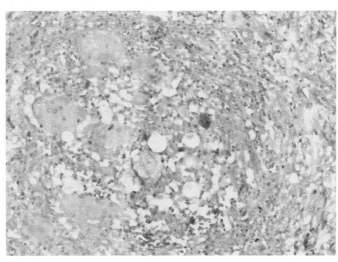

隐球菌性肉芽肿（cryptococcal granuloma）

在多核巨细胞内可见隐球菌。证明隐球菌除做PAS和六胺银染色外，黏液卡红染色对隐球菌具有特征性诊断意义，因隐球菌有一层含黏多糖的厚膜，故黏液卡红染色时，菌体外膜染成鲜红色。而在其他真菌无黏多糖膜。

Cryptococcus locate within multinucleated giant cells. Proven cryptococcal in addition to PAS and PASM staining, carmine stain method shows characteristic diagnostic significance. Because cryptococcus contain a layer thick mucopolysaccharides, so bacterial outer membrane is dyed bright red with mucus carmine stain-method but in other fungi without mucopolysaccharides membrane.

11-5 肺组织胞浆菌病 Histoplasmosis，lung

组织胞浆菌病常导致肉芽肿性改变。具有上皮样细胞和多核巨细胞相似于结核结节。菌体通常在泡沫样吞噬细胞内，很少在细胞外，菌体小，圆或卵圆形。

Histoplasmosis often lead to granulomas with epithelioid cell and multinucleated giant cell response, similar to tuberculosis. Bacteria usually locates within phagocytosis foamy cells, small, round or oval, rarely outside the cells.

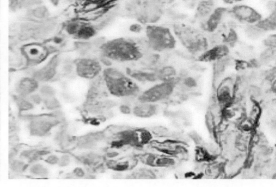

用甲基绿染色在泡沫样吞噬细胞内可检测到组织胞浆菌。

Application of methyl green dye staining, intracellular bacteria can be more clearly seen.

11-6　肺放线菌病 Actinophytosis，lung

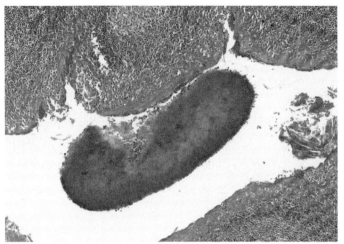

放线菌病，为一种机会性肺感染，多发生于免疫抑制、化疗、激素使用后，镜下呈灶性支气管炎，伴微脓肿和境界不清的肉芽肿形成。

Nocardia actinomycosis，an opportunistic pulmonary infections occur in immunosuppression，chemotherapy，hormone use，microscopy shows focal bronchitis，with microabscesses and state of confusion of granuloma formation.

硅肺伴放线菌感染（silicosis with ray fungi）

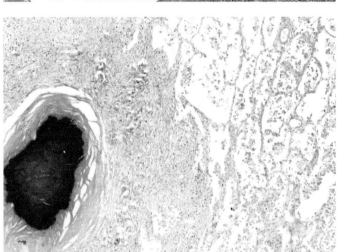

肺组织中见大小不等的硅结节；硅结节周围可见碳末沉积及巨噬细胞浸润；结节中央可见到放线菌。

Varying sizes of silicon nodules are seen in the lung tissue，coal clust deposition and macrophage infiltration in silicon nodules around；in the center of the nodules silica dust deposition and actinomycosis infection can also be seen.

11-7　肺曲菌感染 Aspergillus infection （Aspergillosis），lung

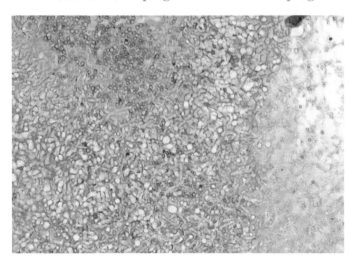

支气管腔内黏液分泌物中可见曲菌感染的真菌菌丝，呈细长，略呈串珠型的分支锐角竹节状。

Aspergillus fungal hyphae visible in bronchial mucus materials，slender，slightly beaded type of branch bamboo-like bacilli.

11-8　获得性免疫缺陷综合征 Acquired immune deficiency syndrome

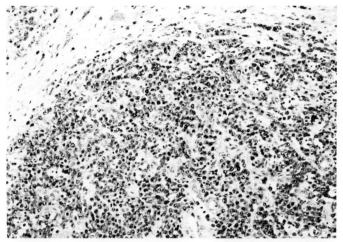

淋巴结中 T- 区细胞成分缺失，滤泡结构消失。

In lymph node the depletion of cellularity in T-zone as well as disappearance of follicular structures.

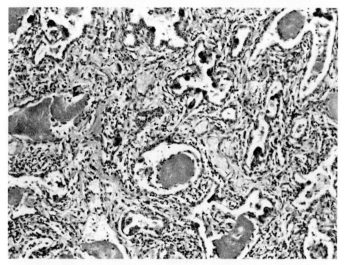

肺间质增厚，肺泡内泡沫状分泌物，提示卡氏肺孢子虫感染。

Lung interstitial thicken and intraalveolar fomay exudate representing pneumocystis carinii infection.

11-9　Kaposi 肉瘤 Kaposi's sarcoma

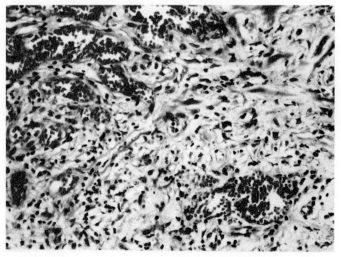

异型梭形细胞和血管瘤样增生的血管混合在一起，伴有红细胞漏出。

Atypical spindle cells are intermingled with angiomatous proliferation of vessels，with Rbc leakage.

11-10　移植肾排斥反应 Rejection of transplant kidney

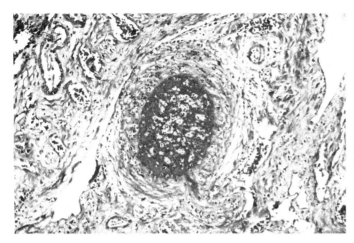

急性排斥反应（acute rejection）

移植肾急性排斥反应中的血管炎，可见血栓和细胞浸润。

Vasculitis in acute rejection of kidney, showing thrombosis and cellular infiltration.

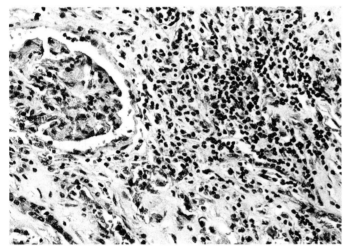

慢性排斥反应（chronic rejection）

移植肾慢性排斥反应中可见肾小管明显萎缩，间质纤维化加重，单核细胞浸润。肾小球毛细血管壁呈缺血性增厚。

In chronic rejection of transplant kidney, there is marked tubular atrophy, increased interstital fibrosis, and mononuclear cells infiltration. The glomorulus shows ischemic axial thickening.

第十二章 泌尿系统疾病
Chapter 12　Diseases of the Kidney and its Collecting System

12-1　肾发育不良 Renal dysplasia

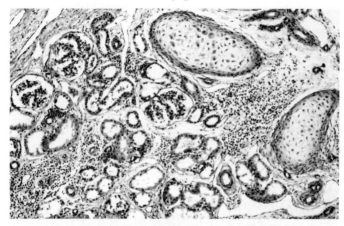

可见原始发育不全肾小球、肾小管和软骨岛，扩张的淋巴管和间质中淋巴细胞浸润。

Primitive tubules and glomeruli, and islands of dysplastic cartilage are seen，dilated lymphatic vessels and lymphatic infiltrates in the intersitium are observed.

12-2　先天性多囊肾 Congenital polycystic kidney

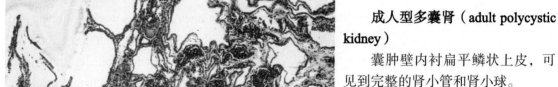

成人型多囊肾（adult polycystic kidney）

囊肿壁内衬扁平鳞状上皮，可见到完整的肾小管和肾小球。

The cyst walls are lined with flatten squamous epithelium，and intact renal tubules and glomeruli are also seen.

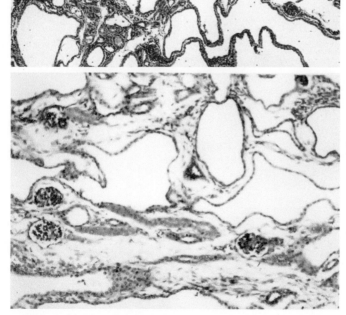

婴儿型多囊肾（infantile polycystic kidney）

囊肿壁内衬肾小管和集合管来源的立方上皮。

The cyst walls are lined with renal tubules and collecting tubes derived from cuboidal epithelium.

12-3 肾小球肾炎 Glomerulonephritis（GN）

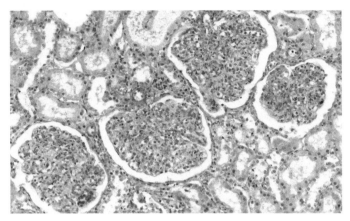

急性肾小球肾炎（acute GN）

肾皮质中肾小球广泛受累。肾小球体积增大，毛细血管丛的细胞数明显增多，主要为内皮细胞、系膜细胞，伴中性粒细胞和单核细胞浸润。

A number of glomeruli in renal cortex are affected. Glomeruli are enlarged, the number of capillary plexus cells proliferate significantly, mainly including endothelial cells, mesangial cells, with inflammation of neutrophils and monocytes.

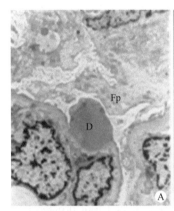
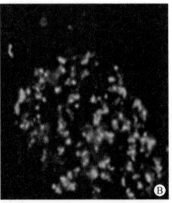

A：电镜示"驼峰"状电子致密物集中分布于毛细血管襻上皮下区，D示电子致密物，Fp示足突。B：免疫荧光显示肾小球内有颗粒状荧光。

A：Electron microscopy shows humps-like electron dense deposits located in the subepithelial region. D：humps-like electron dense, Fp：Foot process. B：Immunofluorescence shows granular patten in the glomerulus.

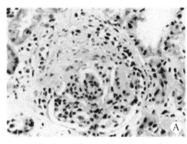
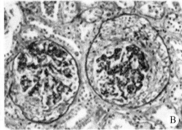
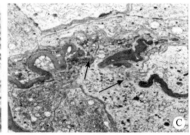

新月体性肾小球肾炎（crescentic GN）

A：H&E 染色可见到受压萎缩的肾小球毛细血管丛和新月形结构，新月体由肾球囊壁层上皮细胞、单核巨噬细胞和纤维素等组成。肾小球球囊腔变窄或闭塞，并压迫毛细血管丛，可出现节段性坏死、弥漫或局灶性内皮细胞增生或系膜细胞增生等改变。B：PAS 染色。C：电镜下新月体性肾小球肾炎基底膜局灶性缺损和断裂（箭头所示）。

A：H&E staining showed the compressive atrophy of the glomerular capillary plexus and crescent structure, mainly composed of capsule epithelial cells, with macrophages-monocytes and fibrin. Bow man's capsule show narrowing or occlusion, and oppress capillary plexus, there may be segmental necrosis, diffuse or focal endothelial cell or mesangial cell proliferations and other changes. B：PAS staining. C：Focal deficiency and rupture of basement membrane of crescentic glomerulonephritis under electron microscopy（arrow）.

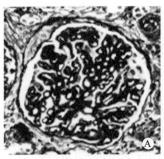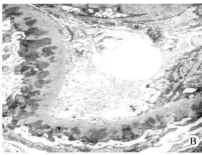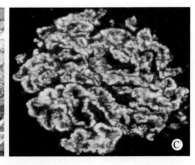

膜性肾炎 [membranous GN（MGN）]

A：PAS 染色，显示弥漫性毛细血管壁增厚但没有细胞数目的增加。B：电子显微镜显示免疫球蛋白的电子致密物沉积于肾小球基底膜的上皮下。C：免疫球蛋白 IgG 颗粒性免疫荧光特征性的沿肾小球基底膜沉积。

A：PAS staining showed diffuse capillary wall thickening，but no increase in cell number. B：Electron microscopy showed that the electron dense of immunoglobulin was deposited in the subepithelial of glomerular basement membrane. C：Immunoglobulin IgG granularly immunofluorescence deposition along glomerular basement membrane.

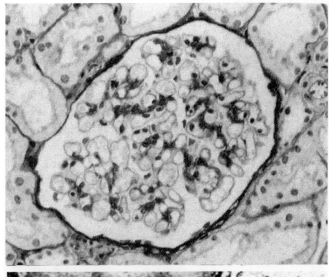

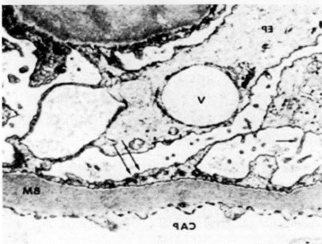

微小病变性肾小球病 [minimal change disease（MCD）]

又称为足突病（foot process disease）或者脂性肾病（lipoid nephrosis）

PAS 染色，近曲小管上皮细胞内出现大量脂质空泡和玻璃样小滴。

电镜下可见上皮细胞足突融合、消失（双箭头所示），上皮细胞胞浆内可见空泡形成（V）。

In PAS stain，tubule cells appeared large lipid vacuoles and hyaline droplets. Electron microscopy showed fusion and disappearance of epithelial foot processes（double arrows），and vacuoles（V）were formed in the cytoplasm of epithelial cells.

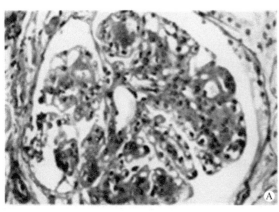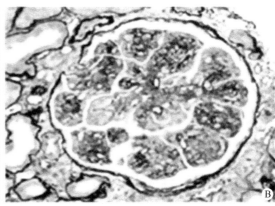

膜增生性肾小球肾炎 [membranoproliferative GN（MPGN）]

A：小叶增多，弥漫性系膜细胞增生，毛细血管壁增厚。

B：显示有系膜细胞增殖，基质增加（银染呈黑色），基底膜因而增厚伴局部分隔，呈"叶"状。

A：Lobular hyperplasia，diffuse mesangial proliferation and thickening of the capillary walls. B：The proliferation of mesangial cells，increased stroma（silver staining black），thickening of basement membranes and with partial septa as a "lobe" shape.

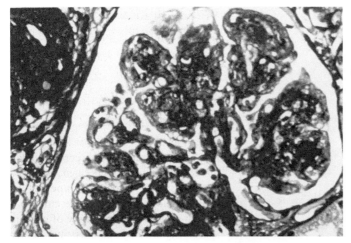

系膜增生性肾小球肾炎 [mesangial proliferative glomerulonephritis（MsPGN）]

PAS- 银染显示毛细血管壁基底膜双轨模式。

PAS- silver staining showed dual track patterns of capillary wall basement membrane.

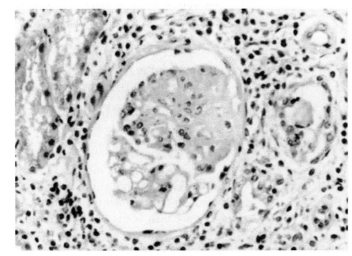

局灶性节段性肾小球硬化 [focal segmental glomerulosclerosis（FSG）]

病变显示肾小球内部分毛细血管襻系膜基质增加，基膜崩解，玻璃样物质沉积和脂质小滴。

The lesions exhibit increased mesangial matrix，collapsed basement membranes in part of the capillary trip of glomeruli，deposition of hyaline masses and lipid droplets.

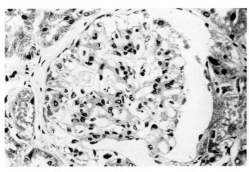
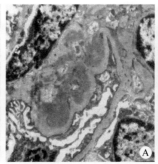
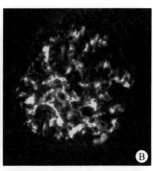

IgA 肾病（IgA nephropathy）

系膜区弥漫增大伴系膜细胞增生和系膜基质增多。A：电镜检查显示系膜区有电子致密沉积物。B：免疫荧光检测见 IgA 的沉积特征，主要位于系膜区。

There is diffuse mesangial regions enlargement with mesangial cell proliferation and mesangial matrix increasing. A：Electron microscopy shows the presence of electron-dense deposits in the mesangium regions. B：Characteristic deposition of IgA，principally in mesangial regions，detected by immunofluorescence.

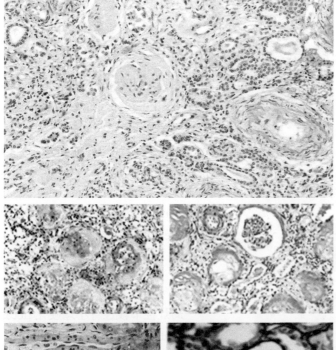

慢性肾小球肾炎（chronic GN）

大部分肾小球发生纤维化和玻璃样变，相应肾小管萎缩消失，代之以间质的纤维化。病变较轻区肾单位出现代偿性改变，表现为肾小球体积增大，肾小管扩张，腔内可出现各种管型。肾间质纤维结缔组织明显增生，内见慢性炎症细胞浸润。

A number of glomerular lesions show fibrosis and hyalinization，corresponding tubular atrophy and disappeared，replaced by interstitial fibrosis. Compensatory changes show glomerular size enlarge，tubular dilation with a variety of casts in spaces. Significant renal interstitial fibrous connective tissue hyperplasia，visible chronic inflammatroy cells infiltration.

狼疮性肾小球肾炎（lupic glomerulonephritis）

A：肾小球中节段性系膜细胞增生伴坏死或核碎片，可见苏木素小体。B：PAS 染色显示肾小球中有几个线圈状病灶。

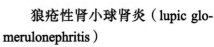

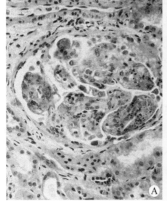
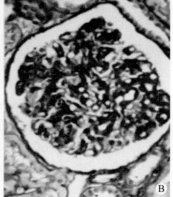

A：Segmental mesangial cell hyperplasia in the glomerulus with necrosis or nuclear debris. Hematoxylin body are also seen. B：PAS staining revealed several wire-loop like lesions in the glomerulus.

12-4　肾盂肾炎 Pyeloriephritis

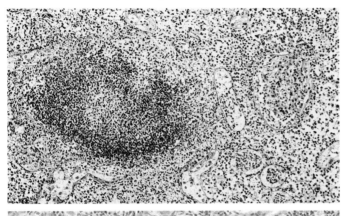

急性肾盂肾炎（acute pyelon-ephritis）

可见局部大量脓细胞（中性粒细胞）聚集，实质成分丧失。

Focal heavy collection of pus cells（neutrophlis）and loss of parenchyma are seen.

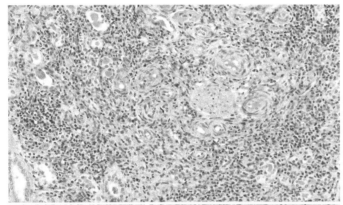

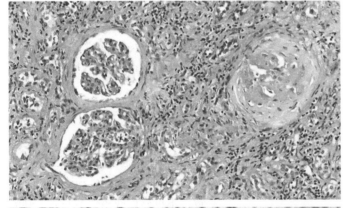

慢性肾盂肾炎（chronic pyelo-riephritis）

肾间质内局灶性的淋巴细胞、浆细胞浸润和间质纤维化。部分肾小管的萎缩引起肾小球萎缩、玻璃样变，临近肾小球代偿性增生。代偿扩张的肾小管内可充满胶样管型类似甲状腺外形（甲状腺化）。

Focal infiltration of lymphocytes，plasma cells and interstitial fibrosis.Part tubules atrophys，causing a corresponding change in glomerular atrophy and hyaline. Neighboring glomeruli compensatory hypertrophy，which is filled with thyroid-like glue-like tube（thyroid-based）.

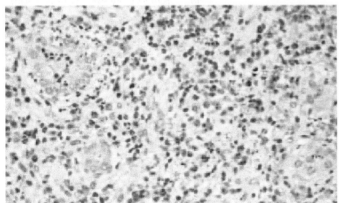

药物诱导性间质性肾炎（drug-induced interstitial nephritis）

病变显示大量嗜酸性粒细胞和单核细胞浸润。

The lesion exhibits prominent eosinophilic and mononuclear cell infiltration.

12-5 过敏性急性小管间质性肾炎 Allergic tubulo-interstitial nephritis

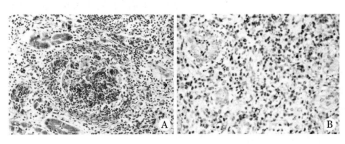

A：肾间质水肿、炎症细胞浸润，并有肾小球和球囊套的形成。B：病变显示大量嗜酸性粒细胞和单核细胞浸润。

A：Renal interstitial edema, inflammatory cells infiltration, and glomerular and its sheath formation. B：The lesion showed extensive infiltration of eosinophils and monocytes.

12-6 肾透明细胞癌 Renal clear cell carcinoma

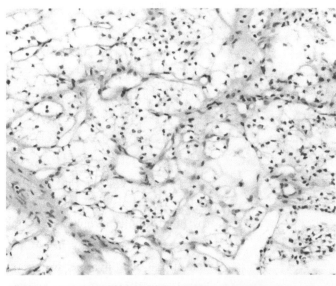

肿瘤细胞体积较大，呈圆形或多角形，胞质丰富，透明或颗粒状，核小，常被推到基底侧，胞质特殊染色后可见含有糖原和脂质。间质具有丰富的毛细血管和血窦。

Tumor cells are larger, round or polygonal, with abundant cytoplasm, clear or granular, small nuclei is often pushed to the base side, after special staining cytoplasm shows visible glycogen and lipids. Interstitial capillaries and sinusoids are abundant.

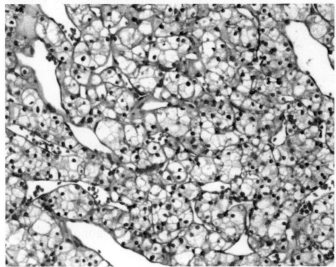

Ⅰ级（grade Ⅰ）

肿瘤细胞胞浆丰富、透亮或少量嗜酸性，胞膜清楚，核圆，大小较一致，不见核仁或核仁不明显。肿瘤中有小薄壁血管构成的网状间隔。

The neoplastic cytoplasm is rich and clear, focally eosinophilic surrounded by a distinct cell membrane. The nuclei are round and uniform, nucleoli are absent or inconspicuous. The tumors typically contain a regular network of small thin-walled blood vessels.

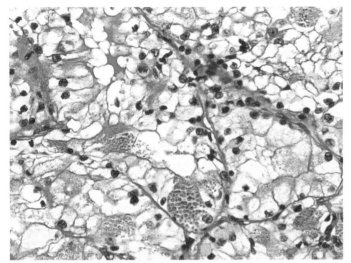

Ⅱ级（grade Ⅱ）

细胞类似于Ⅰ级，但核仁明显。

The cellular morphology is similar to grade Ⅰ, but nucleoli are con- spicuous.

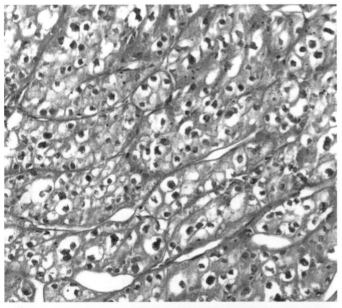

Ⅲ级（grade Ⅲ）

此型中核仁更明显，核异型。

The nucleoli are more conspicuous in this type.

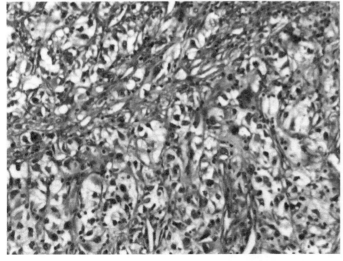

Ⅳ级（grade Ⅳ）

肿瘤细胞胞浆丰富、透亮，胞膜清楚，核多形性，大小不一，核仁明显。

The neoplastic cytoplasm is rich and clear surrounded by a distinct cell membrane. The pleomorphic nuclei in different size，which nucleoli are more conspicuous.

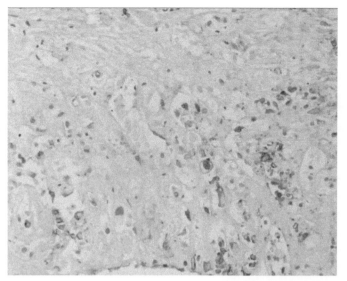

肝肾细胞癌转移（renal cell carcinoma metastasis to the liver）

肿瘤细胞胞浆丰富、淡红或透亮，核多形性，大小不一，免疫组化结果显示肾细胞癌常用标记 CD10 阳性。

The cytoplasm of neoplastic cells is rich, pale red or clear with pleomorphic nuclei in different size. Immunohistochemistry is positive for CD10, a marker for renal cell carcinoma.

12-7 乳头状肾细胞癌 Papillary renal cell carcinoma

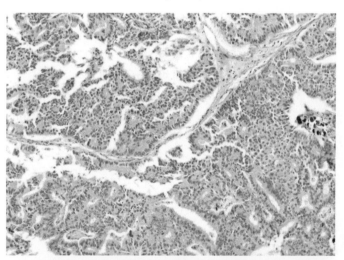

肿瘤细胞呈立方状或矮柱状，乳头状排列。乳头中轴间质内常见砂粒体、泡沫细胞、血管纤维轴索结构，并可发生水肿。

Tumor cells are cuboidal or low columnar, with papillary arrangement. Papilla axis stroma commonly contains psammama bodies, foam cells, vascular fiber axonal structure, and edema.

Ⅰ（Ⅰ type）

肿瘤具有乳头状结构，乳头有纤细的纤维血管轴心。乳头表面被覆单层排列的小细胞，胞浆稀少、淡染。

The tumor has papillary architecture that contains a delicate fibrovascular core and the papillae are covered by small cells with scanty and pale cytoplasm, arranged in a single layer on the papillary surface.

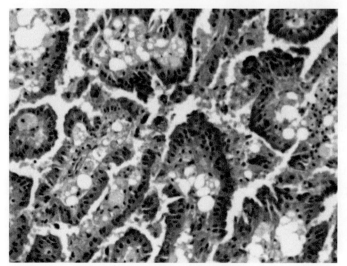

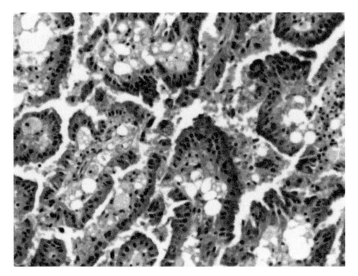

II型（II type）

肿瘤具有乳头状结构，乳头有纤细的纤维血管轴心。乳头表面被覆假复层排列的细胞，核高级别，胞浆丰富、嗜酸性。

The tumor has papillary architecture that contains a delicate fibrovascular core and the papillae is covered by cells with higher nuclear grade, rich and eosinophilic cytoplasm, arranged in a pseudostratified layer on the papillary surface.

12-8　嫌色性肾细胞癌 Chromophobe renal cell carcinoma

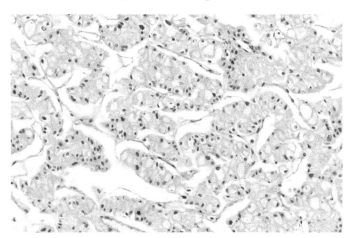

肿瘤细胞大小不一，细胞膜较明显，胞质淡染或略嗜酸性，核周常有空晕。

Tumor cells show varying sizes, cell membranes more obvious, lightly stained cytoplasm or slightly eosinophilic, perinuclear light staining area.

12-9　集合管癌 Collecting-duct carcinoma

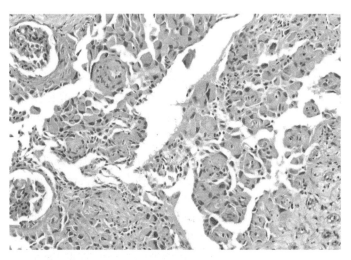

癌细胞立方状，胞浆嗜酸性、嗜碱或嫌色性，细胞核大，核仁明显，高度恶性。癌细胞呈小管状或乳头状排列，少数呈肉瘤样结构。纤维性和胶原性间质多。

Cube-like cancer cells show eosinophilic, basophilic or chromophobe cytoplasm, large nuclei, prominent nucleoli, highly malignant. Carcinoma cells arrange small tubular or papillary patterns, a few are sarcoma-like structure. Fibrous and collagenous stroma are plenty.

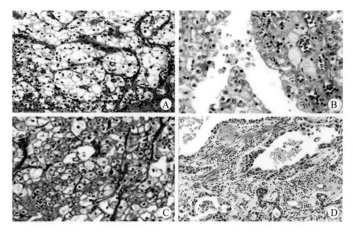

肾细胞癌的细胞学类型（histologic types of renal carcinoma）

A：透明细胞癌；B：乳头状癌；C：嫌色细胞癌；D：集合管癌。

A：clear cell carcinoma；B：papillary carcinoma；C：chromophobe cell carcinoma；D：collecting duct carcinoma。

12-10　肾母细胞瘤 Nephroblastoma

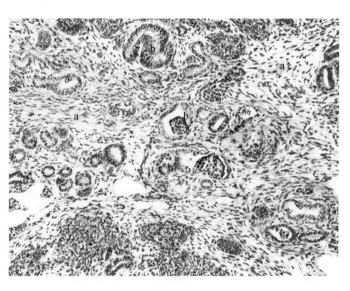

肿瘤由间叶细胞、上皮样细胞和幼稚的胚基组织细胞构成。上皮样细胞体积小，可形成小管或小球样结构，可出现鳞状上皮分化；间叶细胞多为纤维性或黏液性，可出现横纹肌、软骨、骨或脂肪等分化；胚基幼稚细胞为原始细胞，胞质少。

Tumor is composed of mesenchymal cells, epithelial cells and immature embryo-based tissue cells. Epithelial cells can form a small tube or a small ball-like structures, and squamous differentiation; Most mesenchymal cells are fibrous mesenchymal cells or mucinous, may show striated muscle, cartilage, bone or fat differentiation; embryo group blasts are small round or oval blasts, with less cytoplasm.

12-11　低度恶性潜能的多房性囊性肾细胞肿瘤 Multilocular cystic renal neoplasm of low malignant potential

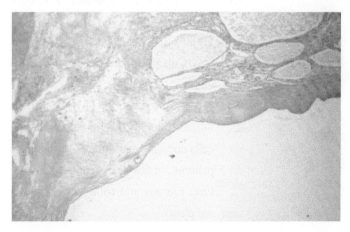

肿瘤完全由囊腔构成，腔壁内衬单层扁平上皮，胞浆透亮或淡染，胞核小而圆，核仁不明显，囊腔间隔由纤维组织构成。

The tumor composes entirely of numerous cysts, which are lined by a single layer of flat epithelial cells with clear to pale cytoplasm, their nuclei are small and round without nucleoli. The septa of cysts consist of fibrous tissue.

12-12　肾血管平滑肌脂肪瘤 Angiomyolipoma（AML），renal

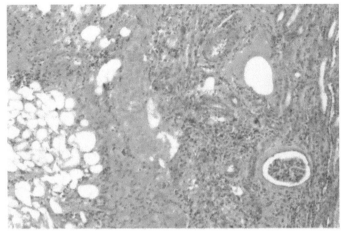

　　AML 与周围肾实质界限清楚，由多少不等的成熟脂肪组织、厚壁不规则血管和平滑肌构成。

　　AML is distinct bound with the surrounding renal parenchyma, consisting of bundles of smooth muscle, mature fat and thick walled blood vessels.

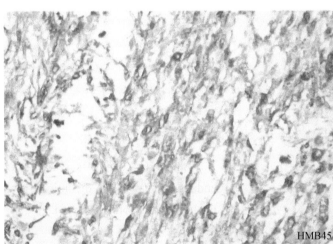

HMB45

　　AML 表达黑色素细胞（HMB45、HMB40、Melan A）和平滑肌（SMA MSA 和 Calponin）的标记，也可有 CD68、NSE、S100、ER 和 PR 的表达，但不表达上皮标记物。

　　AML expressed melanocytes（HMB45，HMB40，Melan A）and smooth muscle（SMA，MSA and Calponin）markers，and expressed CD68，NSE，S100，ER and PR，but no expressed epithelial markers.

12-13　腺性和囊腺性膀胱炎 Cystitis of glandularis and cystica

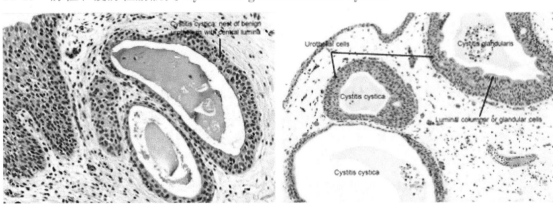

　　膀胱黏膜固有层多数 Brunn 巢增生，伴慢性炎症细胞浸润。部分 Brunn 巢呈腺样结构，内层柱状，外层基底细胞样，腔内可见黏液。

　　Most of the bladder mucosa lamina propria presents Brunn nests proliferation with chronic inflammatory cell infiltration. Some of the Brunn nests are glandular structures with an inner column and an outer basal cells，mucus is visible in the lumen.

12-14 膀胱软斑病 Malacoplakia，bladder

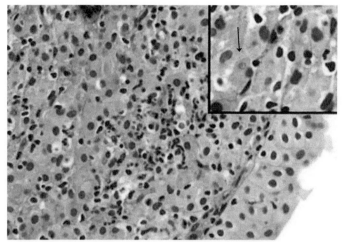

上皮下大量组织细胞聚集，胞浆富含嗜酸性颗粒。

Subepithelial，a large number of histocytes accumulate and its cytoplasm contains rich eosinophilic granules.

12-15 内翻性移行细胞乳头状瘤 Inverted transitional cell papilloma

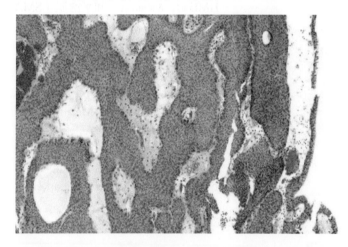

细胞巢索向内膜下呈内生性生长，肿瘤细胞无异形性。

The nests of cells showed an endogenous growth to the intima，and the tumor cells without atypia.

12-16 膀胱尿路上皮（移行细胞）肿瘤 Urothelial（transitional cell）tumor，bladder

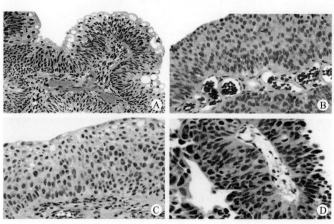

世界卫生组织（WHO）和国际泌尿病理学会（ISUP）关于尿路上皮肿瘤的分类 [classification of urothelial tumor named by World Health Organization（WHO）and International Society of Urological Pathology（ISUP）]

A：尿路上皮乳头状瘤；B：低恶性潜能尿路上皮乳头状瘤；C：低级别尿路上皮乳头状癌；D：高级别尿路上皮乳头状癌。A：urothelial papilloma；B：papillary urothelial neoplasm of low malignant potential；C：low-grade papillary urothelial carcinoma；D：high-grade papillary urothelial carcinoma.

12-17 膀胱的乳头状移行细胞癌 Papillary transitional cell carcinoma, blader

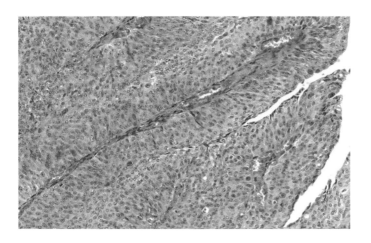

分化好的肿瘤中瘤细胞虽有一定异型性，但近似于正常的移行细胞，核分裂像少见，细胞层次增多至七层以上，乳头状向下浸润生长。分化差的肿瘤中部分细胞排列紊乱，层次增多，核深染，核分裂像较多。

In well-differentiated tumors, tumor cells present certain atypia, but similar to normal transitional cells, rare mitotic figures, cells proliferate to seven layers, or more, papillary grows downward infiltration. In poorly differentiated tumor, tumor cells arranged disorder, cell overproliferation is more than seven layers, with nuclear hyperchromatism and more nuclear mitosis.

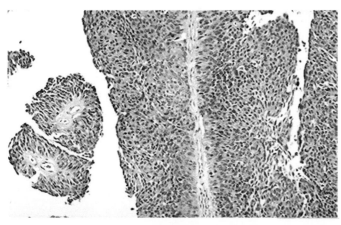

Ⅰ级，肿块由分支状排列的移行细胞团块组成，其中有许多血管的纤细的基质。

Grade Ⅰ, the tumor consists of branching masses of transitional cells supported by delicate stroma containing many blood vessels.

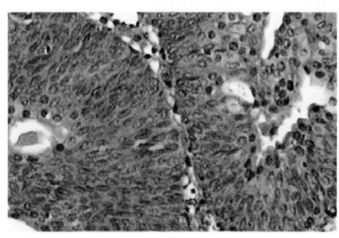

Ⅱ级，癌细胞排列似移行上皮，但细胞大小形状不一，排列极性紊乱。

Grade Ⅱ, cancer cells arranged in similar to transitional cells, but shows greater variability in cell size, shape, and loss of polarity.

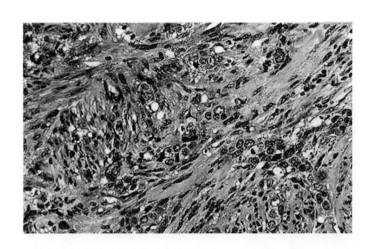

Ⅲ级，细胞高度异型，并侵入肌层。

Grade Ⅲ, tumor cells are high atypia, and muscle layer invasion.

第十三章 内分泌系统疾病
Chapter 13 Disorders of the Endocrine System

13-1 垂体腺瘤 Pituitary adenoma

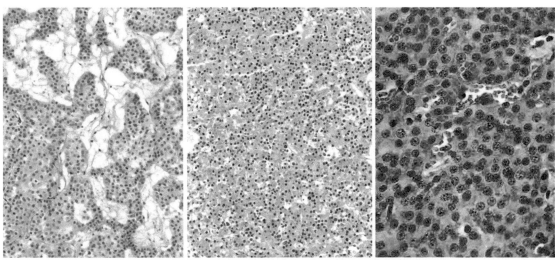

瘤细胞似正常前叶细胞或稍大，核圆或卵圆形，有小核仁。瘤细胞排列成片块、条索、巢状、假腺样或乳头状，有的瘤细胞可有异型性但核分裂罕见。瘤细胞巢之间为血管丰富的纤维间质，但缺乏网状纤维。垂体前叶腺瘤分类应根据组织学、免疫组化、超微结构、临床内分泌功能、影像学和手术所见综合考虑。

Tumor cells are like normal cells in the anterior lobe or slightly larger, with round or oval nuclei, small nucleoli. Tumor cells are arranged in pieces, cords, nests, false adenoid or papillary, and some tumor cells may have atypia but mitotic figures are rare. Vascular-rich fibrous stroma between tumor cell nests. Note also the absence of reticulin network.The classification of anterior pituitary adenoma should be overall considered according to the histological, immunohistochemical, ultrastructure, clinical endocrine functions, imaging and surgery.

13-2 弥漫性非毒性甲状腺肿（地方性甲状腺肿）Diffuse nontoxic goiter（Endemic goiter）

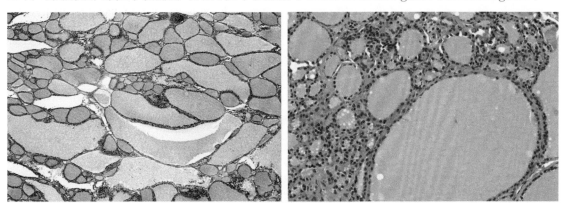

病理分为增生期、胶质贮积期和结节期：此例为胶质贮积期：滤泡大小不等，充满胶质。较大滤泡内衬被压扁的上皮。

Pathological stages：proliferative stage, colloid storage stage and nodules stage. Here this case is colloid storage stage：follicular of various sizes, filled with colloid. Large follicles lined by flattened epithelium.

13-3 弥漫性毒性甲状腺肿 Diffusetoxic goiter

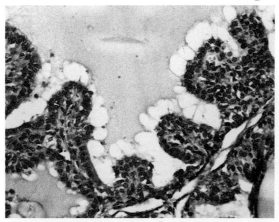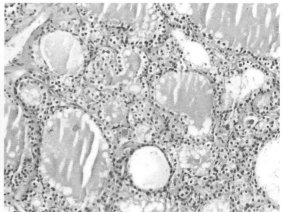

组织学上三个特征：①滤泡上皮增生呈高柱状，核位基底，可有核分裂，但无不典型性，有的呈乳头样增生，并有小滤泡形成。②滤泡腔内胶质稀薄，周边上皮细胞出现吸收空泡。③间质血管丰富、伴淋巴细胞浸润或形成淋巴滤泡。

There are three characteristic histological changes：① Follicular epithelium hyperplasia with high columnar, nuclei located in base, which can have nuclear mitosis, but no atypia, or papillary hyperplasia, or small follicles. ② Follicular cavity contains thin colloid, follicular lining epithelial cells appear absorb vacuoles. ③ Interstitial is rich vessels with lymphocytic infiltration and lymphoid follicles formation.

13-4 亚急性甲状腺炎 Subacute thyroiditis

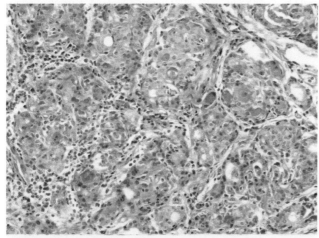

病变呈灶性分布，范围大小不一，发展不一致，部分滤泡被破坏，胶质外溢，引起类似结核结节的肉芽肿形成伴异物巨细胞反应，较多的炎症细胞浸润，可形成微小脓肿，但无干酪样坏死。

Lesions are focally distributed, ranging from different sizes, the development is inconsistent, some follicles are destroyed, colloid spills cause granuloma formation similar to tubercles with foreign body giant cell reaction. Varying amounts of inflammatory cells can form a small abscess, but no caseous necrosis.

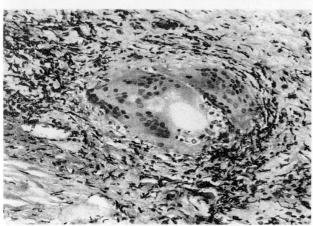

纤维化，滤泡萎缩伴多核巨细胞、炎细胞浸润。

Fibrinous, follicular atrophy and multinucleated giant cells along with inflammatory cells infiltration.

13-5　慢性淋巴细胞性甲状腺炎（桥本甲状腺炎）Chronic lymphocytic thyroiditis（Hashimoto's thyroiditis）

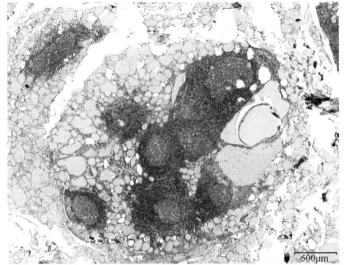

甲状腺组织内大量淋巴细胞形成许多有生发中心的淋巴滤泡。滤泡上皮转化为嗜酸性细胞或许特莱细胞（Hürthle cell）"桥本氏"细胞，胞浆丰富，具有嗜酸性颗粒，核异型明显，但无核分裂。纤维组织增生，有时可出现多核巨细胞。

There is a large number of lymphocytes forming many lymphoid follicles with germinal centers in the thyroid tissue. Follicular epithelium transfered into eosinophilic Hürthle cells or "Hashimoto's" cells, having abundant cytoplasm with eosinophilic granules, nuclei may be heterotypes or atypia, but no nuclear mitosis. There is fibrosis, and sometimes multinucleated giant cells.

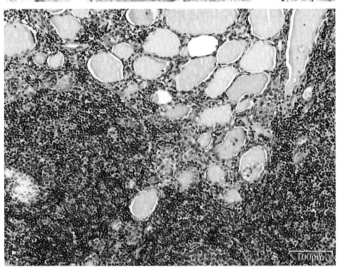

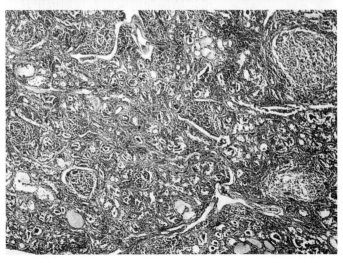

可见淋巴滤泡形成，甲状腺滤泡萎缩伴滤泡上皮嗜酸性变。

Lymphoid follicle formation and atrophic thyroid follicles with oxyphlilic change of the follicular epithelium are seen.

13-6 甲状腺腺瘤 Adenoma，thyroid

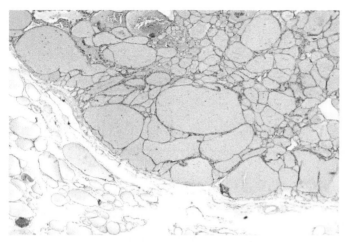

腺瘤常有完整的纤维性胞膜。与周围组织分界清楚。

The adenoma had complete capsule with sharp demarcation from adjacent parenchyma by a fibrous "capsule"．

结节性甲状腺肿与甲状腺腺瘤的鉴别要点：

①腺瘤一般为单发，增生结节多见于多结节性甲状腺肿，也可单发；②腺瘤具有完整包膜且常较厚，增生结节包膜较薄且多不完整；③腺瘤的内部结构单一，增生结节则常见两种或两种以上结构的混合存在；④腺瘤周围常是被挤压萎缩的正常甲状腺组织，增生结节周围常是弥漫性甲状腺肿组织，不见压迫性萎缩。

The Identification between nodular goiter and thyroid adenoma：

① Adenoma usually solitary，hyperplastic nodules found in multinodular goiter，or solitary；② The adenoma had complete thick capsule，nodular hyperplasia capsule is thin and not complete；③ The internal component of adenoma is single，nodular hyperplasia is common a mixture of two or more kinds of components；④ The normal thyroid tissue around adenoma is usually squeezed to atrophy，the tissues around nodules hyperplasia around are often diffuse goiter，without atrophy.

13-7 甲状腺滤泡型腺瘤 Follicular adenoma，thyroid

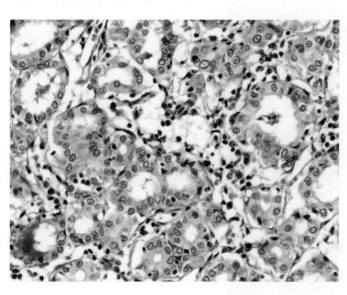

虽然有多种组织学类型，但无特殊临床意义。典型的滤泡腺瘤由厚薄不等的纤维包膜包裹。肿瘤的组织结构和细胞形态与周围甲状腺组织不同。最常呈滤泡性或梁状。继发性病变有间质纤维化、透明变性、出血、钙化、软骨化生、囊性变等。

Though there are a variety of histological types，but have no special clinical significance. The typical follicular adenoma is covered by varying thickness fibrous capsule. The structure and morphology of the tumor cells different from the surrounding thyroid tissue. The most common forms of follicular or trabecular shapes. Secondary lesions have interstitial fibrosis，hyaline degeneration，hemorrhage，calcification，cartilage metaplasia，cystic changes etc.

13-8 甲状腺嗜酸细胞腺瘤 Oncocytic adenoma，thyroid

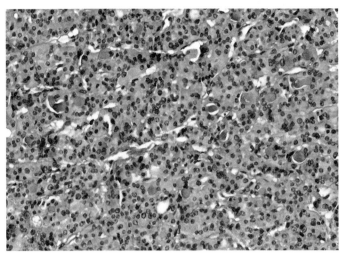

亦称许特莱细胞腺瘤，由大的嗜酸性细胞构成，核大，异型性明显。瘤细胞胞浆有富含大量线粒体的嗜酸性颗粒。瘤细胞排列成小梁状，偶尔可形成滤泡、或实体性结构。内含少量胶质。

Oncocytoma also known as Hürthle cell adenoma. Tumors are formed by large eosinophilic cells，nuclear is large and atypia. Tumor cells cytoplasm have rich eosinophilic particles drived from large number of mitochondria. Tumor cells are arranged in trabecular，occasionally forming follicular or solid structures，containing a small amount of culloid matter.

13-9 甲状腺胎儿型腺瘤 Fetal adenoma，thyroid

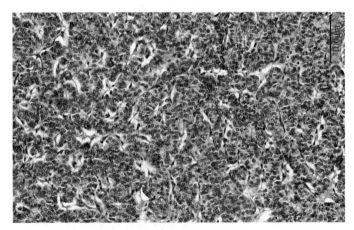

小而一致、仅含少量胶质或没有胶质的微滤泡或梁状结构，伴间质水肿、黏液样，似胎儿甲状腺组织。

Small and consistent，only small amounts of colloid or no colloid，micro follicular or trabecular structures，with interstitial edema，mucus-like，similar to fetal thyroid tissue.

13-10 甲状腺乳头状癌 Papillary carcinoma，thyroid

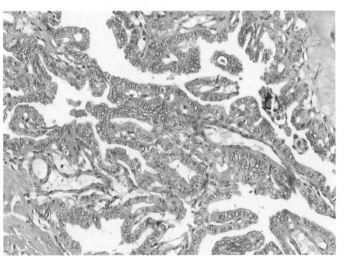

诊断乳头状癌的细胞参数包括毛玻璃样细胞核、核沟和相互重叠的核、砂粒体等。只要存这种细胞形态，不管它是否形成乳头或滤泡或成实性片块或为硬化性均应归入乳头状癌。

The diagnostic cytological parameters for papillary carcinoma are ground glass nuclei，nuclear grooves，overlapping nucleus and psammoma bodies. As long as the memory of this cell morphology，regardless of whether it is the formation of papillary or follicular，or into solid pieces，or sclerosing，it is to be classified as papillary carcinoma.

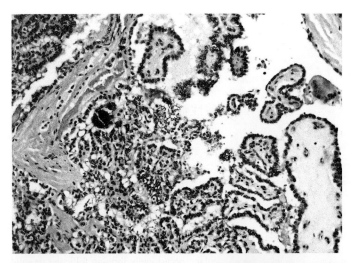

乳头状癌由乳头状间质血管轴心构成复杂的分支树样模式。

Papillary carcinoma shows a complicated branching, treelike pattern outlined by the papilliform axial fibrovascular stroma.

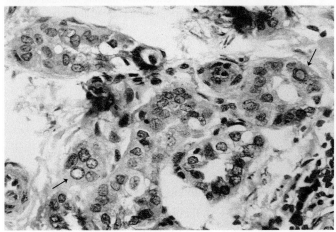

乳头状癌核的特征在于毛玻璃样核，核内假包含体（箭头所示）和核沟。

The nuclear features of papillary carcinoma consist of ground glass nuclei, nuclear pseudoinclusion (arrows) and nuclear grooves.

甲状腺乳头状微小癌（papillary microcarcinoma of thyroid）

乳头状癌直径小于 1cm，包括隐匿型、潜伏型或小乳头癌、无包膜甲状腺肿瘤和隐匿型硬化癌。这类肿瘤发生在儿童具有侵袭性，在成人颈部淋巴结转移。在大体检查时易被漏诊。免疫组化显示 p27 丢失，cyclin D1 上调。

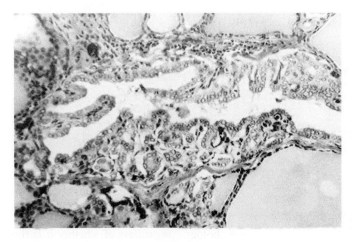

Papillary carcinoma is less than 1 cm in diameter, including cryotype, latent or small papillary carcinoma, without coated thyroid tumor and cryotype sclerosis carcinoma. This cancer occurs in children with invasive, in adult occasionally neck lymph node metastasis. When gross check is susceptible to misdiagnosis. Immunohistochemical shows p27 is losting, cyclin D1 upregulating.

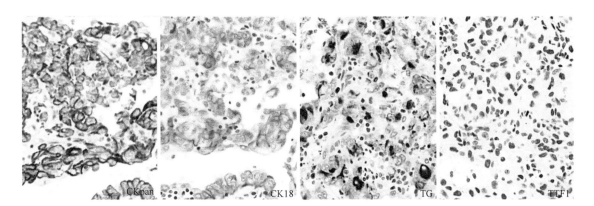

免疫组化显示 CKpan，CK18 阳性表达在肿瘤细胞胞质。甲状腺球蛋白（TG）阳性表达在肿瘤细胞胞核和质。TTF1 阳性表达在肿瘤细胞胞核。

Immunohistochemical CKpan, and CK18 positive cytoplasmic/membranous expression in tumor cells. Thyroglobulin（TG）positive nuclear and cytoplasmic expression in tumor cells. TTF1 positive nuclear expression in tumor cells.

13-11 甲状腺滤泡性癌 Follicular carcinoma，thyroid

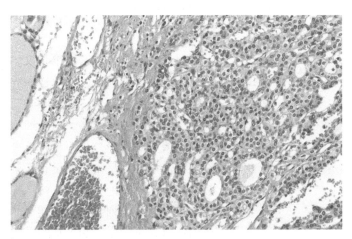

肿瘤组织形态从分化极好像正常甲状腺的滤泡结构到明显恶性的癌。分化好的滤泡癌很难与腺瘤区别，注意是否有包膜和血管侵犯而进行鉴别。分化差的呈实性片巢状，瘤细胞异型性明显，滤泡少而不完整。

Seemingly very normal thyroid follicular structure，but obvious malignant cancer，there have been all sorts of transition from differentiation. Distinguish follicular carcinoma with adenoma is difficult to distinct，pay attention to whether the capsule and vascular invasion. Poorly differentiate showed solid piece nests，tumor cell atypia，small and incomplete follicules.

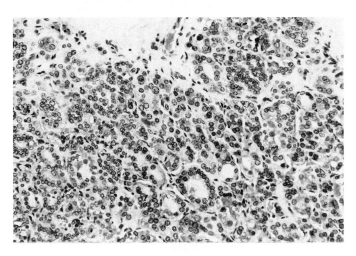

异型滤泡不规则增生，滤泡细胞核深染，染色质粗块样。

Irregular proliferation of atypical follicles are noted，and nuclei of the follicular cells show hyperchromatism and coarse chromatin patterns.

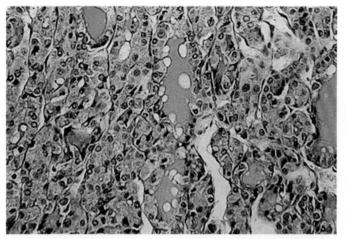

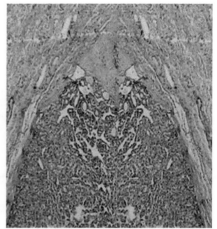

通常滤泡较小，间质内含丰富的薄壁血管，有时形成血窦样结构。癌组织内无乳头形成，也无砂砾体。

The follicles are usually small and contain abundant thin wall vessels, sometimes forming sinusoids. There is no papillary formation and psammoma body in the cancer tissue.

包膜和血管浸润是诊断滤泡癌的重要依据。

It is important basis that capsule membrane and vascular invasions for diagnosis of follicular carcinoma.

13-12　甲状腺髓样癌 Medullary thyroid cancer（MTC）

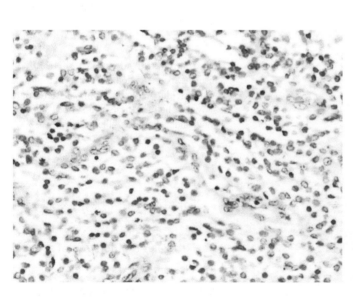

来源于分泌降钙素的甲状腺滤泡旁细胞（C 细胞），是神经内分泌细胞。该肿瘤位列甲状腺肿瘤第三位（约占 3% ～ 12%）。癌细胞核圆形或卵圆形、核仁不显，核分裂罕见。瘤细胞呈实体片巢状、梁状或乳头状、滤泡状排列。梭形细胞常呈漩涡状排列或呈肉瘤样。间质内常有大量的血管和丰富的透明变性胶原和淀粉样物质沉着。

MTC originates from the parafollicular cells（C cells）, which produce the calcitonin. Medullary tumors are the third most common of all thyroid cancers. They make up about 3% ～ 12% of all thyroid cancer cases.

Cancer cells nuclei are round or oval, nucleolus is not significant, mitotic figures are rare. Tumor cells are solid piece nests, trabecular or papillary, follicular arrangements. Spindle cells often have a swirling arrangement or sarcomatoid. The stroma of tumor often contains a large number of blood vessels and rich hyalin degeneration collagen, amyloid deposition.

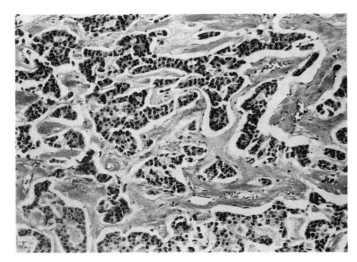

甲状腺髓样癌中可见淀粉样基质和单一的肿瘤细胞呈实心岛状排列。

Amyloid stroma and solid island of monotonous tumor cells are seen in MTC.

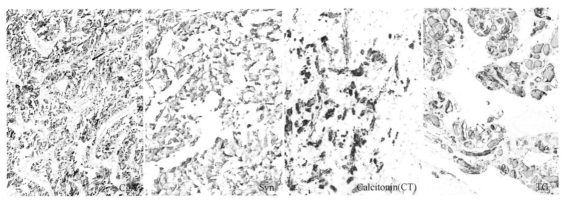

CgA　　　　Syn　　　　Calcitonin(CT)　　　　TG

肿瘤细胞表达神经内分泌标记 CgA，Syn 和降钙素（CT）。肿瘤细胞不表达甲状腺球蛋白（TG），而周围正常甲状腺滤泡上皮表达 TG。

The tumor cells were positive for neuroendocrine markers CgA，Syn and Calcitonin（CT），and negative for TG，while the normal thyroid follicular epithelial cells were positive for TG（IHC stain）.

13-13　甲状腺未分化癌 Undifferentiated carcinoma，thyroid

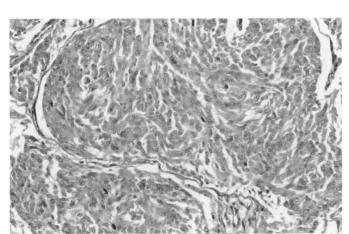

癌细胞大小、形态、染色不一，核分裂象多。形态表现：①小细胞癌，应与淋巴瘤鉴别；②梭形细胞肉瘤样癌；③大多型细胞和巨细胞癌等。

There are various cancer sizes，shapes，coloring and more mitotic figures. Histological patlerns show a variety of types：① Small cell carcinoma，and lymphoma is identified；② Spindle cell sarcomatoid carcinoma；③ Larger pleomorphic cells and giant cell carcinoma，and so on.

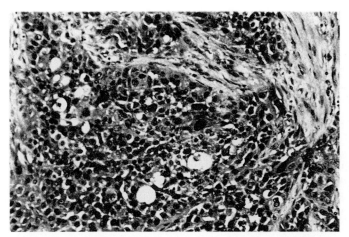

在致密的纤维基质中可见实性巢状和片状多型性肿瘤细胞，伴鳞状上皮样分化。

Solid nests and sheets of pleomorphic tumor cells with squamoid differentiation are seen in dense fibrous stroma.

13-14　甲状腺癌肉瘤 Carcinosarcoma，thyroid

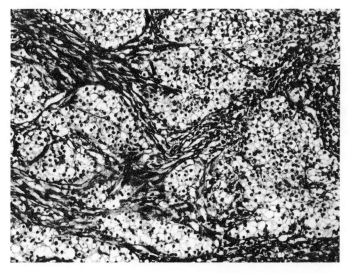

肿瘤有两种细胞成分：一种是呈巢状分布的具有透明胞浆的癌细胞。癌细胞界限清楚，胞浆内富含糖原，核常中位或偏位；另一种是将癌细胞分隔呈巢的梭形细胞。梭形细胞核大、深染，呈束状排列，类似于纤维肉瘤或平滑肌肉瘤。

The tumor has two components：one is carcinoma cells which have well-defined boundaries，cytoplasm rich in glycogen with clear and centrically or eccentrically placed nuclei，growing in the nests. The other is spindle cells which have enlarged，hyperchromatic nuclei，dividing cancer cells into nests and growing in an interlacing arrangement，is similar to fibrosarcoma or leiomyosarcoma.

13-15　甲状旁腺囊肿 Parathyroid cyst

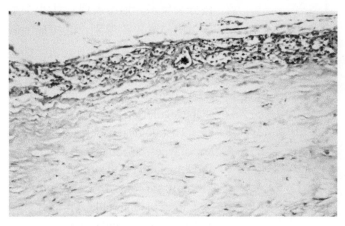

在纤维性囊壁上有受压的甲状旁腺组织。

It shows compressed paeathyroid tissue in the fibrous wall.

13-16 甲状旁腺腺瘤 Parathyroid adenoma

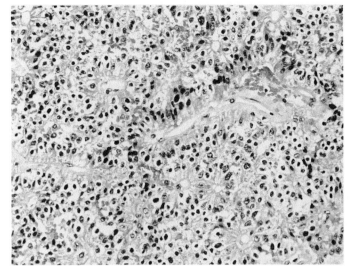

小圆细胞增生常伴有透明胞浆，形成的小腺体伴有中央腔。

The proliferation of small round cells often accompanied with clear cytoplasm, formed small glands central lumens.

13-17 甲状旁腺癌 Parathyroid carcinoma

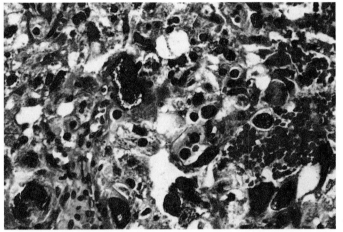

肿瘤细胞显著的多形性，常见瘤巨细胞。

There are a marked pleomorphism of tumor cells and tumor giant cells are frequent seen.

13-18 肾上腺皮质腺瘤 Adrenal cortical adenoma

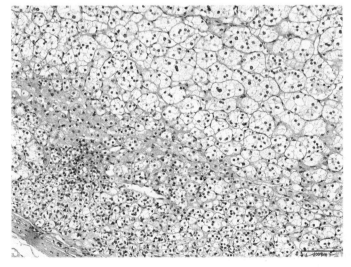

由球状带和束状带区细胞混合组成，细胞排列呈小网状，腺泡状，部分呈束状，通常由不同比例的伴丰富胞浆内脂滴的亮细胞和含脂质稀少的嗜酸性胞浆的暗细胞构成。

The cells are mixed by the zona glomerulosa and zona fasciculata, the cells are arranged in small reticular, acinar, partly fascicular. Tumors are mainly composed of lipid-rich light cells and minority cytoplasm of tumor cells containing less lipid, eosinophilic dark cells.

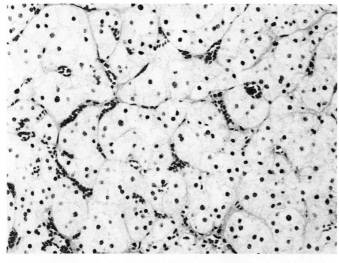

瘤细胞与正常皮质细胞相似，核较小，富含脂质。肿瘤细胞排列成索状或束状，由富含毛细血管的少量纤细的纤维间隔所分隔。

Tumor cells are similar to normal cortical cells, nuclear is small, lipid-rich arranged in cords or clusters separated by delicated fibrous septa with rich interstitial capillaries.

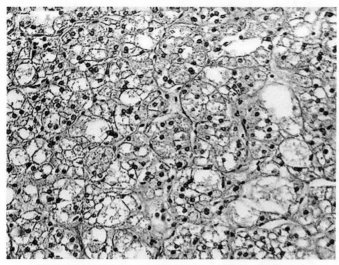

肿瘤可呈脂肪瘤样或髓脂肪瘤样化生，但没有临床意义。免疫组化表达 C17 或 17α - 羟化酶。

It can be lipomaloid or medullary lipoma metaplasia, but it has no clinical significance. C17 or 17 alpha hydroxylase were expressed by immunohistochemistry.

肾上腺皮质腺瘤与皮质增生的鉴别：

①增生结节常为双侧、多发，较小常直径≤1cm，包膜无或不完整，腺瘤多为一侧，单个较大，直径＞1cm；包膜完整。

②腺瘤结节内外组织结构不一样，有压迫现象，腺瘤外的皮质及对侧肾上腺皮质多萎缩，增生结节则无压迫现象，结节内外组织结构相似，对侧肾上腺多同时增生。

③腺瘤细胞排列不规则，可见怪异核细胞，增生结节细胞排列较规则，一般不见核怪异细胞。

Identification between adrenocortical adenoma and hyperplasia：

① Hyperplastic nodules are often bilateral, multiple, often smaller diameter ≤ 1cm, no envelope, or incomplete, Adenoma is a single large in the side, diameter ＞ 1cm; the complete capsule.

② The internal and external structures of adenoma nodules are different, there is oppressive phenomenon, outside the adenoma and contralateral adrenal cortex often atrophy. Nodular hyperplasia without compression, the internal and external structures of the nodules are similar, contralateral adrenal gland is more simultaneous hyperplasia.

③ The adenoma cells are irregular arrangement, visible bizarre nuclear cells, hyperplastic nodule cells were regular, generally not see weird nuclear cells.

13-19　肾上腺皮质腺癌 Adrenal cortical carcinoma/ adenocarcinoma

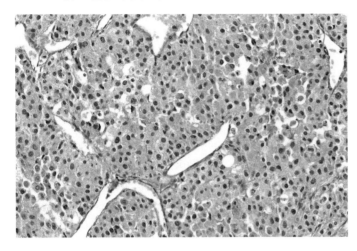

癌细胞呈透明细胞和致密细胞，并按不同比例混合，癌细胞排列成索、巢或腺泡状，异型性明显，核分裂多少不等。易侵犯淋巴管和血管。

Cancer cells are dense cells and clear cells, with mixed in different proportions, cancer cells are arranged in the clusters, nest or acinar. The cells appear atypia, mitotic figures of varying amounts, easily invading lymphatic tubules and blood vessels.

肾上腺皮质癌与皮质腺瘤的鉴别：

①皮质癌常见广泛出血、坏死，腺瘤很少见坏死。

②皮质癌常侵犯包膜、侵入血管及周围组织。

③皮质癌常较多核分裂，核分裂多＞2/10HPF，腺瘤核分裂较少见。

④广泛而明显的核异型、多核巨细胞、较大的核仁及核内包涵体多见于皮质癌。

Identification between adrenal cortical carcinoma and cortical adenoma：

① Cortical carcinoma is common with extensive hemorrhage and necrosis, adenoma is rare necrosis.

② Cortical carcinoma often have invasions capsule, vascular and surrounding tissues.

③ Cortical carcinoma often have more nuclear mitosis, ＞2/10HPF, adenoma mitosis is rare.

④ Extensive and distinct nuclear atypia, multinucleated giant cells, larger nucleoli and intra-nuclear inclusions are common in cortical carcinomas.

13-20　肾上腺嗜铬细胞瘤 Adrenal pheochromocytoma

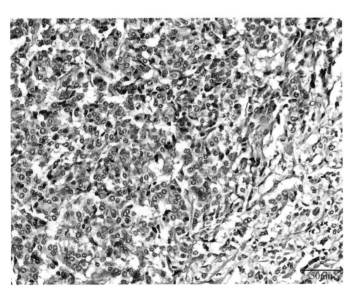

瘤细胞异型性明显，呈大多角形细胞，少数为梭形或柱状细胞，并有一定程度的多形性，可出现瘤巨细胞。瘤细胞胞质内可见大量嗜铬颗粒。瘤细胞呈索状、团状排列；间质为血窦结构。属于副神经节瘤范围。

Tumor cells show obvious pleomorphism, such as large polygonal cells, a few for the spindle or columnar cells with a certain degree of polymorphism, tumors giant cells. The cytoplasm of tumor cells contain a large number of chromaffin granules. Tumor cells arrange in cord or mass; The stroma of tumor appears sinus struc-tures. This tumor belongs to the scope of paraganglioma.

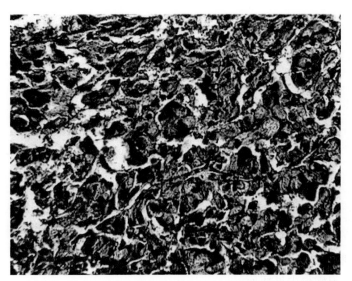

嗜铬细胞瘤的细胞核大小形态很不规则，常见深染核和怪异核，核分裂像罕见。应注意嗜铬细胞瘤出现核的异型性与其生物学行为无关，不应视为诊断恶性嗜铬细胞瘤的形态依据。

The nuclear sizes and shapes of tumor cells are irregular, and the nuclei are dark and bizarre, nuclear mitosis is rare. It should be noted that the atypia of pheochromocytoma doesn't relate to its biological behavior, and should not be regarded as the morphological basis for the diagnosis of malignant pheochromocytoma.

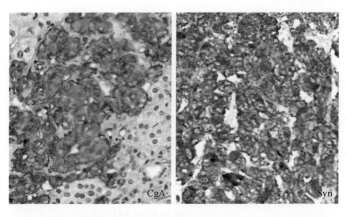

CgA   Syn

免疫组化显示CgA、Syn、S100阳性表达在肿瘤细胞胞质。

Immunohistochemical CgA, Syn, S100 positive cytoplasmic expression in tumor cells.

恶性嗜铬细胞瘤组织学标准，包括：①包膜侵犯；②血管侵犯；③扩散到肾上腺周围组织；④膨胀的、大的、融合性细胞巢；⑤弥漫性生长；⑥坏死；⑦细胞成分增加；⑧肿瘤细胞呈梭形；⑨细胞和核的重度多形性；⑩瘤细胞的单一性（通常是小细胞和高的核浆比率）；⑪核深染；⑫大核仁；⑬核分裂增多；⑭任何非典型核分裂像；⑮缺乏透明球。

Histological criteria of malignant pheochromocytoma including：① Capsule invasion；② Vascular invasion；③ Diffusion into the surrounding tissue of the adrenal gland；④ Expansion, big, and fusion cell nests；⑤ Diffuse growth；⑥ Necrosis；⑦ Increased cell components；⑧ Spindle tumor cells；⑨ Cells and nuclear with severe pleomorphism；⑩ Tumor cells uniformity（usually small cell and high karyoplasmic ratio）；⑪ Hyperchromatic nuclei；⑫ Big nucleolus；⑬ Nuclear mitcsis increase；⑭ Any atypical mitosis；⑮ Lack transparency balls.

13-21 胰岛细胞瘤 Islet cell tumor，pancreas

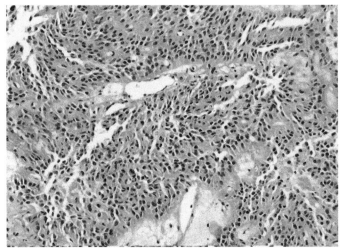

胰岛细胞瘤合成和释放激素进入血液，如胰岛素和胰高血糖素，引起各种症状。胰岛细胞瘤可以是良性的或恶性的（癌）。

Islet cell tumor manufactures and releases hormones，such as insulin and glucagon，into the bloodstream. which cause a variety of symptoms depending on the type of hormone that it produces. Islet cell tumor can be benign or malignant（carcinoma）.

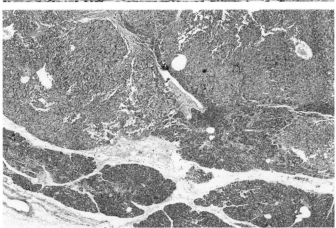

肿瘤交界处上方为胰岛细胞瘤，下方为正常胰腺。

In the junction of tumor and normal tissues，islet cell tumor presents in up of Fig，normal pancreatic tissues is in Fig down.

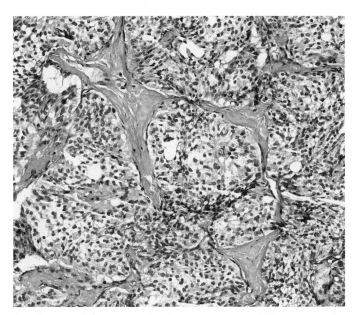

瘤细胞排列形式多样，呈岛片状（似巨大的胰岛）或腺泡和腺管状等。其间为毛细血管及多少不等的胶原纤维分隔瘤组织，并可见黏液、淀粉样变性、钙化等继发性改变。瘤细胞形似胰岛细胞，形态较一致，染色质细颗粒状，可见小核仁。核分裂像少见。

Tumor cells are arranged in various patterns，the island，sheet（like a huge islets）or acinar and duct shapes，etc. The capillaries and collagen fibers varying amounts separated tumor. Secondary changes are mucus，amyloidosis and calcification and so on. Tumor cells are similar to islet cells，shape is more consistent with finely granular chromatin and small nucleoli. Mitotic figures are rare.

13-22 胰岛细胞癌 Islet cell carcinom，pancreas

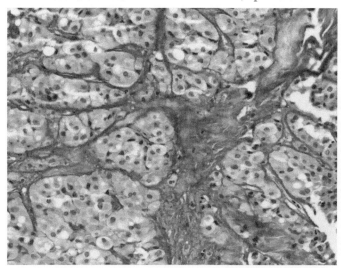

瘤细胞与正常胰岛细胞相似，核不同程度的异型性，但核分裂罕见。高柱状或立方形的瘤细胞排列成 3 种类型：①花带、小梁或脑回状，有丰富的血窦分隔；②腺泡样、腺样或菊形团样；③实性团块或弥漫成片。

Tumor cells are similar to normal islet cells，with significantly different degrees of nuclear atypia，but mitotic figures are rare. High columnar or cuboidal tumor cells arranged in three types：① Flower zone，trabecular or gyrus-like，separated by abundant sinusoids；② Acinar-like，adenoid or rosettes；③ Solid mass or diffuse sheets.

13-23 糖尿病的胰腺 Diabetic pancreas

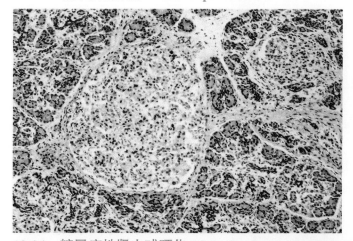

糖尿病母亲分娩的婴儿胰岛增生可能是代偿性增生的结果。有些病例中可见胰岛纤维化或被淀粉样物质取代。

Hyperplasia of islet may be a consequence of compensatory hyperplasia in infants of diabetic mother. Some cases shows fibrosis or amyloid replacement of islets.

13-24 糖尿病性肾小球硬化 Diabetic glomerulosclerosis

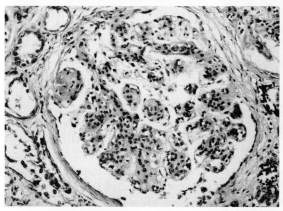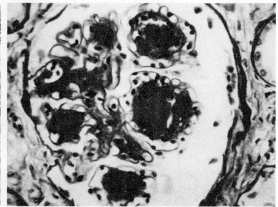

肾小球呈弥漫增厚，系膜基质增多，系膜细胞增生。PAS 染色显示圆形均质、嗜伊红的结节，伴周围毛细血管动脉瘤样扩张。

The glomerulus show diffuse thickening，increase in mesangial matrix and proliferation of mesangial cells. PAS stain shows a round，homogeneous eosinophilic nodule with an aneurysmaloid dilatation of the surrounding capillaries.

第十四章 生殖系统和乳腺疾病
Chapter 14 Diseases of the Genital System and Breast

14-1 宫颈上皮内病变 Cervical intraepithelial lesion（CIN）

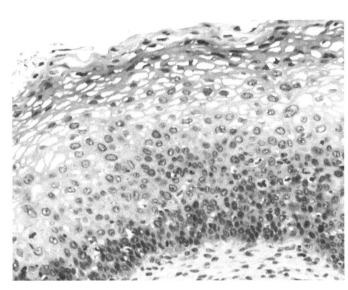

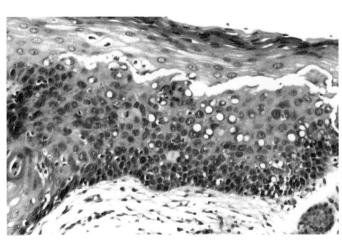

宫颈低级别鳞状上皮内病变 [low-grade squamous intraepithelial lesion of uterine cervix（CIN Ⅰ级）]

基底层细胞/副基底层细胞增生，不超过上皮层下 1/3。细胞境界清楚，极性保持，细胞核增大，略深染，异型性小，核分裂少。上 2/3 层细胞成熟。

CIN Ⅰ：A proliferation of basal/parabasal-like cells is at most extends no more than down one-third of the whole epithelium layer. The cells have well-defined boundary，maintained polarity，enlarged and hyperchromatic nucleus with minimal atypia and little mitotic activity. Cell maturation can be seen in the upper two-thirds of the epithelium layer.

CIN Ⅱ级

基底层细胞/副基底层细胞增生，扩展至上皮的中 1/3 层。上 1/3 层细胞成熟。

CIN2：A proliferation of basal/parabasal-like cells is at extends up into the middle two-third of the epithelium. The cells have obvious dysplasia and mitotic activity and increased cytoplasm-nuclear ratio. Cells maturation can be seen in the upper one-third of the epithelium.

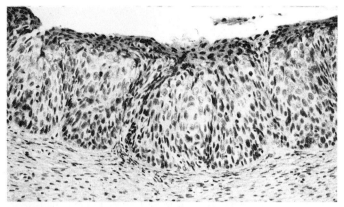

CIN Ⅲ级

核深染、拉长的细胞垂直排列，累及鳞状上皮全层2/3，基底膜完整。

CIN Ⅲ：Hyperchromatic elongated cells are arranged perpendicular and involves more than two thirds to full thickness of squamous epithlium with intact basement membrane.

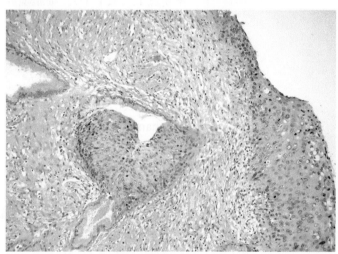

宫颈高级别上皮内病变累及腺体（high-grade squamous intraepithelial lesion of uterine cervix involved glands）

正常颈管腺体被 CIN3 的鳞状上皮所取代。

The normal cervical gland is replaced by the squamous epithelium with CIN3.

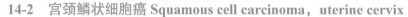

14-2　宫颈鳞状细胞癌 Squamous cell carcinoma，uterine cervix

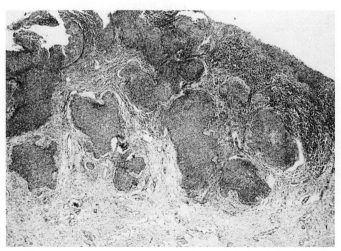

宫颈微小浸润癌（microinvasive carcinoma，uterine cervix）

原位癌累及腺体的背景中可见早期浸润性鳞癌。

Micro invasion of squamous cell carcinoma is seen in the background of carcinoma in situ involved glands.

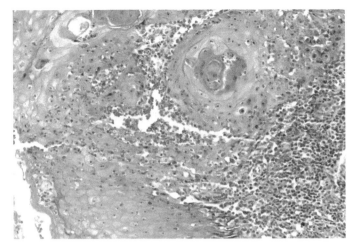

Ⅰ级（well differentiated）

肿瘤细胞以角化成分为主，可见角化珠形成。肿瘤细胞片状排列，核分裂活性低。

There is prominent keratinization，with squamous pearls formation. Tumor cells are arranged in sheets and mitotic counts are lower.

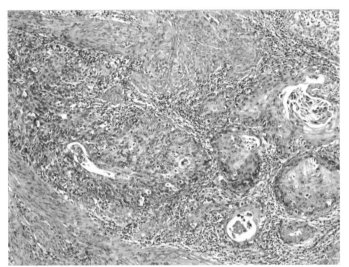

Ⅱ级（moderately differentiated）

肿瘤细胞具有鳞状细胞分化，一般没有角化珠形成。肿瘤细胞片状排列。

The tumor cells have squamous-cell differentiation. Generally，keralinized pearls are absent. Tumor cells are arranged in sheets

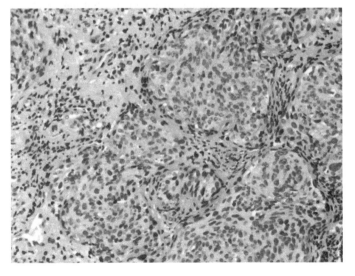

Ⅲ级（poorly differentiated）

肿瘤主要由基底样细胞形成大小不等癌巢构成。细胞核分裂增加。

The tumor is composed of the predominant basal-like cells forming large and small various nests. The mitotic counts are higher.

14-3 宫颈原位腺癌 Cervical adenocarcinoma in situ

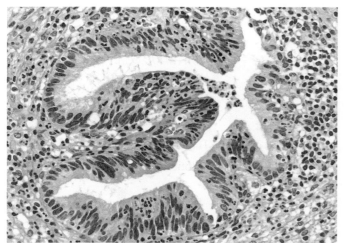

宫颈腺体形态不规则，核染色质增加排列拥挤出现核分裂活性，但间质浸润。

Glands were irregular shapes and densely packed with nucleolus, chromatin increased with mitotic activity, but no invasion.

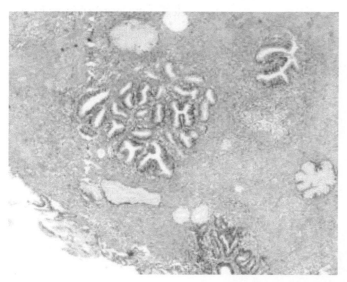

宫颈原位腺癌病变局限于正常腺体的水平，不超过未受累腺体隐窝。腺体拥挤，尽管局灶可有乳头和 / 或筛状结构，大部分腺体仍保持正常的分叶状结构。

依据细胞核的非典型性、复层程度、核分裂像 / 凋亡进行诊断。

Lesions were confined to the normal glandular depth, not exceeding the crypt of the uninvolved gland. Although the focal gland crowded, may have papillary and / or cribriform structure, most of the glands still maintain normal lobulated structures. The diagnosis was according to the dysplasia, the extent of the gland structure complex, the nuclei mitotic image and apoptosis index.

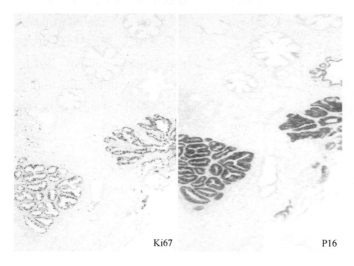

免疫组化结果显示 Ki67 阳性比例大于 30%。上皮细胞 P16 阳性。

Immunohistochemistry stains show Ki67 is more than 30%, P16 positive, apoptosis index increase.

Ki67　　　　　　　　　　P16

14-4 宫颈腺癌 Cervical adenocarcinoma

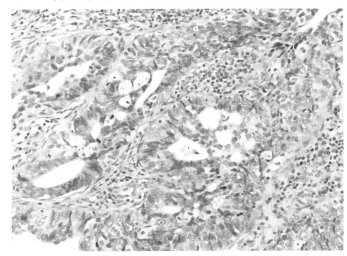

癌细胞呈腺管样结构，管腔形态不规则，细胞层次不等，胞质内含有黏液。分化差时癌细胞排列成实体癌巢，癌细胞异型性大，可见黏液湖形成。

Cancer cells are glandular structures, irregular cavities, layers disordered, the cytoplasm contains mucus. Poor differentiated cancer cells are arranged in solid nests with obvious atypia, forming mucous lake.

14-5 宫颈腺鳞癌 Adenosquamous carcinoma, uterine cervix

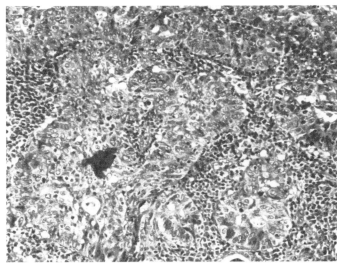

肿瘤由两种细胞成分组成，一种为排列成不规则腺样结构的上皮细胞（下方），另一种为排列成巢状的具有鳞样分化的上皮细胞（上方）。

The tumor is composed of two kinds of cell components, one kind of epithelial cells are arranged in irregular glandular structures（below）and the other kind of epithelial cells are arranged in nests with squamous differentiation（upper）.

14-6 子宫内膜增生症 Endometrial hyperplasia

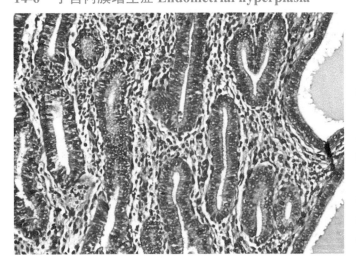

单纯性增生（simple pattern）

无非典型性子宫内膜增生。（endometrial hyperplasia without atypia）

腺体过度增生，大小形态不规则，腺体和间质比例增高，但没有细胞学非典型性。

The glands in irregular size and shape are over proliferation with increasing the glands to stroma ratio, but without cytological atypia.

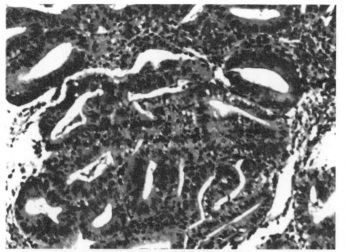

非典型子宫内膜增生/子宫内膜样上皮内瘤变（atypical hyperplasia/endometrioid intraepithelial neoplasia）

管状腺体或分支腺体排列拥挤，伴有细胞学改变。细胞核增大、圆形，极性消失，核仁明显。

The disease is composed of crowded arrangement of tubular or branching glands with cytological changes. The nuclear atypia includes enlargement，loss of polarity and prominent nucleoli.

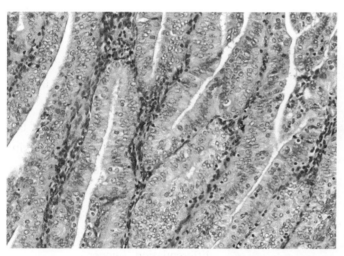

非典型复杂性增生（atypic complex type）

子宫内膜腺体拥挤呈巢状，高柱状腺上皮可向腺腔内呈乳头状或向间质内出芽样生长。上皮细胞异型性，细胞极性紊乱，体积增大，核浆比例增加，核染色质浓聚，核仁明显，伴核分裂象。

Endometrial glands are crowded as nests，some high columnar epithelial cells grow papillary to the glandular cavity or to interstitial sprouting. Epithelial cell show atypia，polarity disorder，the size increase，nuclear cytoplasm ratio increase，nuclear chromatin condensilion，prominent nucleoli，increase mitotic figures.

14-7 子宫腺肌症 Adenomyosis，uterus

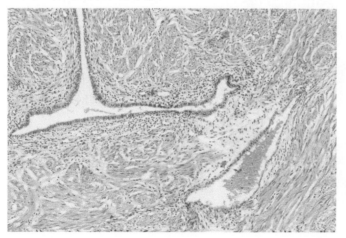

子宫内膜腺体和间质异位于子宫肌层中（距子宫内膜基底层 2mm 以上）。

The endometrial glands and stroma are located in the myometrium（2mm or more from the basal layer of the endometrium）.

14-8 卵巢子宫内膜异位症 Endometriosis，ovary

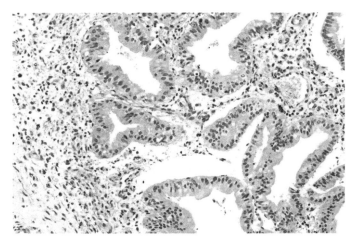

卵巢内出现与正常子宫内膜相似的子宫内膜腺体、子宫内膜间质及含铁血黄素；少数情况下，因时间较久，可仅见增生的纤维组织和含有含铁血黄素的巨噬细胞。

Some endometrial glands，endometrial stroma and hemosiderin are ectopical present in ovary. Few cases，due to a longer time，only show proliferation of fibrous tissues and macrophages containing hemosiderin.

14-9 子宫内膜样腺癌 Endometrioid carcinoma，uterus

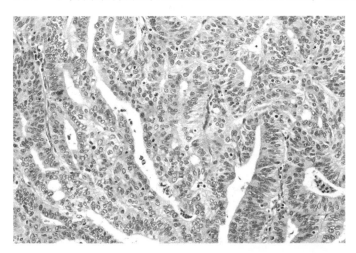

宫内膜腺癌（Ⅰ级）[endometrial adenocarcinoma（Ⅰ）]

肿瘤呈腺性或绒毛腺性结构，部分融合，缺乏分隔间质。肿瘤细胞核大、深染，胞浆嗜酸、颗粒状。

The tumor cells have enlarged，hyperchromatic nuclei and eosinophilic，granular cytoplasm and display glandular or villoglandular architecture with some areas where the glands are confluent and lack of intervening stroma.

宫内膜腺癌（Ⅱ级）[endometrial adenocarcinoma（Ⅱ）]

明显的腺管样结构背靠背、共壁等改变。管腔形态不规则，细胞层次不等，胞质内含有黏液。癌细胞异型性，核分裂较多。

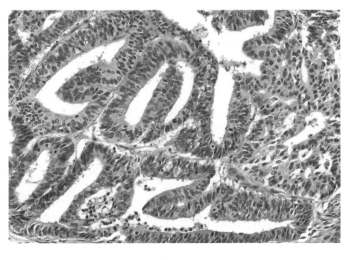

Obvious glandular structures with back to back，co-walls and other changes. Irregular lumen，polarity and layers disorder，the cytoplasm contains mucus. Cancer cells are atypia and more mitotic figures.

14-10 子宫平滑肌瘤 Leiomyoma，uterus

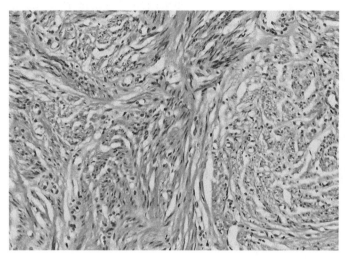

肿瘤推挤式生长，与周围正常平滑肌界限清楚。瘤细胞形态与正常子宫平滑肌细胞相似，梭形，束状或旋涡状排列，胞质红染，核呈长杆状，两端钝圆，核分裂少见，缺乏异型性。

The tumor shows a push-type growth, and the boundaries are clear with normal smooth muscle surrounding. Tumor cells morphology are similar to normal uterine smooth muscle cells, spindle bundles or vortex-like arrangements. The tumor cells show eocinophilic cytoplasmic staining, nuclear elongated rod-shaped, rounded at both ends, mitotic figures rare, lacks atypia.

14-11 子宫平滑肌肉瘤 Leiomyosarcoma，uterus

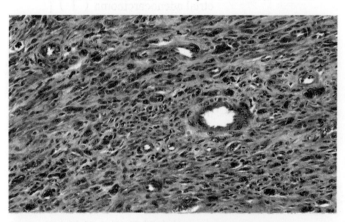

平滑肌肉瘤细胞梭形有明显异型性，核分裂数＞5个/10HPF，核的显著多形和多核瘤巨细胞。可见由凝固性瘤细胞坏死形成的鬼影细胞。

Leiomyosarcoma cells have significant atypia, mitosis count ＞ 5/10 HPF, obviously pleomorphic nuclei and tumor giant cells. Ghost cells are seen from the coagulation necrosis of tumor cells.

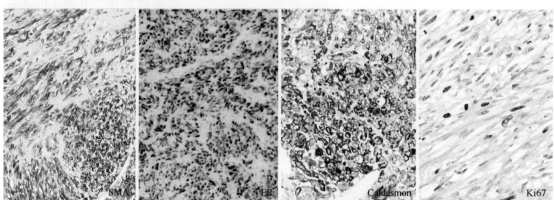

SMA 阳性表达在肿瘤细胞胞质。Caldesmon 阳性表达在肿瘤细胞膜/质。ER、Ki67 阳性表达在肿瘤细胞胞核。

SMA positive cytoplasmic/membranous expression in tumor cells，Caldesmon positive cytoplasmic/membranous expression in tumor cells. ER and Ki67 positive nuclear expression in tumor cells.

14-12 子宫间质肉瘤 Stromal sarcoma，uterus

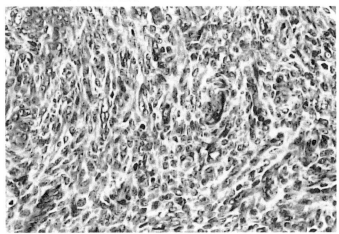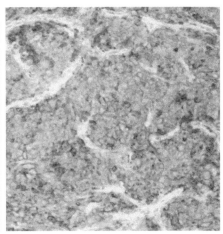

肿瘤由小圆形或短梭形细胞构成，呈致密巢状排列，核分裂像多见。免疫组化结果显示CD10 阳性。

The tumor is composed of small round or short spindle cells with brisk mitotic activity and arranges tight nests. Immunohistochemistry is positive for CD10.

14-13 子宫癌肉瘤 Carcinosarcoma，uterus

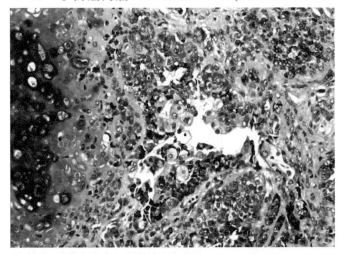

为混合分布的恶性上皮和间叶成分。恶性上皮成分为核大、深染、排列成腺样结构的子宫内膜样癌；恶性间叶成分可以为淡染疏松黏液背景中的梭形细胞，也可以为软骨肉瘤。

The tumor is mixed of malignant epithelial and mesenchymal components. The malignant epithelial components are endometrial carcinoma with enlarged，hyperchromatic nuclei in an gland-like structure. The malignant mesenchymal cells can be either spindle cells in the background of lightly stained loose mucus or chondrosarcoma.

14-14 卵巢癌 Ovary carcinoma

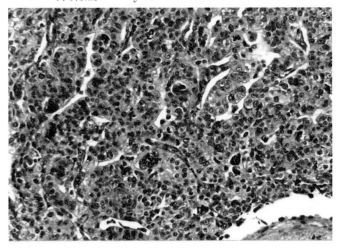

肿瘤组织呈低分化腺癌形态，核大、深染，核浆比增高，可见多形性核。

The tumor morphologically is poorly differentiated adenocarcinoma with large，hyperchromatic, polymorphic nuclei and increased nucleus cytoplasm ratio.

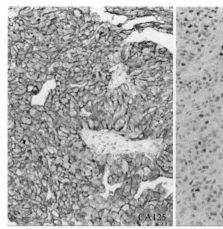
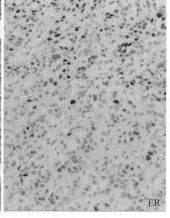

免疫组化结果显示卵巢特异性标记CA125阳性，雌激素受体（ER）阳性。

Immunohistochemistry is positive for CA125，one marker of ovary carcinoma and estrogen receptor （ER） positive.

14-15　葡萄胎 Hydatidiform mole

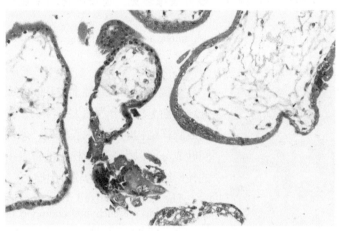

①绒毛因间质高度疏松水肿黏液变性而增大；②绒毛间质内血管消失，或见少量无功能的毛细血管，内无红细胞；③滋养层细胞有不同程度增生。

① Villi are enlarged because of highly interstitial edema with mucoid degeneration；② Capillaries disappear or few non-functioning vessels without red blood cells in stroma；③ Different degrees of trophoblast proliferation.

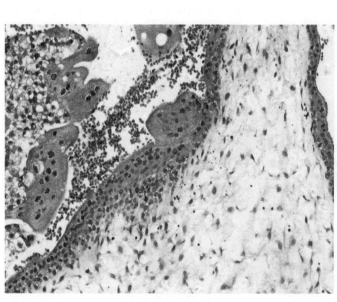

绒毛滋养层细胞增生包括细胞滋养层细胞（朗格汉斯细胞）位于正常绒毛内层，呈立方或多边形，胞质淡染，核圆居中，染色质较稀疏。合体滋养层细胞位于正常绒毛的外层，细胞体积大而不规则，胞质嗜酸呈深红色，多核，核深染。

The proliferation of trophoblast include cytotrophoblasts （Langerhans cells） at villi lining, cubic or polygonal, lightly stained cytoplasm, round nuclei located in the cells center with relatively sparse chromatin. Syncytiotrophoblast at the outside of villi, large size and irregular, eosinophilic cytoplasm condensed, multinuclei, nuclear stained relatively dark.

14-16　子宫绒毛膜癌 Choriocarcinoma，uterus

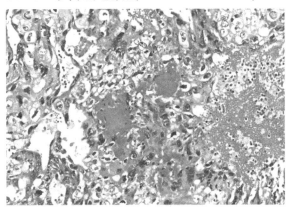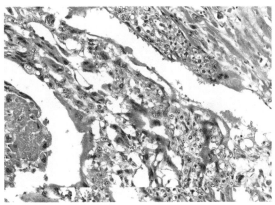

　　肿瘤由分化不良的细胞滋养层和合体滋养层两种瘤细胞组成，两种细胞混合排列成巢状或条索状，细胞异型性明显，核分裂象多见。癌组织和周围正常组织有明显出血、缺血性坏死，继发性炎症细胞浸润。瘤组织中无绒毛，无肿瘤间质，无血管间质。

　　Tumor is composed of poorly differentiated cytotrophoblasts and syncytiotrophoblasts，with two types of cells are mixed in nests or cords arrangements，significant cellular atypia and mitotic figures are common. Cancerous tissue and surrounding normal tissues have significant bleeding，ischemic necrosis，secondary inflammatory cells infiltration. Cancer cells do not form villi，nor stromal vascular and nor tumor stroma.

14-17　卵巢浆液性腺癌 Serous adenocarcinoma，ovary

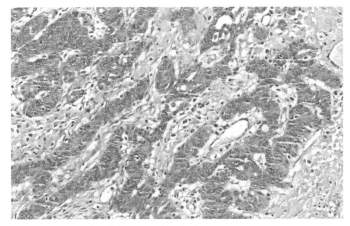

　　癌细胞腺样排列，浸润性生长，伴肿瘤间质增生。

　　Cancer cells show adenoid arrangement，invasive growth，with the proliferation of tumor stroma.

14-18　卵巢浆液性乳头状腺癌 Serous papillary adenocarcinoma，ovary

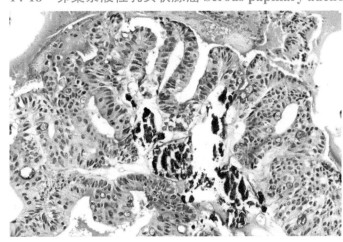

　　癌细胞乳头状排列，浸润性生长，伴肿瘤间质增生，含有同心圆钙化的砂粒体。癌细胞具有显著的异型性或未分化细胞。

　　Cancer cells show papillary arrangement，invasive growth，with the proliferation of tumor stroma. Cancer cells show significant atypia or undifferentiated cells with concentric calcified psammoma bodies.

14-19 卵巢黏液性囊腺瘤 Mucinous cystadenoma, ovary

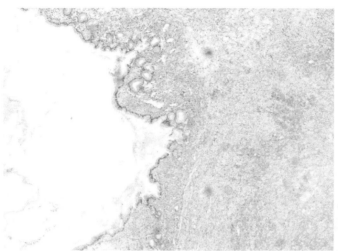

瘤细胞为缺乏纤毛的高柱状上皮细胞伴有细胞顶端黏液空泡。肿瘤细胞排列腺样，多囊，囊内含粉红色黏液。可发生于子宫内膜组织异位的基础上，称为"苗勒氏黏液性"囊腺瘤，类似于子宫内膜上皮或宫颈上皮。

Tumor cells are lacking cilia high columnar epithelial cells with cell top mucus vacuoles. Tumor cells are arranged in adenoid, polycystic form, intracyst contains pink mucus. It occurs in the foundation of the ectopic endometrial tissue called "Mullerian mucinous" cystadenoma, similar to the endometrial epithelium or cervical epithelium.

14-20 卵巢黏液性乳头状腺癌 Mucinous papillary adenocarcinoma, ovary

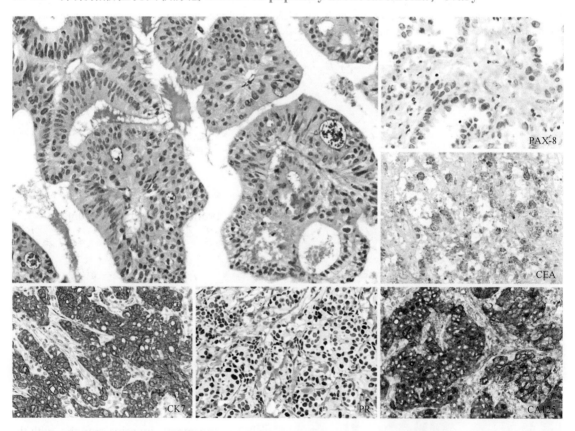

癌组织呈乳头状生长伴黏液分泌。免疫组化显示 PAX-8、孕激素受体（PR）阳性表达在肿瘤细胞胞核。CEA、CK7、CA125 阳性表达在肿瘤细胞胞质。

Tumor grows with papillary or solid with mucus secretion. Immunohistochemical PAX-8 and PR positive nuclear expression in tumor cells CEA, CA125 and CK7 positive cytoplasmic/membranous expression in tumor cells.

14-21 输卵管低分化腺癌 Poorly differentiated adenocarcinoma，salpinx

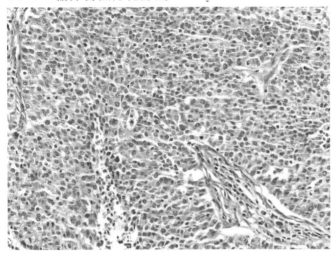

原发于输卵管的癌，少见，镜下肿瘤为不同分化程度的浸润性乳头状腺癌。有多种变型，主要为浆液性、宫内膜样、腺棘皮癌样、浆液黏液混合性或黏液样、移形细胞癌或透明细胞癌等。

Cancer originated in the fallopian tube is rare. Microscopic tumor is differentiation for different levels of invasive papillary adenocarcinoma. There are many variations, mainly serous, endometrioid, echinoderms, serous mixing mucus or mucus, transitional cell carcinoma or clear cell carcinoma, etc.

14-22 卵巢粒层细胞瘤 Granulosa cell tumor，ovary

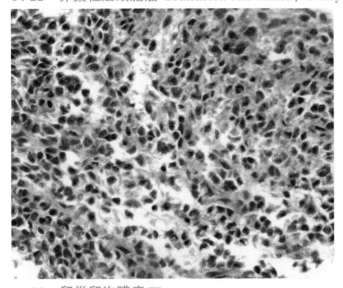

瘤细胞体积较小，椭圆形或多角形，细胞质少，细胞核常见核沟，呈咖啡豆样外观。瘤细胞排列成弥漫型、岛屿型、梁索型，分化较好的瘤细胞常围绕一腔隙，排列成卵泡样的结构，中央为粉染的蛋白液体或退化的细胞核，称为 Call-Exner 小体。

Tumor cells are smaller, oval or polygonal, less cytoplasm, visible nuclear grooves, like coffee beans appearance. Tumor cells arrange in diffuse, island types, beam cable types, well differentiated tumor cells often around a lacuna, arranged in follicle-like structure, the center is the protein with light stain or degradation nuclei, known as Call-Exner bodies.

14-23 卵巢卵泡膜瘤 Thecoma，ovary

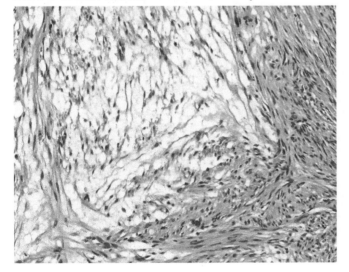

瘤细胞由成束的短梭形细胞组成，核卵圆形，胞质由于含脂质而呈空泡状。玻璃样变的胶原纤维可将瘤细胞分割成巢状。瘤细胞黄素化时，细胞大而圆，核圆居中，与黄体细胞相像，称为黄素化的卵泡膜细胞瘤。

Tumor cells are composed of short spindle cells, nuclear is oval, due to lipid-content, showing cytoplasmic vacuolization. Hyaline collagen fibers can divide tumor cells into nests. When tumor cells are luteinized, cells are large and round, with a round nuclear center, and similar to the luteal cells, called luteinizing thecoma.

14-24 卵巢硬化性间质瘤 Sclerosing stromal tumor，ovary

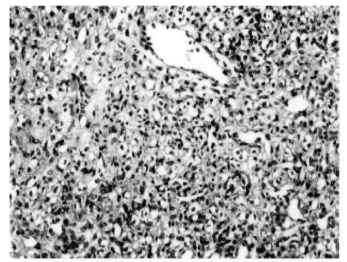

细胞稀少的致密胶原区与细胞丰富的水肿区分隔成小叶状。薄壁小血管，伴有不同程度的硬化，其中混合有类似于纤维母细胞的梭形细胞和类似于黄素化的卵泡膜瘤细胞。

A dense region with fewer cells and dense collagen and a edema region with rich cells mixed and divided into small lobes. Thin-walled small vessels present in stroma with varying degrees of sclerosis, The ca cells are similar to luteinized mixed with spindle cells similar to fibroblasts.

14-25 卵巢支持 - 间质细胞肿瘤 Sertoli-stromal cell tumors，ovary

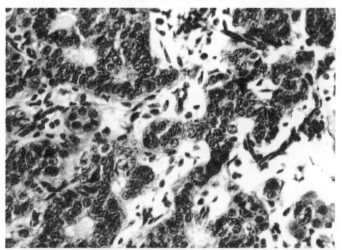

支持细胞形成小管或条索，在纤细或水肿的纤维间质中含间质细胞。间质细胞呈梭形，细胞浆稀少，细胞核浓染，可含有空泡、脂质或 Reink 结晶。

Sertoli-cells form tubules or cords，with stromal cells in slender or edematous fibrous stroma. Stromal cells are spindle shaped with scant cytoplasm and dense nuclei，which may contain vacuoles，lipids，or Reink crystals.

14-26 卵巢无性细胞瘤 Dysgerminoma，ovary

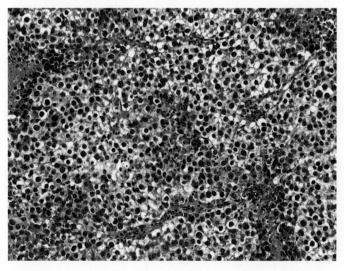

癌细胞体积大而一致，胞膜清晰，胞质空亮充满糖原，核居中，1～2个明显的核仁，核分裂多见。瘤细胞排列成巢或条索状。瘤巢周围常有淋巴细胞浸润，并可有结核样肉芽肿。约 15% 的无性细胞瘤含有合体细胞滋养层成分。

The tumor cells are large and consistent，prominent cell membrane，cytoplasm light，full of glycogen，the nucleus center with 1 ～ 2 prominent nucleoli，and mitotic figures are common. Tumor cells are arranged in nests or cords. lymphocytes frequent interval around cancer nest，and may associated with tuberculoid grannuloma. Approximately 15% of dysgerminoma contain syncytiotrophoblasts components.

14-27 卵巢胚胎性癌 Embryonal carcinoma，ovary

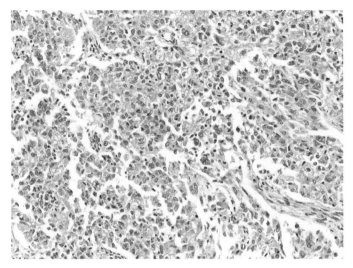

肿瘤细胞排列成腺管、腺泡或乳头状，分化差的细胞则排列成片状。肿瘤细胞形态呈上皮样，细胞大，显著异型，细胞之间界限不清，细胞核大小形态不一，核仁明显，常见核分裂像和瘤巨细胞。

Tumor cells arrange in tubular, acinar or papillary，poor differentiated cells arrange in sheets. Tumor cells show epithelioid morphology，large，ill-defined，significantly atypical with varying size and shape，prominent nucleoli，and mitotic figures，tumor giant cells are common.

14-28 卵巢卵黄囊瘤 Yolk sac tumor，ovary

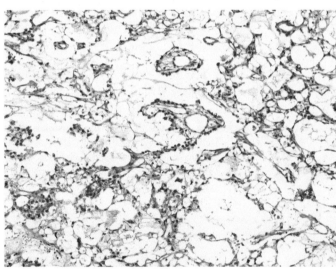

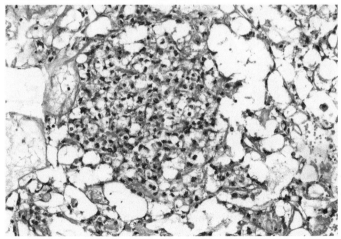

肿瘤中可见多种组织形态：①疏网状结构，是最常见的形态，相互交通的间隙形成微囊、乳头和腺管结构，内衬立方或扁平上皮，背景呈黏液状。②S-D 小体：由生殖细胞围绕的纤维血管，类似肾小球样结构。③多泡性卵黄囊结构，形成与外胚层卵黄囊相似、大小不等的囊腔，内衬扁平上皮、立方上皮或柱状上皮，囊之间为致密的结缔组织。④细胞外嗜酸性玻璃样小体也是常见的特征性结构。⑤有肝细胞样分化。

A variety of morphologies are seen in tumor tissue：① Loosen netword structure is the most common form，the each transport forms the microcyts，papillary and glandular structures，lining cubic or flattened epithelia，mucus-like background. ② S-D（Schiller-Duval）bodies：fibrovascular surrounded by germ cells，similar to the glomerular structures. ③ Multivesicular yolk sac structure is similar to the cysts of the ectoderm yolk sac tumor with varying sizes，lined squamous，cuboidal or columnar epithelia，between the cysts is dense connective tissues. ④ Excellular eosinophilic hyaline bodies is a common characteristic structure. ⑤ May present hepatocyte-like differentiation.

14-29 卵巢甲状腺肿 Struma ovary

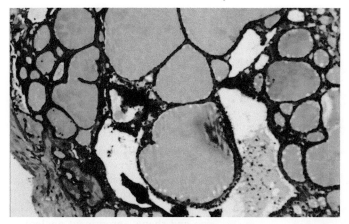

属于单胚层畸胎瘤，肿瘤由充满胶质的腺泡组成，类似于正常位置的甲状腺。腺泡由单层、低立方、核圆、胞浆嗜酸的细胞组成。

The tumor is classsified to monodermal teratoma and composed of acnini filled with colloid, resembling eutopic thyroid. The acinic cells are single layer, low cuboidal with round nuclei and eosinophilic cytoplasm.

14-30 卵巢畸胎瘤 Teratoma, ovary

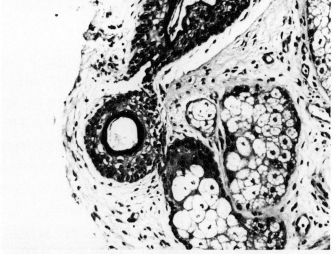

成熟性囊性畸胎瘤（mature cystic teratoma）

肿瘤起源于2个或3个胚层（外胚层、中胚层、内胚层）。肿瘤常呈囊性，囊壁由成熟的组织如外胚层起源的鳞状上皮及附属器毛囊和皮脂腺等组成。

The tumor is derived from two or three germ layers（ectoderm, mesoderm and endoderm）and usually cystic. The cyst wall is composed of mature tissues such as ectodermal derivatives represented by squamous epithelium and other adnexal structures（e.g. hair follicle and sebaceous glands）.

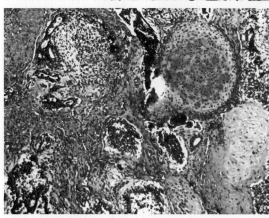
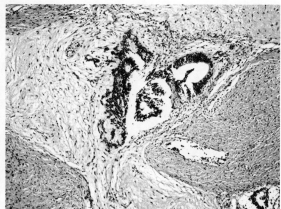

未成熟性畸胎瘤（immature cystic teratoma）

肿瘤组织中可见未成熟胚胎组织。图正中所示原始神经管。

There are immature embryoid tissues. There are primitive neuroectodermal tubules（central）in the tumor.

14-31 腺瘤样瘤 Adenomatoid tumor

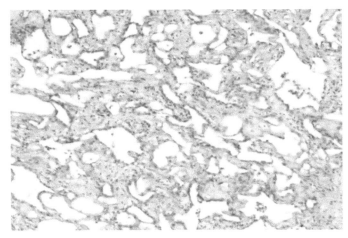

由嗜酸性间皮细胞构成实性条索以及扩张的小管。泡状胞质是其特点。间质纤维化，也可有大量平滑肌成分。

Eosinophilic mesothelial cells consists of solid cords and dilated tubules. Vesicular cytoplasm is characterized by its cytoplasm. Interstitial fibrosis is associated large amounts of smooth muscle components.

14-32 乳腺增生 Breast hyperplasia

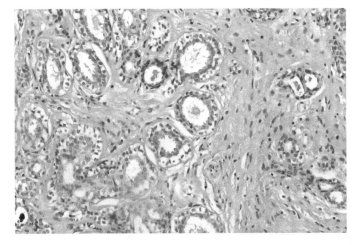

乳腺小叶增生（lobular hyperplasia of breast）

乳腺小叶增生，囊肿形成、间质纤维增生外，伴有末梢导管和腺泡上皮的增生。上皮增生使层次增多，并形成乳头突入囊内，乳头顶部相互吻合，构成筛状结构。

Breast lobular hyperplasia, cyst formation, interstitial fibrosis are often associated the peripheral ductal and acinar epithelial hyperplasia. The epithelial hyperplasia form the papillary projecting into the cysts, the top of the papillary fuses, constituting acribriform patterns.

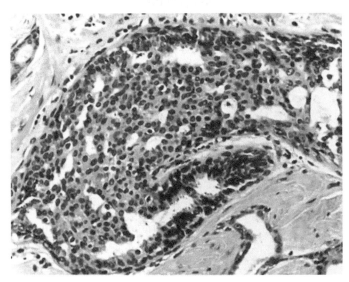

导管增生（ductal hyperplasia）

腺体形态各异、排列紊乱,边窗。细胞边界清楚,均匀,核卵圆、核沟、假包涵体，流水排列，有时混有分泌细胞。ER 表达异质性。

Glands disorderly vary in size and shape, and arrange disorders with side-windows. Cells often have indistinct borders and unevenly spaced. Nuclei are often oval with grooves and pseudoinclusions. Nuclei show streaming pattern. Some apocrine cells admixed in tumor.

ER is heterogeneous expression.

14-33　乳腺纤维腺瘤 Fibroadenoma，breast

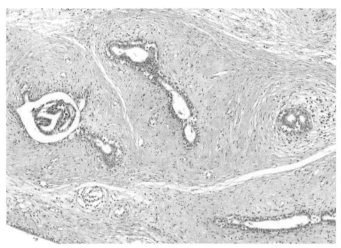

　　肿瘤主要由增生的纤维和腺体组成。腺体圆形或卵圆形，或被周围的纤维结缔组织挤压呈裂隙状；间质通常较疏松，富于黏多糖，也可较致密，发生玻璃样变或钙化。

Tumor is mainly composed of hyperplastic fibrous and glands. Glands are round or oval, or slit-like squeezed by fibrous connective tissues surrounding; Stroma usually loose, rich in mucopolysaccharides, also more dense with connective tissue hyaline degeneration or calcification.

14-34　导管原位癌 Ductal carcinoma in situ，breast

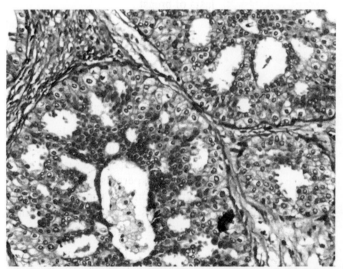

低级别（low grade）

　　肿瘤细胞小、单一性，细胞核大小一致，染色质均匀，核仁不明显，核分裂罕见，呈筛状，腔圆。

The tumor cells are small and monotonous uniform with monomorphic nuclei, homogeneous chromatin, inconspicuous nuclei and scant mitotic activity, growing in rounded, cribriform patterns.

高级别（high grade）

　　乳腺粉刺癌（comedocarcinoma of breast）

　　肿瘤细胞形成实性巢状结构，核大小不一，极性紊乱，染色质粗大，管腔内见粉刺样坏死。

The tumor cells have variable size, poorly polarized nuclei with coarse, clumped chromatin and grow in solid nests pattern. Comedoid necrosis exists in duct lumina.

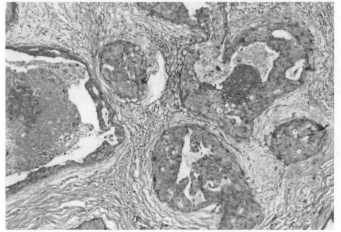

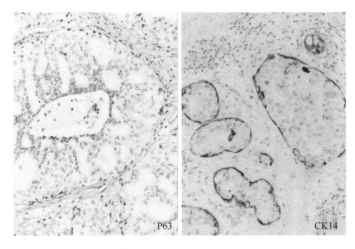

免疫组化结果显示导管肌上皮标记 P63 和 CK14 阳性。

Immunohistochemistry is positive for P63 and CK14, a markers of myoepithelial cells.

14-35 乳腺浸润性导管癌 Infiltrating duct carcinoma，breast

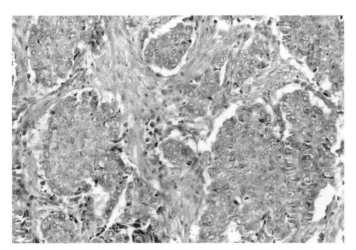

癌细胞排列为条索状、实性细胞巢状或伴有少量腺样结构，散布于丰富的致密的纤维性间质中。肿瘤细胞大小形态各异，异型性明显，核分裂象多见，伴局部肿瘤细胞坏死。

Cancer cells are arranged in cords, solid nests or a small amount of adenoid structures, spread to the dense fibrous stroma. Tumor cells show various sizes and shapes, atypia, mitotic figures are common, with local tumor cell necrosis.

浸润性癌Ⅰ级，非特殊类型（invasive carcinoma of no specific type，gradeⅠ）

肿瘤由明显的腺管组成，细胞较小，形态较一致，核分裂罕见。免疫组化结果显示 HER2 和 ER 弱阳性。

The tumor is composed of distinct glandular tubules with small, regular uniform cells and scant mitotic counts. Immunohistochemistry is weakly positive for HER2 and ER.

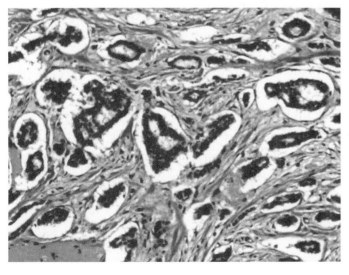

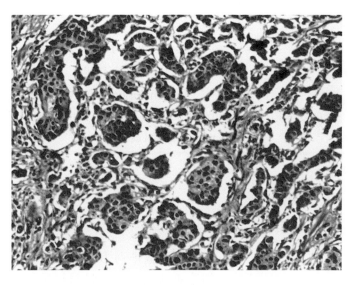

浸润性癌 Ⅱ 级，非特殊类型（invasive carcinoma of no specific type，grade Ⅱ）

肿瘤细胞呈条索状或不规则腺管排列、细胞小到中等大，形态较一致，核分裂可见。

免疫组化结果显示 HER2 中等阳性和 ER 强阳性。

The tumor cells are small to medium in size and regular uniform with a few nuclear mitoses，growing in cords or irregular ducts structures.

Immunohistochemistry is moderately positive for HER2 and strongly positive for ER.

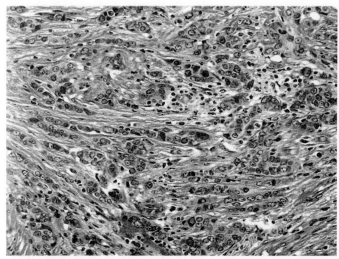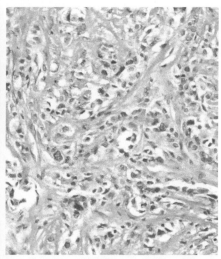

浸润性癌 Ⅲ 级，非特殊类型（invasive carcinoma of no specific type，grade Ⅲ）

肿瘤细胞呈实性巢状分布，无明显腺管样结构，细胞胞浆丰富，核大小不一，核分裂像多见。免疫组化结果显示 HER2 强阳性和 ER 阴性。

The tumor cells have rich cytoplasm and variable nuclei in size with visible mitotic activity，arranged in solid nests without obviously glandular tubule structures. Immunohistochemistry is strongly positive for HER2 and negative for ER.

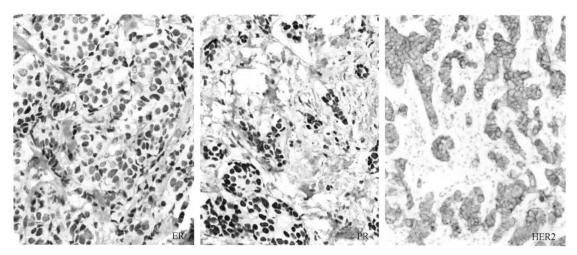

侵润性乳腺导管癌免疫组化显示 ER、PR 阳性表达在肿瘤细胞核。肿瘤细胞 HER2 膜阳性。

Immunohistochemical ER and PR positive nuclear expression in tumor cells. HER2 positive membrane expression in tumor cells.

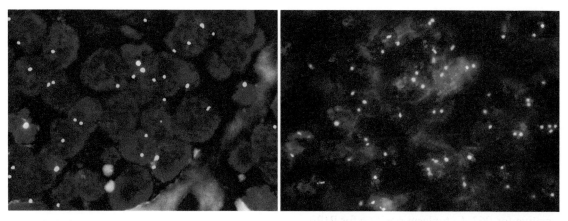

乳腺癌 FISH 检测：HER2（红）/CEP17（内对照探针绿）正常在 1.8～2.2 之间，平均每个细胞核 HER2/CEP17 信号比＞ 2.2，提示 HER2 基因扩增。左图 HER2 基因扩增阴性。右图 HER2 扩增阳性。

Fluorescence in situ hybridization（FISH）for HER2：HER2（red）/CEP17（control probe in green）. The normal value is between 1.8 ～ 2.2，the average ratio of HER2/CEP17 is more than than 2.2 in the nucleus，suggesting that HER2 gene amplification.

The left figure is negative for HER2 amplification. The right figure is positive for HER2 gene amplification.

14-36 乳腺小叶原位癌 Lobular carcinoma in situ，breast

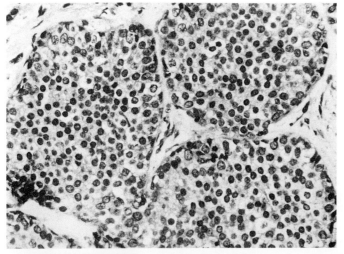

仍可见完整的小叶结构，小叶内几乎所有的腺泡膨胀，代之排列松散、细胞核一致增生的小细胞。

Lobular architecture is maintained on low-power examination，most of acini of a lobular unit are distended by a dispersive proliferation of cells with small，uniform nuclei.

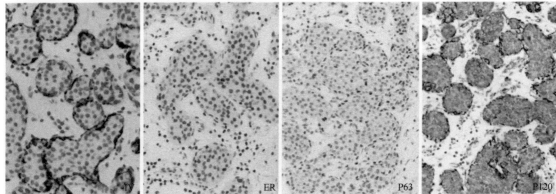

免疫组化结果显示 IV 胶原基底膜阳性。ER 弱阳性。导管肌上皮标记 P63 阳性。P120 胞浆阳性。

Immunohistochemistry is positive for Type IV Collagen and weakly express ER. Myoepithelial positive for P63. Cytoplasm positive for P120.

14-37 乳腺浸润性小叶癌 Infiltrating lobular carcinoma，breast

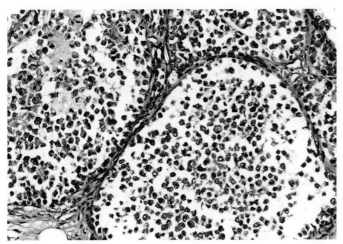

癌细胞较小，界限清楚，黏附性差。胞质少，嗜酸性或淡染，常有胞质内小空泡甚至呈印戒细胞样，胞质空泡内常可见嗜酸性包涵体样小球（AB/PAS 阳性）。核圆-卵圆形、核仁不明显，核分裂象少见。

The cancer cells are small，boundaries clear，poor adhesion. Less cytoplasm less eosinophilic or lightly stained，small cytoplasmic vacuoles inside often even showing signet ring cell-like，eosinophilic inclusions（AB / PAS-positive）are in the cytoplasm. Nuclear is round-oval，inconspicuous nucleoli，and mitotic figures are rare.

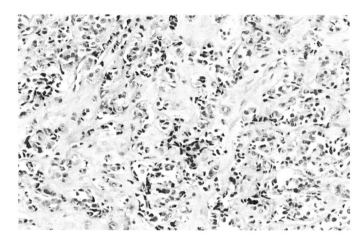

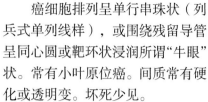

癌细胞排列呈单行串珠状（列兵式单列线样），或围绕残留导管呈同心圆或靶环状浸润所谓"牛眼"状。常有小叶原位癌。间质常有硬化或透明变。坏死少见。

Cancer cells, arranged in a single row beaded (Pvt style singleline-like), around the catheter or target residual cluctal infiltration shows in concentric circles or target circles, so-called "bull's eye" shape mode. Often accompanied by lobular carcinoma in situ. Interstitial often become hardened or hyaline degeneration. Necrosis is rare.

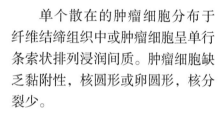

单个散在的肿瘤细胞分布于纤维结缔组织中或肿瘤细胞呈单行条索状排列浸润间质。肿瘤细胞缺乏黏附性，核圆形或卵圆形，核分裂少。

Tumor cells either appear individually dispersed through a fibrous connective tissue or arrange in single linear invaded the stroma. The tumor cells lack cohesion with round or ovoid nuclei and a little mitotic activity.

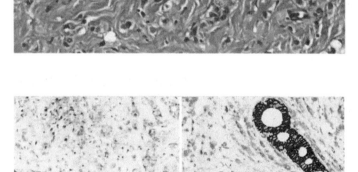

HER2 P120

免疫组化结果显示 E-cad 阴性，ER 阴性，HER2 和 P120 中等阳性。

Immunohistochemistry is moderately positive for HER2 and P120, but negative for E-cad and ER.

14-38 乳腺髓样癌 Medullary carcinoma，breast

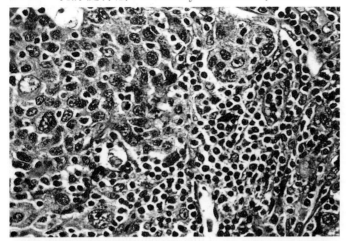

可见巨大的上皮细胞巢，无腺样结构，癌细胞体积大，多形，合体状，癌中和癌周伴有中等到显著程度的淋巴细胞、浆细胞浸润，提示了宿主对肿瘤的反应。

Large epithlial nests without glandloid structure. Cancer cells are large, multi-shaped, syncytioid, inside and periphery of the cancer show infiltration of significant lymphocytes and plasma cells, suggesting the host response to the tumor.

14-39 乳腺黏液癌 Mucinous carcinoma（乳腺胶样癌 Colloid carcinoma），breast

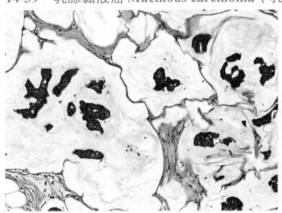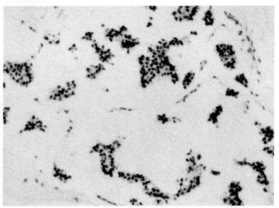

大量细胞外黏液中漂浮簇状增生的肿瘤细胞，细胞较小、一致。
免疫组化结果显示 HER2 阴性和 ER 强阳性。
Clusters of generally small and uniform proliferating tumor cells float in large amounts of extracellular mucin. Immunohistochemistry is strongly positive for ER and negative for HER2.

14-40 乳腺 Paget's 病 Paget's disease，breast

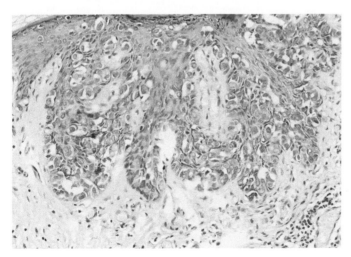

表皮内见 Paget 细胞，其体积大，圆或卵圆形，胞界清楚。胞质丰富，淡染或透明。核大，圆形，染色质细粒状，核仁清楚。核分裂象易见。Paget 细胞可散在或成群出现于表皮内各层。可见病变深部的导管内癌。约 1/3 有浸润性癌。

Paget cells are seen within the epidermis. Its bulky, round or oval, boundaries clear. Cytoplasm is rich, lightly stained or transparent. Nuclear is large, round, thin chromatin, nucleolus prominent. Mitotic figures are easily seen. Paget cells can be scattered or in groups present in all layers of the epidermis. Intraductal carcinoma is always visible in deep lesions, about one-third with invasive cancer.

14-41　肝乳腺癌转移 Breast cancer metastasis，liver

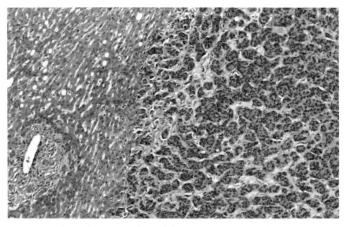

正常肝组织（左侧）旁见大量呈巢状排列的上皮细胞团，胞浆淡红，核深染（右侧）。

There are a large number of epithelial cell clusters in nests（right）near normal liver tissue（left）. These epithelial cancer cells present light staining cytoplasm and hyperchromatic nucleus.

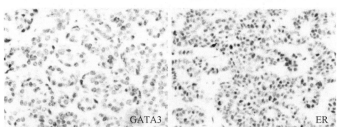

GATA3　　　　ER

免疫组化结果显示乳腺癌常用标记 GATA3 和 ER 阳性。

Immunohistochemistry is positive for GATA3 and ER usually used in breast cancer.

14-42　前列腺增生 Prostatic hyperplasia

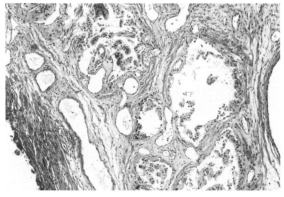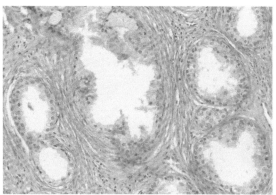

　　前列腺增生中包括分泌细胞、基底细胞，以及原始间叶、成纤维细胞及平滑肌细胞的增生，形成结节。增生的腺上皮可形成不规则乳头，但仍保留正常腺体的两层细胞特点：内层腺上皮细胞，外层基底细胞，周围有完整的基底膜包绕。前列腺增生有多种形态：①纤维肌腺瘤样；②腺瘤样型；③纤维肌型；④肌型；⑤纤维血管型。上述各型结节可在同一病例中混合存在。增生性结节可同时伴发基底细胞增生，筛状增生，萎缩后增生，腺瘤样增生，硬化性腺病等。

　　Prostate hyperplasia includes secretry cells，basal cells，primitive mesenchymal cells，fibroblast and smooth muscle cells components，which formates nodules. Epithelial hyperplasia can form irregular papillary，but still retains the characteristics of normal gland cell layers：the inner layer is epithelial cells，the outer layer is basal cells，basement membrane surrounding a complete package around. Prostate hyperplasia presents a variety of forms：① adenomatous muscle fiber；② adenomatous type；③ muscle fiber type；④ muscular；⑤ fibrovascular type. These various types of nodules can be mixed in the same cases. Hyperplastic nodules can also be associated with basal cell hyperplasia，cribriform pattern hyperplasia，after atrophy hyperplasia，adenomatous hyperplasia，sclerosing adenosis and so on.

14-43 前列腺癌 Prostatic carcinoma

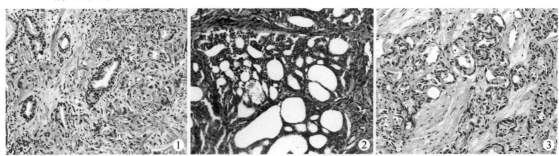

①核间变，出现一个或多个大而明显的核仁（诊断前列腺癌重要的指标）；②腺体结构异常筛网状结构；③间质浸润。

① Nucleus anaplasia refers to prostate ducts and acinar epithelial. one or more large and prominent nucleoli（an important indicator of diagnosis of prostate cancer）；② Abnormal glandular structures, cribriform or network patterns；③ Interstitial invasions.

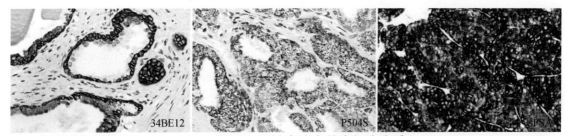

免疫组化显示 34BE12、P504S 和 PSA 阳性表达在肿瘤细胞胞质。

Immunohistochemical 34BE12，P504S and PSA positive cytoplasmic/membranous expression in tumor cells.

14-44 精原细胞瘤 Seminoma

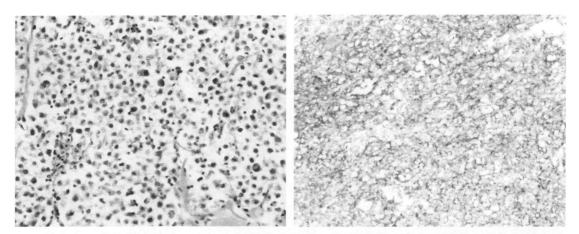

形态为一致的肿瘤细胞，瘤细胞圆形或多角形，胞质透明，核大而规则，明显的核仁呈棒状，核分裂象数目不等。纤维分隔伴有淋巴细胞浸润，也可形成淋巴滤泡。免疫组化显示 PLAP 阳性表达在肿瘤细胞胞质

Tumor cells are round or polygonal with uniform shape，clear cytoplasm，large and regular distinct nucleoli appear rods with some mitotic figures. There is with lymphocytic infiltration and lymphoid follicles formation in fibrous sepla. Immunohistochemical show that PLAP positive in cytoplasmic/membranous expression in tumor cells.

第十五章 神经系统疾病
Chapter 15 Diseases of the Nervous System

15-1 流行性脑脊髓膜炎 Epidemic cerebrospinal meningitis （急性化脓性脑膜炎 Acute suppurative meningitis）

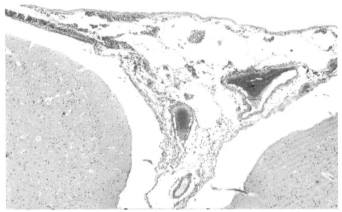

蛛网膜下腔增宽，血管扩张充血，大量中性粒细胞、浆液及纤维素渗出和少量淋巴细胞、单核细胞浸润。邻近的脑皮质可有轻度水肿。

Subarachnoid space widened, vascular dilatation and hyperemia, a large number of neutrophils, serious and fibrinous exudations, a small amount of lymphocytes and mononuclear cell infiltration. Adjacent cortex may show mild edema.

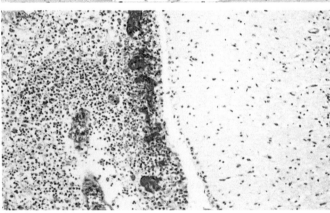

软脑膜急性化脓性炎症，可见大量中性粒细胞浸润和淤血（脓性渗出）。

Acute suppurative inflammation is seen in leptomeninges. Heavy infiltration of neutrophils and congestion （suppurative exudates） are seen.

15-2 脊髓灰质炎 Poliomyelitis

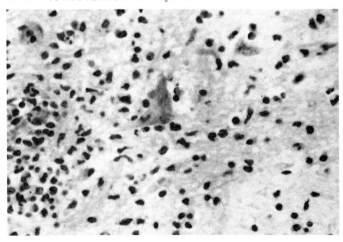

脊髓束切面显示前角细胞发生变性，并可见卫星现象和周围胶质细胞增生。

Spinal cord section shows anterior horn cells undergoing degeneration, statellitosis and surrounding glial cell proliferation.

15-3　脑脓肿 Intracerebral abscess

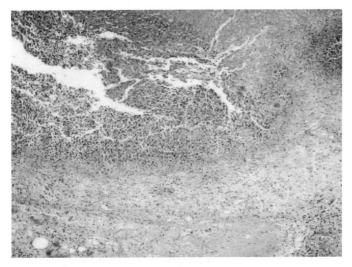

图左上角是炎细胞和脑组织坏死区，其外围有"脓肿膜"包绕，依次是肉芽组织和炎细胞浸润。

The upper left part of the field is an area of inflammatory cells and cellular debris of brain tissue necrosis. This area is surrounded by a developing "capsule", composed of granulation tissue and inflammatory cells.

15-4　流行性乙型脑炎 Epidemic encephalitis B （病毒性脑炎 Viral meningitis）

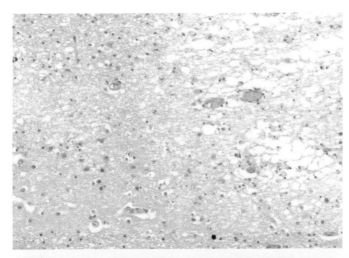

组织学上五种基本病变：①脑实质血管周围炎症反应，淋巴细胞套形成。②噬神经细胞现象。③神经细胞卫星现象。④筛状软化灶。⑤小胶质细胞结节。

Five basic histological lesions：① parenchymal perivascular inflammation, the formation of lymphocytic vascular cuff. ②neuronophagia. ③ satellitosis. ④ cribriform malacia. ⑤ microglial nodules.

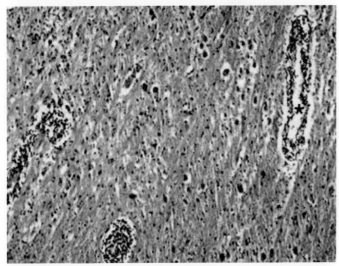

血管周围炎症反应（perivascular inflammatory reaction）

淋巴细胞围绕小血管浸润（＊表示血管腔）。

Clusters of lymphocytes typically surround cerebral blood vessels. A blood vessel lumen is identified by the asterisk（＊）.

15-5　海绵状脑病 Spongiform encephalapathy

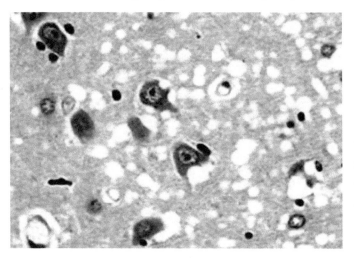

克罗伊茨费尔特 - 雅各布病（creutzfeldt-Jacob disease）

大脑灰质海绵状改变，神经毡内和神经元呈小泡样结构。

The development of spongiform change in affected areas of gray matter. The spongiform change is visible as small vacuoles within the neuropil, as well as within the cytoplasm of an occasional neuron.

15-6　脑梗死（急性）Brain infarction（acute）

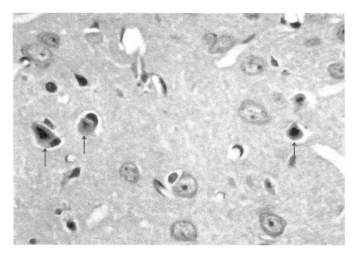

神经元急性坏死（acute necrosis of neuron）

脑梗死区域可见多个"红色神经元"（箭头所示），是神经系统急性坏死的特征性变化。

The cerebral infarcted area contains multiple"red neurons"（arrow），a classic feature of acute necrosis of the CNS.

15-7　阿尔茨海默病 Alzheimer Disease（AD）

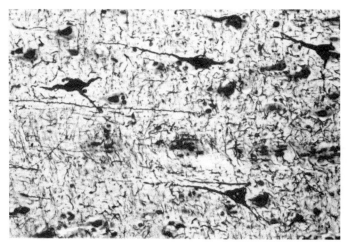

神经原纤维缠结（neurofibrillary tangle）

银染显示几乎所有神经元都呈现神经纤维不规则扭曲。

Almost every nerve cell shows irregular twisting of neurofibrils by silver stain.

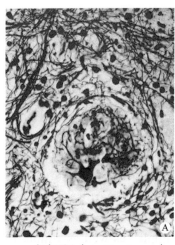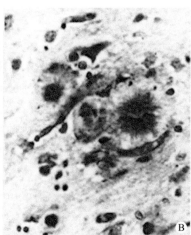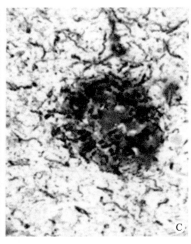

老年斑（senile plaque）

A：神经轴突不规则退变或异常增长（Bodian 染色）。B：大脑皮质中可见两个纤维化的圆形小体，这些放射状的纤维物质经 PAS 染色呈阳性。C：免疫组化双标记染色显示抗 β-淀粉样蛋白在老年斑内（呈红色），而营养不良性神经突起细丝蛋白（呈棕色）。

A：Axons are destroyed irregularly and also abnormally enlarged（Bodian stain）. B：Two round bodies of fibrosis can be found in the cerebral cortex. These radial fibrous substances are positive for PAS staining. C：Immunohistochemical double labeling staining showed that β-amyloid protein was present in the center of senile plaques（red）and dystrophy neurofilament protein（brown）.

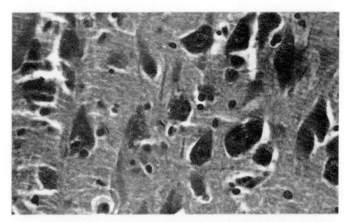

颗粒空泡变性（granulovacuolar degeneration）

顶叶皮层大锥体细胞的胞质中可见较多小颗粒和微小空泡。

Multiple small intracytoplasmic granules and microvacuoles are seen in the cytoplasm of large pyramidal cells of parietal cortex.

15-8 帕金森病 Parkinson's disease（PD）

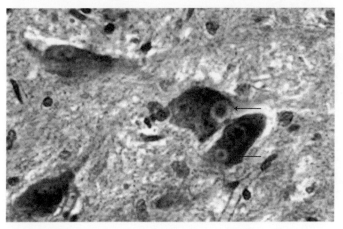

大脑黑质路易小体（lewy bodies in brain substantia nigra）

帕金森病的黑质神经元内路易小体（箭头所示）。

Parkinson disease，Lewy bodies（arrow）in the cytoplasm of pigmented neurons of the substantia nigra.

15-9 原发性脱髓鞘疾病 Primary demyelinating disease

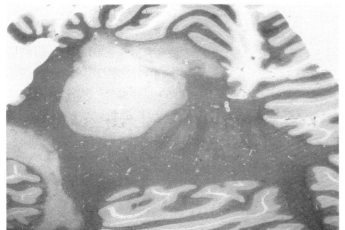

多发性硬化症 [multiple sclerosis（MS）]

脑白质中可见境界清楚的圆形脱髓鞘病变斑（PTAH 染色）。

A round well defined demyelinated plague is seen in cerebellar white matter（PTAH stain）.

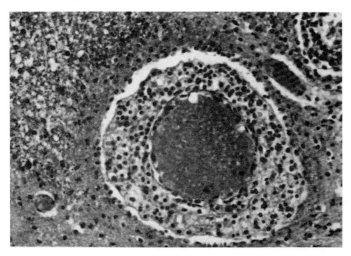

脑白质血管周围单核泡沫细胞聚集伴水肿和反应性胶质细胞增生。

Cerebellar white matter shows perivascular accumulation of mononuclear foam cells with surrounding edema and reactive gliosis.

15-10 毛细胞型星形细胞瘤 Pilocytic asteocytoma （WHO I）

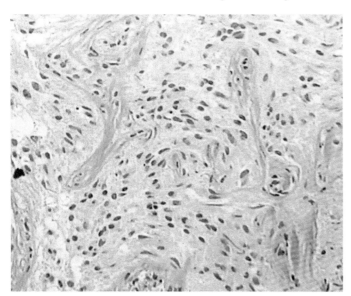

细胞密度低，组织呈致密区和疏松区。

①含 Rosenthal 纤维的梭形细胞构成的胶质纤维，如毛发样修长。可呈螺旋状扭曲，或波浪或旋涡状，相互交错，排列紧密的致密区。②疏松区多极细胞伴微囊和颗粒小体形成为特点。

① The cell density was low, and the tissue consisting of compact and loose with glial fiber and spindle cells of Rosenthal fibers as hairloid slender with spirally twisted, or wavy or swirling, and closely arranged. ② In the loose area, multipolar cells with microcapsules and small particles become characteristic.

15-11 弥漫型星形细胞瘤 Diffuse astrocytoma（WHO Ⅱ）

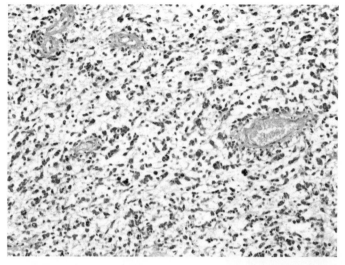

星型胶质瘤Ⅱ级常见的组织学亚型是纤维型星形细胞瘤，瘤细胞不密集，但分布不均。细胞胞浆不多，有轻度异型性，核分布在胶质纤维网上，核分裂很少见，有微囊。

Common histological subtypes of astrocytic tumor Ⅱ is fiber astrocytic tumor, cells are not intensive, but showing the uneven distribution. The cells are small cytoplasm, mild atypia, nuclear distribution of glial fibrillary network, mitotic figures are rare, with microcysts.

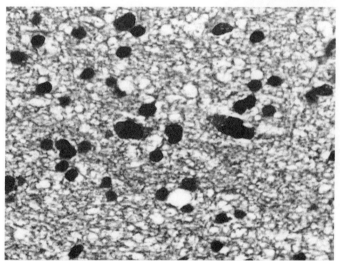

弥漫型胶质瘤（diffuse Glioma）

肿瘤细胞呈多型性，核深染。

Pleomorphism and nuclear hyperchromasia of tumor cells are seen.

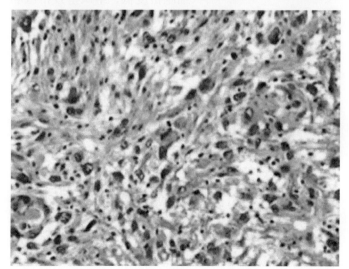

多形性黄色瘤型星形细胞 [pleomorphic xanthoastrocytoma（PXA）]

肿瘤由纤维性、巨大、多核含脂质的肿瘤性星形细胞构成。

The tumor is composed of fibrous, huge, multinucleated containing lipid tumor astrocytes.

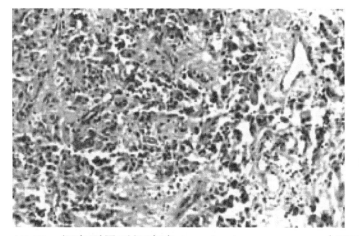

室管膜下巨细胞型星形细胞瘤
（subependymal giant cell astrocytoma）

瘤细胞围绕在小血管周围。

The tumor cells surround the small vessel.

15-12　间变型星形细胞瘤 Anaplastic astrocytoma（WHO Ⅲ）

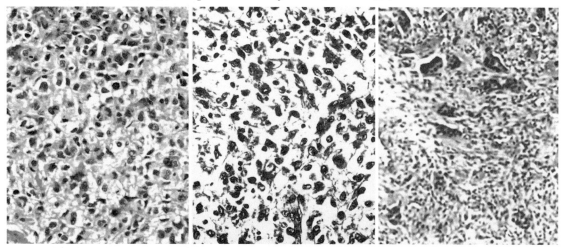

瘤细胞密集，核异型性和多形性，见有多数单核和多核瘤巨细胞。属于 WHO 分类Ⅲ级。若出现肿瘤性坏死灶，说明已经转变成恶性胶质母细胞瘤。

Tumor cells are condensed, pleomorphic, atypia, showing most mononuclear or polynuclear tumor giant cells belong to WHO Ⅲ grade. If there is tumor necrosis, that explains the tumor has been malignant glioblastoma.

15-13　多形性胶质母细胞瘤 Pleomorphic glioblastoma（WHO Ⅳ）

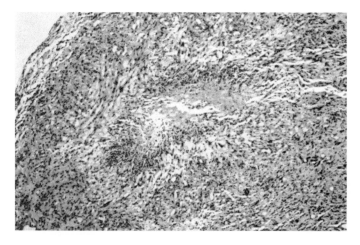

中央可见栅栏状核围绕的坏死（是该肿瘤的重要特征）。

Tumor nuclei pseudopalisading arrangement around the necrosis is seen in the center of figure（It is an important diagnostic feature for this tumor）.

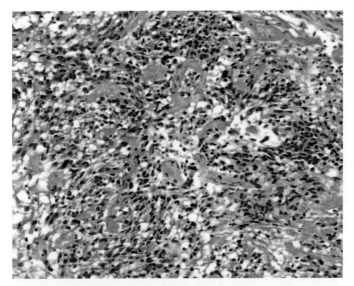

瘤细胞密集，异型性明显，可见怪异的单核或多核瘤巨细胞。出血坏死明显，肿瘤细胞可围绕坏死灶周围呈假栅栏状排列，瘤组织内小血管增生，血管内皮增生。

Tumor cells are condensed, obvious atypia, showing weird mononuclear or polynuclear tumor giant cells. Hemorrhagic necrosis is obvious, Tumor cells with pseudopalisading arrangement surround the necrotic foci, with the proliferation of small blood vessels and endothelia.

胶质母细胞瘤（glioblastoma）

肿瘤细胞密度高、分化差，常呈多形性，明显的核异型和活跃的分裂活性。明显的微血管增生和/或坏死。

Tumor cells have high density and poor differentiation, with pleomorphic, distinct nuclear atypia and mitotic activity. Marked microvascular hyperplasia and/or necrosis.

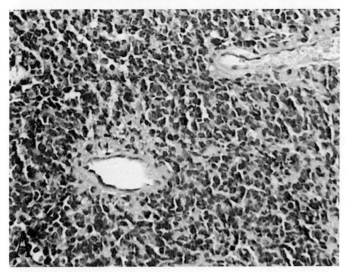

15-14 大脑胶质瘤病 Gliomatosis，cerebri（WHO Ⅲ）

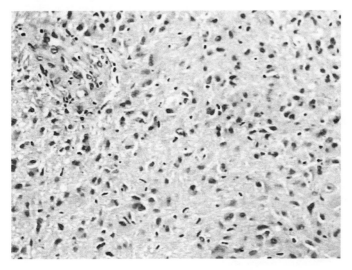

瘤细胞核卵圆形或梭形，染色质深。

The nucleus of tumor is ovoid or spindle with amount chromatin.

15-15 少突胶质细胞瘤 Oligodendroglioma

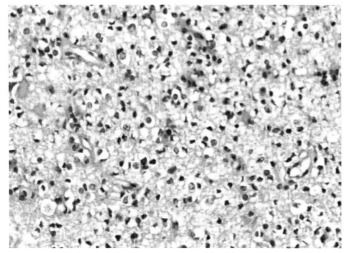

肿瘤弥漫性生长，细胞密度中等，大小一致，核圆形位于中央，核周有空晕，胞质透亮，构成蜂窝状瘤细胞群。

The tumor has diffuse growth, medium cell density and uniform size. The uncleus is located in the center, and perinuclear halo. The cytoplasm is clear, forming a honeycombed tumor cellular group.

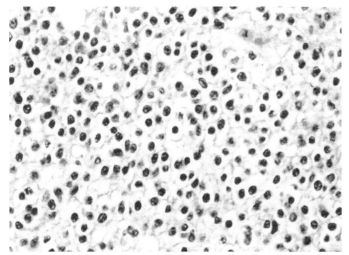

肿瘤细胞形态单一。瘤细胞核圆,位于中央,见特征性的核周空晕,呈煎鸡蛋样外观。

Monotonous round nuclei tumor cells are located in the center. The characteristic perinuclear halo, having fried-egg appearance.

15-16 间变型少突胶质细胞瘤 Anaplastic oligodendroglioma

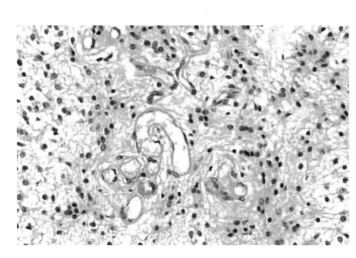

肿瘤弥漫性生长。瘤细胞分化差，异型明显，核分裂活跃。

血管呈丛状结构，多数血管呈枝芽状穿插在瘤细胞群之间，可形成典型的致密鸡爪样分支毛细血管网，与肿瘤钙化及砂砾体的形成有关。

Tumor shows diffuse growth. Poorly differentiated tumor cells, obvious atypia with a lot of mitotic figures. Plexiform vascular structures are interspersed between the tumor cells, which can form a typical chicken claw dense capillary networks, may be associated with calcification and psammoma bodies formation.

15-17 混合型胶质瘤 Mixed glioma

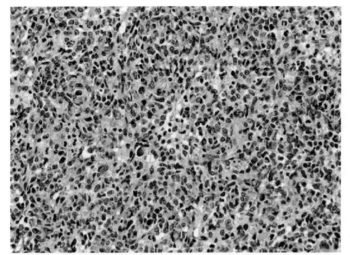

混合型胶质瘤以少突胶质细胞为主，混有小胶质细胞。

Mixed cells gliomas are mainly oligodendrocytes，mixed with microglia.

15-18 室管膜瘤 Ependymoma

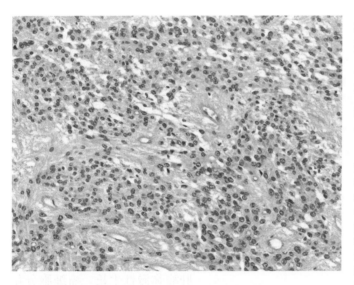

瘤细胞围绕空腔呈腺管状排列形成室管膜菊形团，或围绕血管排列形成假菊形团，并以细胞突起与血管壁相连，有时可形成乳头状结构。当瘤组织中瘤细胞密集，核分裂活跃，并有假栅栏状坏死时，可诊断为间变型室管膜瘤。

Tumor cells arrange around the cavity forming glandular ependymal rosettes, or around the blood vessels forming a false rosettes，and cell processes connected with the vessel wall, and sometimes papillary structures can be formed. When the tumor cells condense，mitotic activity increases，and there is a pseudopalisading around necrosis，which can be diagnosed as anaplastic ependymoma.

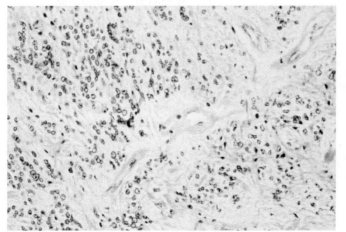

在小血管周围肿瘤细胞呈放射状排列，在血管周围有瘤细胞细纤维突起，这些肿瘤细胞的血管周围排列称为假菊形团。

Around small vessels there are tumor cells arranged in radiating fashion. Fine fibrillary processes are seen in perivascular region. These perivascul arrangements of tumor cells are called pseudorosettes.

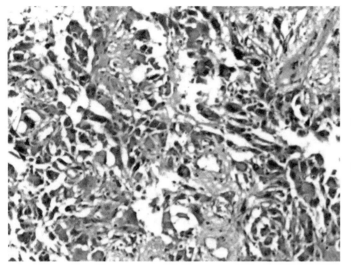

上皮型室管膜瘤形成以血管为中心的菊形团。

The epithelioid ependymoma forms a rosettes mass centered on blood vessel.

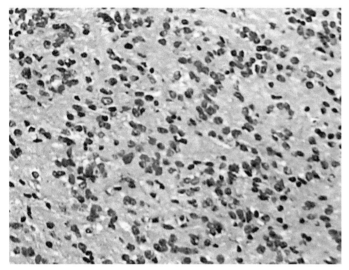

细胞型室管膜瘤（cell type ependymoma）

瘤细胞丰富、细胞界限不清、细胞核均匀成片分布，无间变特征。

The tumor cells are rich, cell boundaries unclear. The nuclei are homogeneous, sheet distribution and without atypical characteristic.

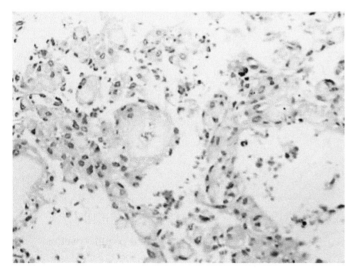

黏液乳头型室管膜瘤（myxopapillary ependymoma）

肿瘤呈乳头状结构，瘤细胞放射状排列在乳头轴心血管周围。黏液聚积在血管和瘤细胞之间和囊腔内。核分裂象少或缺如。

The tumor presents papillary structure. The neoplastic cells are radially arranged around the vascular in the papillary axis. Mucus accumulates bet- ween the blood vessels and the tumor cells and in the cystic cavity. Nuclear mitosis is less or absent.

15-19   间变型室管膜瘤 Anaplastic ependymorna

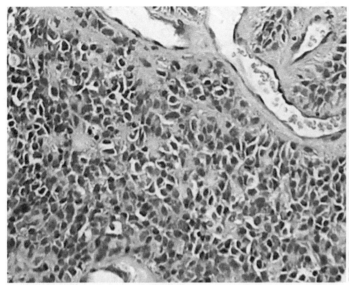

　　瘤细胞丰富、核异形显著、核分裂活性高。常伴微血管增生和假栅栏状坏死和出血。

Tumor cells are rich, obvious nuclear atypia and high mitotic activity. Microvascular hyperplasia and false palisade necrosis and bleeding are common.

　　不典型的血管呈菊形团样。

Atypical blood vessel shaped rosettes.

15-20   室管膜下瘤 Suhependymoma

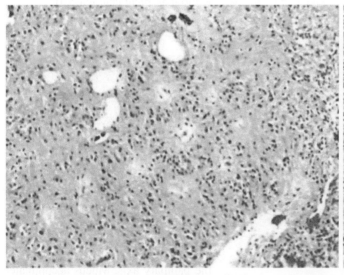

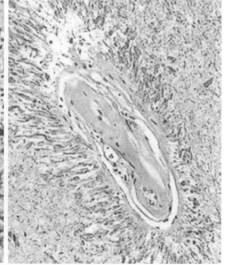

　　簇状细胞核埋入胶质细胞纤维基质中，见小囊腔形成。

The cluster nuclei are embedded in the glial fiber matrix and small cyst is formed.

　　室管膜上假菊形团。

Ependymal pseudorosetles.

15-21　脉络丛乳头状瘤 Choroid plexus papilloma

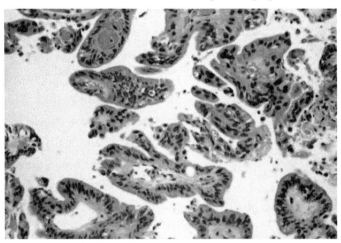

许多分支状乳头，由假复层立方或柱状上皮被覆，中央为纤细的毛细血管轴心，免疫组化：GFAP、S-100 蛋白、CK 和 EMA 标记阳性。

Many branched papillaes are covered by a pseudostratified cubic or columnar epithelium with a central capillary axis. Immunohistochemistry：GFAP、S-100、CK and EMA markers are positive.

15-22　脉络丛癌 Choroid plexus carcinoma

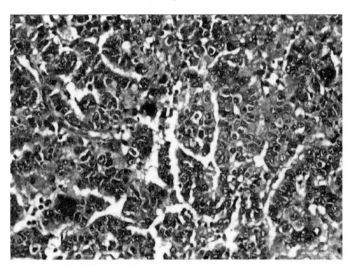

肿瘤呈实体状、片状和筛状，而乳头状结构不明显。瘤细胞多形性，可见多核或瘤巨细胞。核浓染，核分裂象易见伴坏死灶。

The tumors were solid, sheet and cribniform, whereas the papillary structures were not obvious. Tumor cells are pleomorphic with multinucleated or neoplastic giant cells. Nuclear dense, nuclear mitosis and necrotic foci are easily seen.

15-23　起源未定的神经上皮肿瘤 Neuroepithelial tumours of uncertain origin

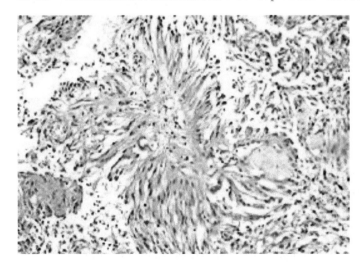

星形母细胞瘤（astroblastma）

星形细胞宽突起放射性围绕在血管周围为特征，血管壁玻璃样变。

Astrocytes are broad, projecting, characterized by radioactivity around the vessel, hyaline degeneration of vessel walls.

15-24 髓母细胞瘤 Medulloblastoma

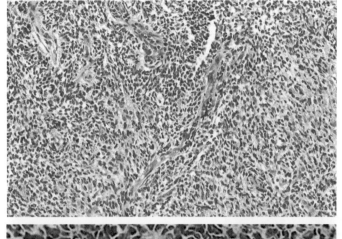

细胞密度高，肿瘤细胞核大深染，染色质多，核分裂多，瘤细胞核圆到卵圆形或雪茄烟样，胞质少。

The cells density is high with large and dense nuclear containing hyperchromatic, mitotically active nuclei, the nuclei are round to oval or cigar like, and very little cytoplasm.

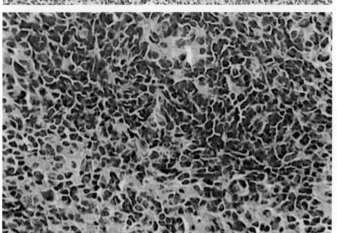

部分瘤细胞环绕神经纤维呈放射状排列形成典型的菊形团结构(称 Homer Wrigh)，具有一定的诊断意义。纤细的纤维间质，血管不多。

Part of the tumor cells surrounding nerve fibers radially form typical rosettes structure (called Homer Wrigh), has a certain significance for diagnosis. Stroma with delicate fiber, not much blood vessles.

15-25 节细胞神经瘤 Ganglioneuroma

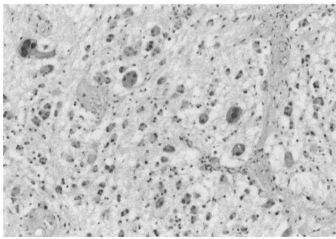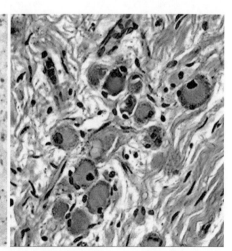

由不规则簇状、大多极神经元和突起构成。瘤细胞分布不规则，单核、双核或多核，可见有核仁和胞质内尼氏小体，瘤组织内混杂有髓鞘和无髓鞘的神经纤维。

Tumor is composed of irregular clusters, most extreme neurons and projections. Tumor cells show irregular distribution, monocytes, dual-nucleo or multi-nucleo, with nucleolus and cytoplasm Nissl bodies, mixed with myelin and myelin-free nerve fibers in the tumor tissue.

15-26 婴儿促纤维增生型星形细胞瘤 / 节细胞胶质瘤 Desmoplastic infantile astrocytoma and gangliogliom

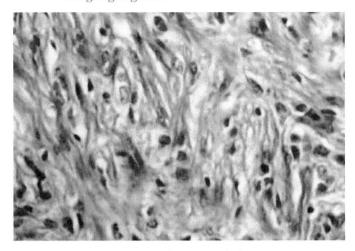

明显的间质纤维增生伴神经上皮成分。

An apparent mesenchymal fibric tissue hyperplasia with neuroepithelial components.

15-27 胚胎发育不良型神经上皮肿瘤 Dysembryoplastic neuroepithelial tumour

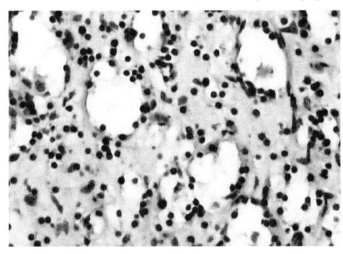

特异性胶质神经元结构，明显的多形性，可见微血管网，血管球形成和黏液变性，神经上皮细胞漂浮在黏液池内。

Specific glioneuronal structures, obvious pleomorphic, visible microvascular networks, glomus formation and mucoid degeneration, neuroepithelial cells floating in the mucus pools.

15-28 中枢神经细胞瘤 Central neurocytoma

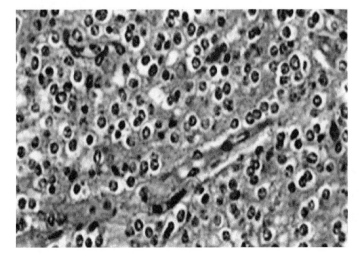

肿瘤由形态一致伴神经元分化的圆形细胞构成，瘤细胞排列成流水状或室管膜瘤样的血管周围假菊形团，可见钙化。

The tumor is composed of uniform round cells with neuronal differentiation, and the tumor cells arrange in the form of flowing water or ependymoma like perivascular pseudorosettes, and calcification is seen.

15-29　小脑发育不良型节细胞瘤 Dysplastic gangliocytoma，cerebellum

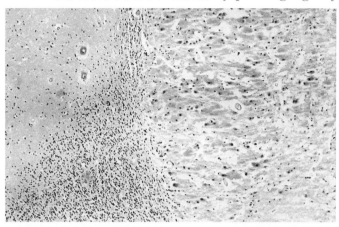

病灶内小脑颗粒层和 Purkinje 细胞层结构改建，代之以外层异常的有髓纤维束和内层大量结构不良和形态异常的神经元。

The structure of the cerebellar granule layer and the Purkinje cell layer in the lesion is reconstructed and replaced by the outer myelinated fibrous bundle and the large number of poorly neurons with structures disorder and morphologically abnormal in inner layer.

15-30　室管膜母细胞瘤 Ependymoblastoma

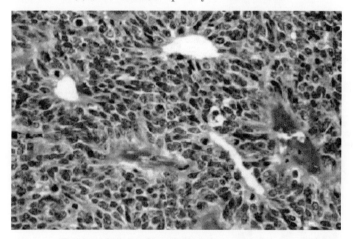

为中枢 PNET 伴多层菊形团，菊形团周围是未分化的神经外胚层细胞。

It is the central nervous system PNET. The tumor forms multilayer rosseles，which surrounding undiffe-rentiated neuroectodermal cells.

15-31　幕上原始神经外胚层肿瘤 Primitive neuroectodermal tumour（PNET），supratentorial

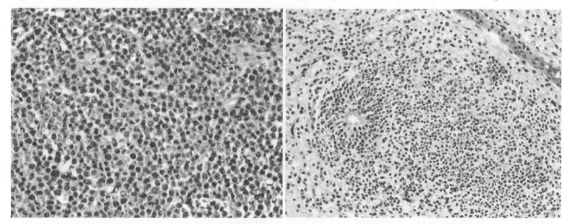

相似小脑髓母细胞瘤，小圆形瘤细胞，核深染，染色丰富，胞浆少或无，可以见到 Homer-Wright 菊形团，出血和坏死灶。

Similar to cerebellar edulloblastoma，small round tumor cells with dark nuclei，rich chromatin，and little or no cytoplasm. Homer-Wright rosseles can be seen with bleeding and necrotic foci.

15-32　脑膜瘤 Meningioma

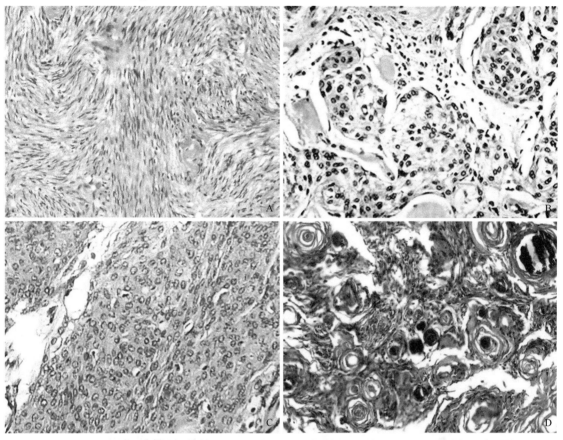

A：纤维型，瘤细胞为长梭形，呈致密交织束状结构，其间可见网状纤维或胶原纤维。B：脑膜细胞型。C：合体细胞型。D：砂粒体型，肿瘤细胞呈大小不等同心圆状或漩涡状排列，其中央的血管壁常有透明变性，以至于钙化形成砂粒体。

A：Fibroblastic-type. Tumor cells are large spindle, showing a dense interwoven bundles structures, in which reticular fibers or collagen fibers are visible. B：Meningotheliomatous. C：Syncytial. D：psammomatius tumor cells show varying sizes arrangement in a concentric or spiral manner, the central vessel walls often show hyaline degeneration, even forming calcified psammoma bodies.

15-33　神经鞘瘤 Neurilemmoma

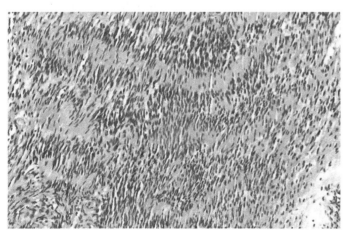

肿瘤细胞梭形境界不清，相互紧密平行排列呈栅栏状或不完全的漩涡状。肿瘤有两种组织形态：一般颅内的神经鞘瘤较多出现 antoni B 型结构，椎管内的神经鞘瘤多以 antoni A 型结构为主，且更易见小囊腔形成。

Spindle tumor cells are closely arranged in parallel palisade or incomplete swirling. There are two kinds of morphology, generally, intracranial schwannomas show more antoni B-type structure, intraspinal schwannoma are mostly antoni A structure, and easier to see the formation of small cysts.

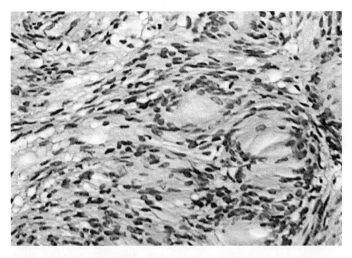

①束状型（antoni A 型），细胞梭形境界不清，相互紧密平行排列呈栅栏状或不完全的漩涡状，后者称 verocay 小体。

① Bundle type（antoni A type），spindle-shaped cells, closely arranged in parallel palisade or incomplete swirling, the latter called verocay bodies.

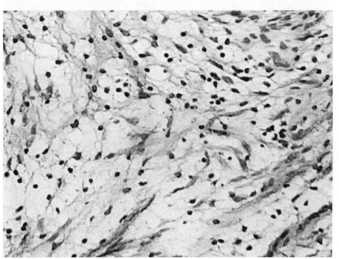

②网状型（antoni B 型），细胞稀少，排列呈稀疏的网状结构，细胞间常有小囊腔形成。

② Network or mesh type（antoni B type），rare cells, arranged in a sparse network structures, intercellular often forming small cysts.

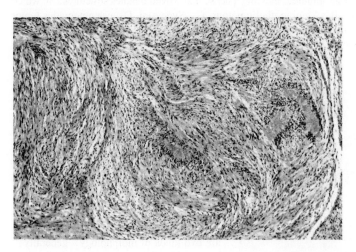

可见施万细胞结节样增生。核呈特征性的栅栏样排列。

Nodular proliferations of schwann cells are seen. Nuclear palisading arrangement is its characteristic.

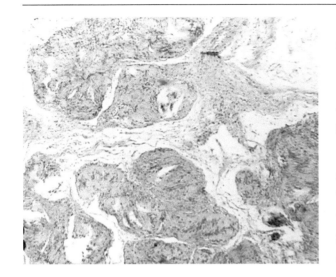

丛状神经鞘瘤（plexiform schwannoma）

肿瘤丛状或多结节状生长，好发于四肢、头颈部皮肤或皮下组织神经丛，与神经纤维瘤病2型有关。颅神经和脊神经很少累及。

Tumor is plexiform or multinodositas growth，occurs in the skin or the subcutaneous tissue nerve plexus of the head and neck and the extremities，related to in the 2 types of neurofibromatosis. It is rarely involved in the cranial nerves and spinal nerves.

黑色素性神经鞘瘤（melanotic schwannoma）

肿瘤境界清楚，含黑色素呈黑色。发病高峰比普通型神经鞘瘤早10岁，有10%以上的病例转化为恶性。该肿瘤分为非砂砾体型和砂砾体，前者易累及脊髓，后者累及肠道、心脏和颅神经，其中50%有carney综合征，以面部雀斑、心脏黏液瘤和内分泌过度为特点。

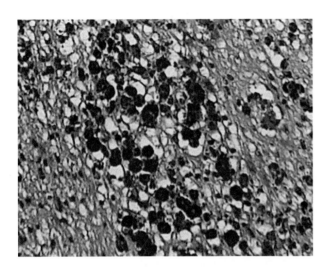

Tumor is well demarcated and black colour with containing melanin. The peak of morbidity is 10 years earlier than the common type schwannoma. More than 10% of the cases turned to malignant. The tumor is divided into non-psammoma body type and psammoma body type，the former is prone to involve the spinal cord，the latter is involved in the intestinal，heart and cranial nerves，50% of these have carney syndrome，which is characterized by face freckle，heart myxoma and excessive endocrines.

15-34 上皮样恶性外周神经鞘瘤 Epithelioid malignant peripheral nerve sheath tumor（MPNST）

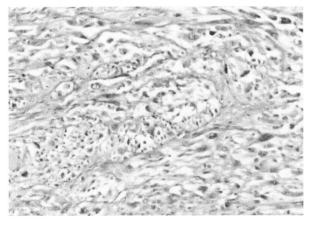

为高度恶性肿瘤。肿瘤形态颇似纤维肉瘤，有较多核分裂象并伴有血管增生和细胞坏死。瘤细胞多型、肥硕、胞浆嗜酸性。

It is a highly malignant tumor. Tumor morphology is resembles fibrosarcoma. There are more mitotic figures accompanied by vascular proliferation and cells necrosis. Tumor cells are pleomorphic and plump with eosinophilic cytoplasm.

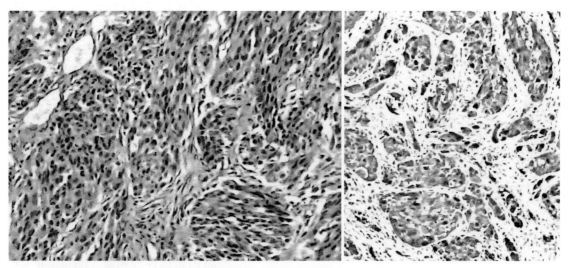

肿瘤细胞呈梭形，形态颇似纤维肉瘤。瘤细胞表达 S-100 蛋白。

The tumor cells are spindle shaped，and they are similar to fibrosarcoma. The tumor cells expressed S-100 protein.

15-35　神经纤维瘤 Neurofibroma

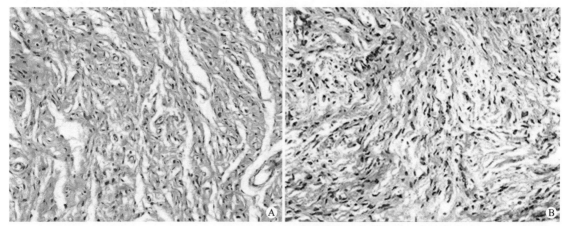

A：肿瘤组织由增生的 Schwann 细胞、神经束膜样细胞和成纤维细胞构成。这些肿瘤细胞交织排列，成小束。瘤细胞细长，棒状核或波浪状核，伴大量网状纤维和胶原纤维及疏松的黏液样基质。若细胞密度增大，核异型并见核分裂像增加，提示恶变。

B：可见束状波浪形拉长的细胞，其核呈鳗鱼样，胶原纤维间隔形成。

A：Tumor tissue are composed of hyperplastic schwann cells，perineurium-like cells and fibroblasts. Tumor cells arranged interwoven into small bundles. Tumor cells are slender，rod-like or wavy-like nuclei，accompanied by a large number of reticular fibers and collagen fibers and loose myxoid stroma. If the cells increase density，nuclear atypia and mitotic figures，suggesting malignancy possibility.

B：There are bundles，wavy elongated cells，the nuclear is eel-like and collagen fibers spacing.

15-36 脑转移性肿瘤 Brain metastatic tumors

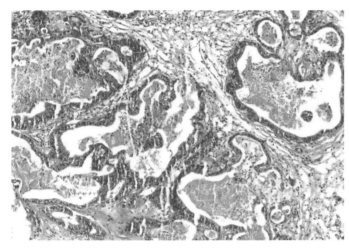

脑转移性腺癌（brain metastatic adnorcarcinoma）

转移腺癌细胞成灶状分布，癌组织和脑组织分界清楚，常伴有淋巴细胞和单核细胞浸润。瘤内和瘤周微血管增生，常见有肿瘤性坏死。

Metastatic adnorcancimoma cells are focal distribution, and tumor nests show clear boundaries with brain tissue, often accompanied by lymphocytes and monocytes infiltration. Intratumoral and peritumoral microvascular proliferation common present tumor necrosis.

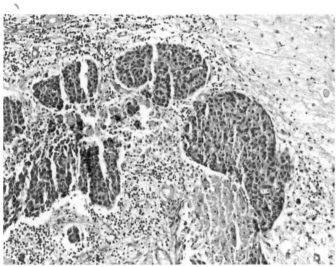

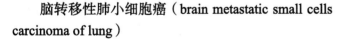

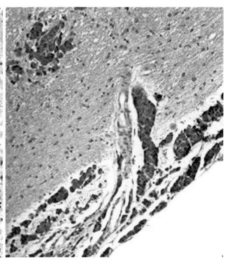

脑转移性肺小细胞癌（brain metastatic small cells carcinoma of lung）

脑和软脑膜见到肿瘤，肺癌发生脑转移很常见，尤其是小细胞癌和腺癌。

Tumor was found in the brain and leptomeninges. Lung cancers occur brain metastases are common especially SCLC and adenocarcinoma.

第十六章 骨 疾 病
Chapter 16　Bone Diseases

16-1　骨瘤 Osteoma

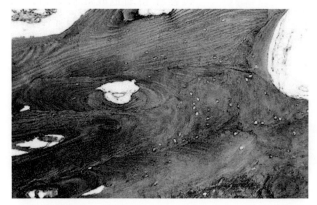

肿瘤由分化良好的骨组织构成。

The tumor is composed of well differentiated bone tissue.

16-2　骨母细胞瘤 Osteoblastoma

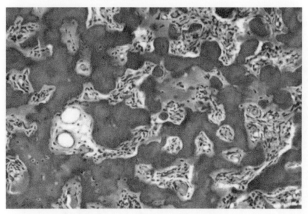

肿瘤由随意、混沌地排列的针状编织状骨或小梁构成，衬覆单层骨母细胞。散布的破骨细胞型多核巨细胞。肿瘤中血管丰富，常见血管外红细胞。

The tumor was composed of random, chaotic array of acicular a braided or trabecular bone spicule, lined with monolayer osteoblast. The osteoclast type multinucleated giant cells were diffused. It often contains rich blood vessels and extravascular red blood cells.

16-3　骨样骨瘤 Osteoid osteoma

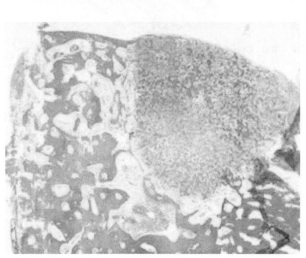

肿瘤的基本的特征：中央区域是富于血管的结缔组织，在骨和骨样组织周边衬覆了分化成熟、增生活跃的骨母细胞。骨母细胞产生骨样基质，有时产生骨。骨样骨瘤一般没有软骨。几乎总有一血管增生的硬化骨区域包围着肿瘤。与其周围的反应性硬化骨之间的界限清楚。

The basic feature of the tumor is that the central region is rich vascular connective tissue, bone and osteoid tissues are surrounded by differentiated mature and actively proliferating osteoblast. The osteoblast produces a osteoid matrix and sometimes produces bone. Osteoid osteoma usually has no cartilage. There is almost a proliferation of sclerotic bone areas surrounding the tumor. The boundary is clear between the reactive sclerotic bone and its surroundings.

16-4 骨肉瘤 Osteosarcoma

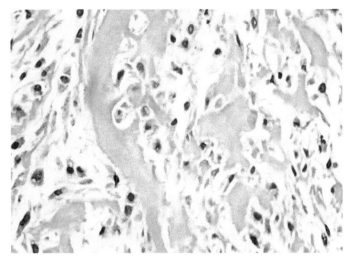

成骨型骨肉瘤（osteoblastic osteosarcoma）

肿瘤主要由少量梭形细胞和大量的骨样基质构成。骨样基质为非钙化的骨基质，嗜伊红，致密，均质。

The tumor is composed of a few spindle cells and a large amount of osteoid matrix that is a non-calcified with eosinophilic staining, dense and homogeneous.

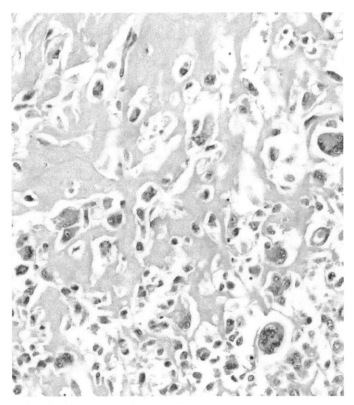

瘤细胞异型性明显，核深染，呈炭块状偏于一端。易见核分裂，细胞胞浆较宽，嗜酸性，细胞周围可见花边状骨样基质即肿瘤成骨。此为诊断成骨肉瘤的重要依据。肿瘤向三个方向分化（骨样分化、软骨样分化和纤维样分化）的表现是成骨肉瘤的特征。

Tumor cells show obvious atypia, nucleus stained darkly, lump charcoal shaped, biased side. Mitotic figures are easy to see, cytoplasm wide, eosinophils, visible osteoid matrix lacy surrounding tumor cells, namely neoplastic osteogenesis. It is the important evidence for the diagnosis of osteosarcoma. Tumor shows three type differentiations (bone-like differentiation, cartilage-like differentiation and fibroma-like differentiation), it is the feature of osteosarcoma.

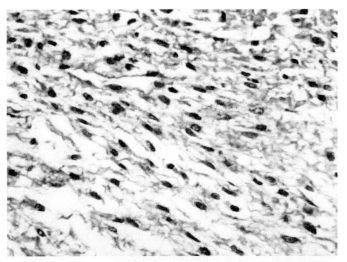

成纤维型骨肉瘤（fibroblastic osteosarcoma）

肿瘤主要由梭形细胞组成，胞浆淡染，核大小不一，核浆比增高，似纤维肉瘤或恶性纤维组织细胞瘤。

The tumor is mostly composed of spindle cells with pale stained cytoplasm, nuclei in various size and increased nuclei-cytoplasm ratio, like fibrosarcoma or malignant fibrous histiocytoma.

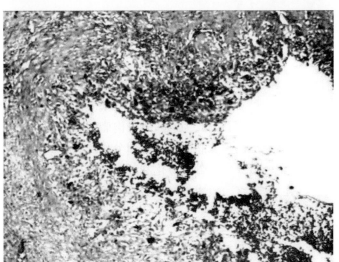

毛细血管扩张型骨肉瘤（telangiectatic osteosarcoma）

低倍镜下可见充满血的囊腔。

Low-power microscopy reveals cystic spaces filled with blood.

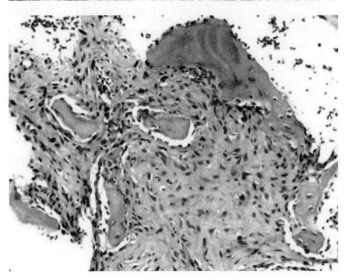

低级别中心性骨肉瘤（low grade central osteosarcoma）

发生于骨髓腔内的低级别骨肉瘤，由轻度不典型性的梭形细胞和骨样基质组成。

The tumor is a low grade malignant, bone forming neoplasm arising in medullary cavity of bone, consist of spindle cells with mild atypia and osteoid productions.

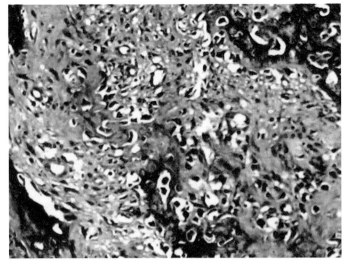

高倍镜下囊壁没有衬覆内皮，可见高度间变的肿瘤性大细胞及骨样组织。

High-power microscopy shows the cystic spaces has no endothelial lining，the highly anaplastic large cells and osteoid tissues are seen.

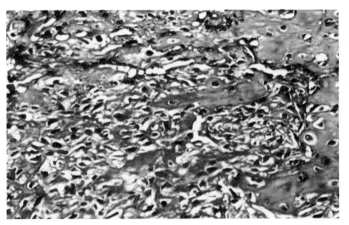

骨旁骨肉瘤（parosteal osteosarcoma）

发生于骨表面的低级别骨肉瘤，由形态良好的骨小梁和梭形细胞组成伴有软骨分化。

The tumor is a low grade malignant bone forming neoplasm arising on the surface of bone，consist of well formed bony trabecula and spindle cells with cartilaginous differentiation.

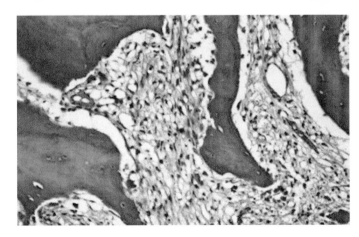

骨旁骨肉瘤（parosteal osteosarcoma）

不规则骨小梁间可见中度不典型的梭形肿瘤细胞浸润。

The infiltration of the moderate atypical spindle cell is seen between the irregular trabecular bones.

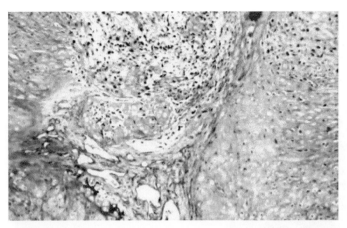

骨膜骨肉瘤（periosteal osteosarcoma）

发生于骨表面的中等分化的成软骨型骨肉瘤，由分叶状的恶性软骨和少量成骨组成。

The tumor is an intermediate grade malignant, cartilage and bone forming neoplasm arising on the surface of bone, consisted of malignant cartilage in lobular structure and a little osteoblast.

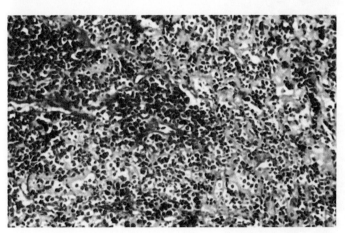

小细胞骨肉瘤（small cell osteosarcoma）

肿瘤由小细胞及其产生的骨样基质组成。

The tumor is consist of small cells with variable degree of osteoid matrix.

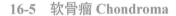

16-5 软骨瘤 Chondroma

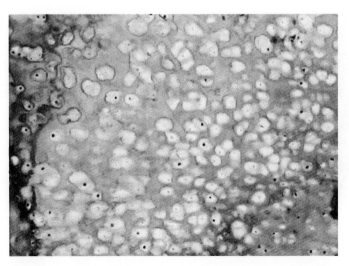

分化成熟的软骨组织，可见明显的软骨陷窝。

The differentiation mature cartilage cells with cartilage lacuna.

16-6 软骨肉瘤 Chondrosarcoma（CHS）

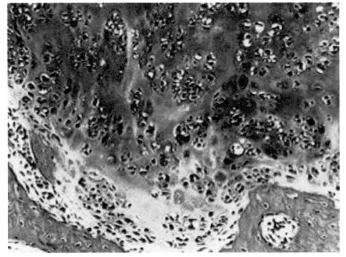

高分化软骨肉瘤（highly differentiated chondrosarcoma）

软骨肉瘤产生丰富的蓝 - 灰色软骨基质，有大小不等、形状不规则的软骨小叶，小叶可被纤维性条索或渗透于其中的骨小梁分隔。

The chondrosarcoma produces a rich blue gray cartilage matrix with unequal and irregularly shaped cartilage lobules，which can be separated by fibrous cords or trabecular bone infiltrated into them.

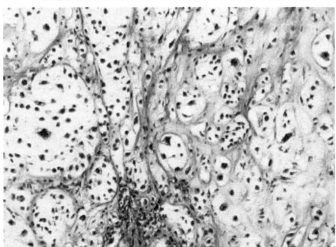

高分化软骨肉瘤中瘤细胞核异型明显。

The cartilage nuclear atypia of highly differentiated chondrosarcoma is obvious.

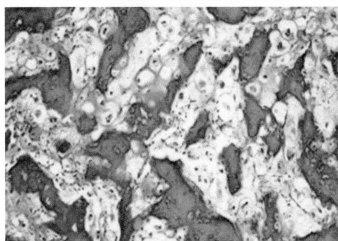

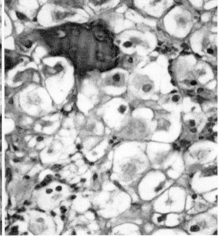

透明细胞软骨肉瘤（clear cell chondrosarcoma）

肿瘤细胞胞浆透亮富有液泡样结构。Tumor cells cytoplasm is clear with rich vacuole structures.

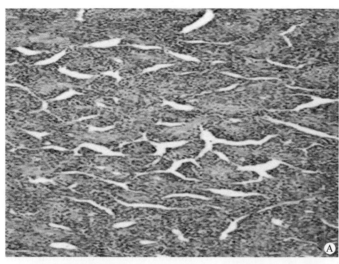

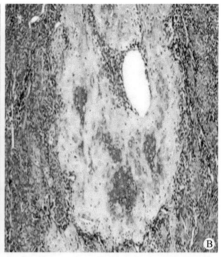

间叶性软骨肉瘤（mesenchymal chondrosarcoma）

A：显示血管外皮瘤样区域。B：间叶性软骨肉瘤中央为分化好的软骨岛。

A：It demonstrates a hemangiopericytomaloid region. B：The central is a well differentiated cartilage island.

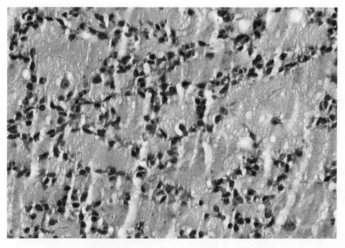

骨外黏液软骨肉瘤（extraskeletal myxoid chondrosarcoma）

瘤组织呈多结节状，瘤细胞形态一致，呈软骨母细胞的特征。瘤细胞排列成索状、线状或巢状，可看到分化好的软骨细胞。细胞外的基质呈浅嗜酸性或呈黏液样。

Tumor tissue shows multiple nodules, consistent tumor cell morphology, showing chondroblastoma features. Tumor cells are arranged in cords, linear or nest, well differentiated chondrocytes may present. The extracellular matrix is weak eosinophilic or myxoid.

软骨肉瘤的分级。

1级：细胞密度中等，核大小一致，肥硕，染色质较深。双核细胞少见。细胞学非常类似内生性软骨瘤。

2级：细胞量、核异型性核体积都更明显增加，染色质浓集。

3级：细胞密度及核的多形性、异型性都超过2级，核分裂易见。

The grade of chondrosarcoma.

1：The density of the cell is medium, the size of nuclear is the same, stout, duck stain. Binuclear cells are rare. The cytology is very similar to that of an endogenous chondroma.

2：Amount of cells, nuclear atypia, nuclear volume were more significantly increased chromatin condensation.

3：Cell density, nuclear polymorphism and atypia are more than grade 2, nuclear mitosis is easy to see.

16-7 骨巨细胞瘤 Giant cell tumor，bone

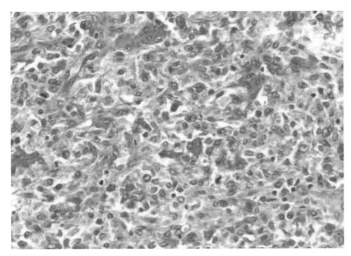

低度恶性潜能肿瘤，由单核基质细胞（主要肿瘤细胞）及多核巨细胞组成。多核巨细胞由单核基质细胞融合而成，常见核分裂，可有成骨现象（见骨和骨样基质沉积）。肿瘤可分为三级，随级别增高，基质细胞增多，异型明显，而多核巨细胞则减少。

Low potential malignancy tumor, composed of stromal monocytes (the primary tumor cells) and multinucleated giant cells. Most of multinucleated giant cells are fromed by mononuclear stromal cells fusion, so mitotic figures are common, Osteogenesis phenomenon can be observed (bone and bone-like matrix deposition). Tumors can be divided into three grades, with grades increase, stromal cells increasing with obvious atypia, and polynuclear giant cells decrease.

16-8 Ewing 肉瘤 Ewing sarcoma

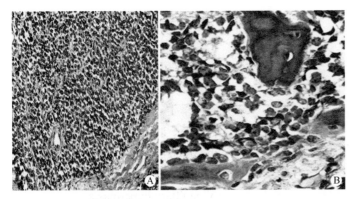

A：小圆形肿瘤细胞弥漫生长，B：肿瘤细胞核染色质细腻，胞浆稀少。浸润骨组织。

A：Small round tumor cells diffusely grow，B：The tumor cell nuclei are fine chromatin with sparse cytoplasm. Invasive bone tissue.

第十七章 皮肤和附件的疾病

Chapter 17　Diseases of the Skin and its Appendages

17-1　角化棘皮瘤 keratoacanthoma

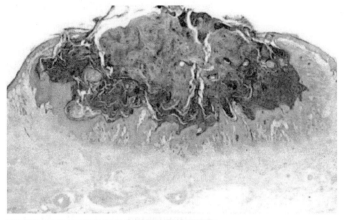

低倍镜下病变呈火山口样外观，内含大量角化物质，两侧为唇样边缘，是由鳞状上皮像真皮深层推进所形成。表面无坏死及真性溃疡形成。

A low power view of the tumor demonstrates a central crateriform lesion filled with a keratotic plug and two flanks of lip like edges consisting of squamous cells pushing into the deep dermis. There is no necrosis and true ulceration on the surface.

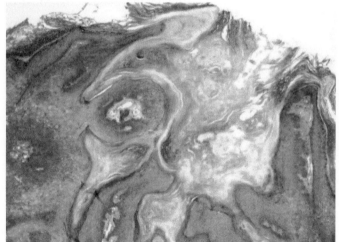

17-2　脂溢性角化病 Seborrhoeic keratosis

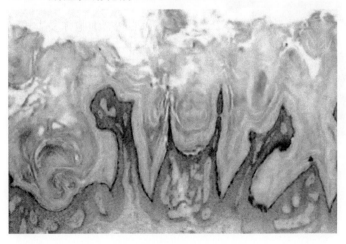

病变边界清楚，3种基本变化：①角化过度。②棘层肥厚。③乳头瘤样增生。

The lesion is well demarcated, and three basic changes：
① hyperkeratosis. ② acanthosis.
③ papillary hyperplasia.

17-3　日光性角化病 Actinic keratosis

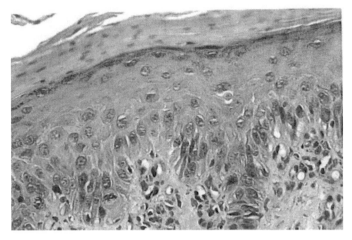

①表皮病变与周围正常表皮部分界限清楚，一般不累及末端毛囊及汗腺导管。②基底层及棘细胞层增生，出现细胞多形、核大不规则、浓染、排列紊乱等变化。③表皮乳头状瘤样增生或扁平增生角化过度、角化不良。④真皮上部常有嗜碱性变性，并有以淋巴细胞为主的炎细胞浸润。

① The epidermal lesions are clearly defined with the surrounding epidermis, and the ends of the hair follicles and sweat ducts are not affected. ② Hyperplasia of basal lamina and prickle cell layer, and cell polymorphism, nuclear irregular, dark dyeing, disorder of arrangement and so on. ③ Superficial papillary hyperplasia or flat hyperplasia, hyperkeratosis, dyskeratosis. ④ The upper part of the dermis often has basophilic degeneration, and there are inflammatory cells infiltrated mainly by lymphocytes.

17-4　鳞状上皮乳头状瘤 Squamous papilloma

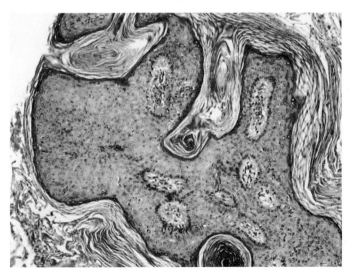

鳞状上皮向外过度生长形成乳头，乳头呈圆形或椭圆形上皮团块，中心含有血管的疏松结缔组织，表面角化亢进。

Squamous epithelium overgrows outward to form papillae with round or oval, loose connective tissues containing blood vessels present in the centre of papillary. There is hyperkeratosis on the surface squamous epithelium.

17-5　鲍温病 Bowen disease

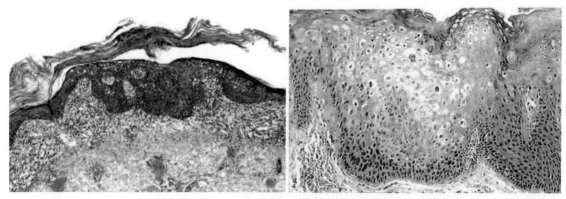

　　一种鳞状细胞原位癌。角化亢进，表皮全层上皮细胞非典型性，排列紊乱，极性消失，细胞的形状、大小不一，核大而深染。真皮上部慢性炎细胞浸润。

　　The tumor is a form of squamous cell carcinoma in situ, with hyperkeratosis, full-thickness of epidermal atypia, disorder and loss of normal polarity. The neoplastic cells are variable in morphology and size and their nuclei are enlarged and hyperchromatic. There is a chronic inflammatory infiltration in the upper dermis.

17-6　皮肤鳞状细胞癌 Squamous cell carcinoma, skin

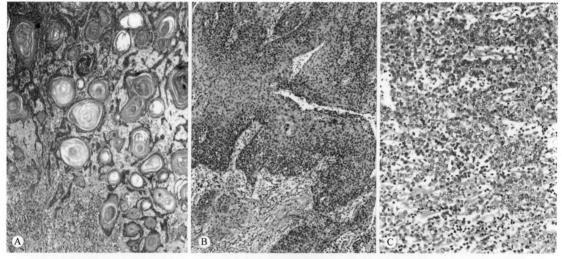

　　A：高分化癌（well differentiated squamous cell carcinoma of the skin）

　　肿瘤细胞以角化成分为主，胞浆粉染或细胞外大量角化珠形成。肿瘤细胞呈小巢状、条索状排列，核分裂低。

　　Tumor cells have prominent keratinization with pink cytoplasm and many extracellular keratinization pearls formation and low mitotic counts, arranged in small nestes or trabecules.

　　B：中分化癌（moderately differentiated squamous cell carcinoma of the skin）

　　肿瘤细胞具有鳞状细胞分化，片状排列，一般没有角化珠形成。

　　The tumor has squamous-cell differentiation and is arranged in sheets. Generally, pearl formation is absent.

　　C：低分化癌（poorly differentiated squamous cell carcinoma of the skin）

　　肿瘤主要由基底样细胞形成大小不等癌巢构成，无明显角化和细胞间桥。

　　The tumor is composed of predominantly of basal-like cells without obvious keratinization and intercellular bridges, forming large and small nests.

17-7 色素性基底细胞乳头状瘤 Pigmented basal cell papilloma

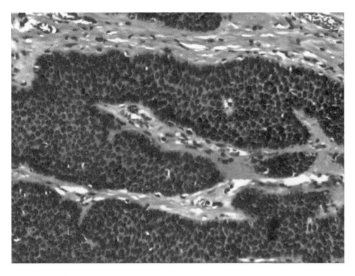

肿瘤由基底细胞样细胞团组成，周边呈栅栏状。肿瘤巢和间质之间无裂隙。肿瘤巢内的基底样细胞排列规则，有极向，核中等大，深染，未见明显核仁及黑色素沉积。

The tumor is composed of basaloid cells with peripheral palisading arrangement. There is no cleft between stroma and tumor nests where the polarity of basaloid cells are ordered with moderate size and hyperchromatic nuclei, undetectable nucleoli and melanin.

17-8 基底细胞癌 Basal cell carcinoma

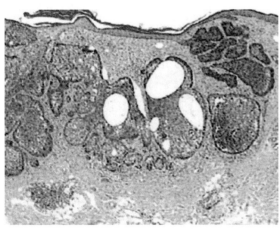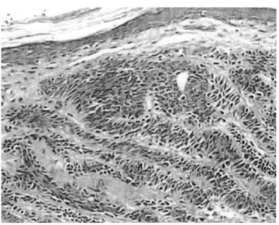

肿瘤由非典型基底细胞样细胞团组成，周边呈栅栏状，呈结节状生长。肿瘤巢和间质之间有裂隙。肿瘤巢内的基底样细胞排列紊乱，极向消失，核大，深染，可见核仁。

The tumor is composed of atypical basaloid cells with peripheral palisading in a nodular pattern. There is cleft between stroma and tumor nests where the polarity of atypical basaloid cells are disordered. Tumor cells are enlarged, hyperchromatic nuclei and visible nucleoli.

17-9　皮肤派杰病 Paget disease，skin

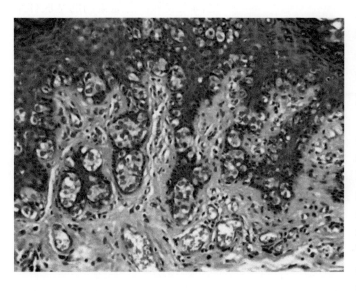

皮肤 Paget's 病属于乳腺外 Paget's 病。镜下形态与乳腺 Paget's 病相似，伴有浸润的病变尤其是深度超过 1～3mm 者，可能有淋巴结转移。表皮内见派杰细胞，细胞体积较大、胞浆丰富淡染、核大、深染，核仁明显，呈单个散在或小簇状分布于表皮内。

Skin Paget's disease belongs to extramammary Paget's disease. Microscopic morphology is similar to Paget's disease of the breast. The tumor associated with invasive disease, especially deeper than 1～3mm who may have lymph node metastasis. The tumor is characterized by Paget cells in large size with abundant pale cytoplasm, and large nuclei, prominent nucleoli scattered throughout the epidermis either as single cells or in small clusters.

17-10　汗管瘤 Syringoma

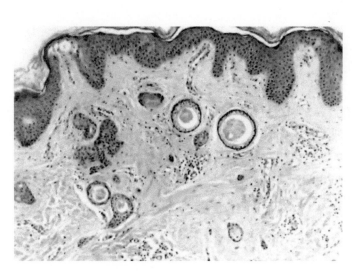

肿瘤位于真皮内，由嗜碱性上皮细胞索和囊状导管嵌于纤维性或硬化的间质内。导管衬以两层上皮细胞，外层细胞扁平，内层细胞呈空泡状，内含糖原。近表皮囊腔内有大量角化物质。间质内肥大细胞增多。

The tumor is located in the dermis and is embedded in fibrous or sclerotic stroma by basophilic epithelial cords and cystic ducts. The ducts is lined with two layers of epithelial cells. The outer layer is flat and the inner cells are vacuolated and contain glycogen. There is a large amount of keratinized substance in the cavity of the near surface epithelium. Interstitial mast cells infiltrate.

17-11 螺旋腺瘤 Spiradenoma

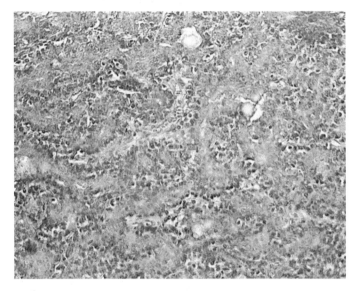

①由基底细胞样细胞构成的单个或多个结节，结节之间常为水肿性间质，其中有扩张的血管。②有大量淋巴细胞散在分布于肿瘤结节内。③深染和浅染的两型肿瘤性上皮细胞，暗细胞为小的基底细胞样细胞，亮细胞大，核呈空泡状，胞浆丰富而浅染，位于细胞簇中央。④衬覆双层上皮细胞的小管。⑤嗜酸性 PAS 阳性小球。

① A single or multiple nodule is composed by basaloid cells, and often surrounded by edematous stroma, with dilated vessels. ② There are a large number of lymphocytes scattered in tumor nodules. ③ With two type of dark staining and light staining of tumor epithelial cells, dark cells are small basaloid cells, light cells are large and nuclei are vacuolated, cytoplasm is rich with pale, locating in the middle of cell clusters. ④ A tubule lined with double epithelial cells. ⑤ Eosinophilic PAS positive globules.

17-12 皮肤汗孔瘤 Poroma，skin

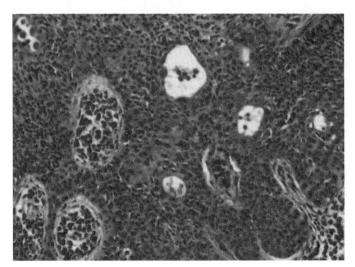

肿瘤细胞由形态较一致的基底细胞样细胞组成，伴有汗孔或汗管分化。

The tumor is composed of basaloid cells in uniform size with porokeratosis or syringocystadenoma differentiation.

17-13 乳头状汗管囊腺瘤 Syringocystadenoma papilliferum

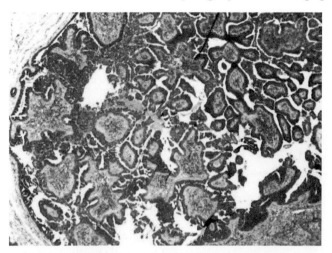

表皮向下延伸至真皮内形成囊性凹陷，囊腔内可见宽的绒毛状突起。囊壁腔面衬覆柱状上皮、胞浆丰富，可见顶浆分泌，周边为立方上皮细胞。乳头间质内见较多浆细胞浸润。

The tumor shows a cystic sag formed by the epidermis extends downwards into the dermis and broad villous projections in cystic walls lined by columnar epithelium toward the lumen which has rich cytoplasm and decapitation secretion, and simple cuboidal epithelium at the periphery. Plasma cells are noted within the papillary stroma.

17-14 汗腺癌 Hidradenocarcinoma

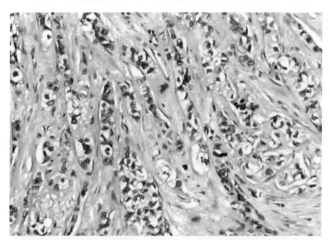

肿瘤细胞呈小巢状、条索状分布，局灶有导管、小管结构，肿瘤细胞浆空泡化。

The tumor cells are arranged in small nests or cords which focally tubular and ductal structures. Tumor cells are cytoplasmic vacuoles.

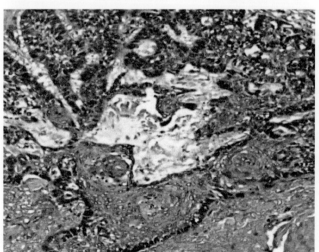

①坏死很常见。②肿瘤一般不与表皮相连，但表面上皮可形成溃疡。③细胞类型与汗腺瘤相同，局灶可见显著的核，多形性及异型性细胞和分裂象，浸润生长。

①Necrosis is very common. ②Generally, the tumor is not connected with the epidermis, but the surface epithelium may form ulcer. ③The cell type is similar to the sweat gland tumor. The tumor cells present nuclei with pleomorphic atypia, cells mitosis, and invasing growth.

17-15 皮脂腺腺瘤 Sebaceous adenoma

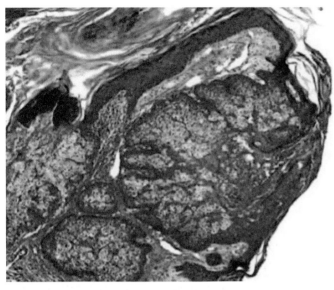

①肿瘤边界清楚，周围胶原受压形成假包膜。②皮脂腺小叶形成。③小皮脂腺导管分化可呈鳞状细胞化生。④皮脂腺外周基底细胞样层次增多，有成熟分化极性。⑤间质内常见淋巴细胞和浆细胞浸润。

① The tumor border was well demarcated and the surrounding collagen was compressed to form a false envelope. ② Sebaceous gland lobules formation. ③ The differentiation of small sebaceous gland ducts may be squamous metaplasia. ④ The peripheral basaloid cells layer of sebaceous glands increased, and the cellular polarity is mature and differentiation. ⑤ Infiltration of lymphocytes and plasma cells is common in stroma.

17-16 皮肤皮脂腺癌 Sebaceous carcinoma，skin

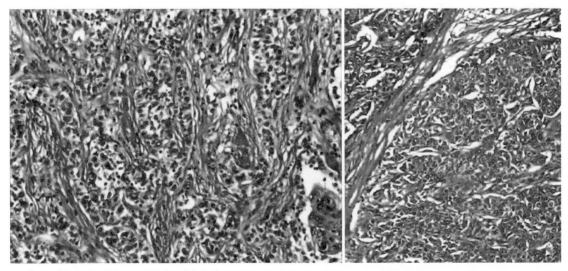

肿瘤细胞呈巢状分布，肿瘤细胞胞浆丰富，部分透亮，细胞核卵圆形，空泡状，核仁明显。

The tumor cells are arranged in nests with rich, focally clear cytoplasm, oval and vesicular nuclei and prominent nucleoli.

17-17　毛母质瘤 Pilomatricoma

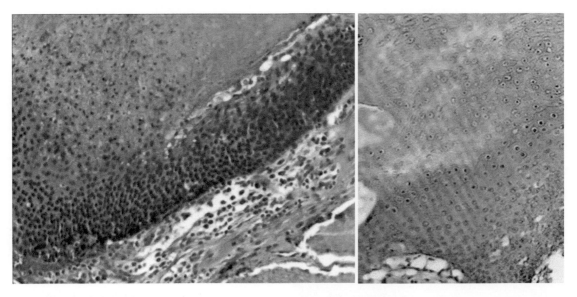

　　肿瘤由两种细胞组成，一种为大小较一致的基底细胞样细胞，核大、圆形或卵圆形，质少，核密集，细胞界限不清，不成栅栏状排列，部分细胞胞浆宽红染，有角化。另一种细胞为影细胞，淡伊红色，细胞界限清楚，核不着色，在胞核部位出现阴影。可看到基底细胞样细胞过渡为影细胞。

　　The tumor is composed of two kinds of cells, one is basaloid cells in uniform size with large, round or oval nuclei, scarce cytoplasm, nuclear dense, indistinct borders and no picked fence, focally wide cytoplasm with red staining and keratosis. The other is shadow cells with light red cytoplasm, distinct borders and undetectable nuclei which are not stained and appear shadows in nuclear site. Basaloid cells transition to shadow cells can be seen.

17-18　外毛根鞘瘤 Tricholemmoma

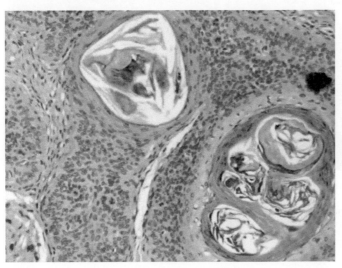

　　肿瘤细胞为棘细胞或基底细胞样细胞，形成不规则团状或巢状，细胞团或巢中央小囊形成，腔内充以角化物质，似毛囊分化。

　　The tumor is composed of prickle or basaloid cells in irregular mass or nests. The central compartment of the cell mass or nest is formed with a microcyst filled with keratin material, which resembles follicular differentiation.

17-19 毛细血管瘤 Capillary hemangioma，skin

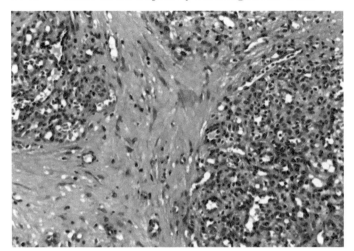

由大小稍不等的毛细血管组成，被纤维组织分隔呈小叶状。

The tumor is composed of capillaries with a slightly ununiformed size，separated by fibrous tissue into lobular structures.

17-20 皮肤肉芽组织型血管瘤 Granulation tissue type hemangioma，skin

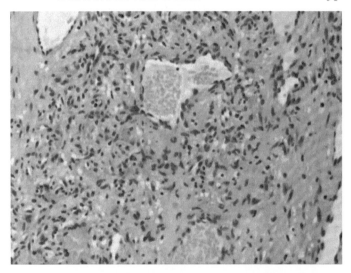

由大小不一的毛细血管和纤维黏液样间质组成。

The tumor is composed of capillaries with an ununiform size and fibrous myxoid stroma.

17-21 皮肤纤维组织细胞瘤 Fibrous histiocytoma，skin

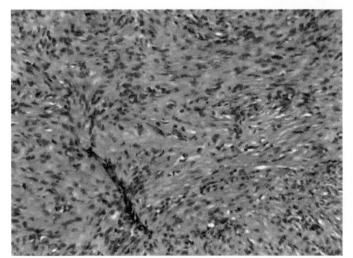

由紧密排列的梭形细胞及少量多核巨细胞组成，肿瘤组织呈编织状排列。

The tumor is composed of closely packed spindle cells and a few multinucleated giant cells with interlacing arrangement.

17-22 皮肤软纤维瘤 Soft fibroma, skin

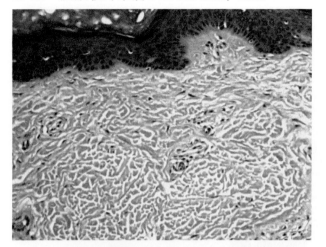

由表皮及其所包围的真皮结缔组织组成。

The tumor is composed of the epidermis and dermal connective tissues surrounded.

17-23 皮肤色素痣 Pigment naevus, skin

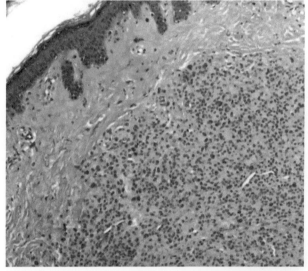

皮内痣（dermal nevus）

痣细胞呈巢状位于真皮内，其上部痣细胞多呈上皮样痣细胞，下部痣细胞多为淋巴细胞样或梭形。在成熟的痣内可见到多核巨细胞，核小而深染。

Nested nevus cells are entirely located in dermis, nevus cells near epidermis have epithelioid cells and far from epidermis in deep have lymphocyte. like or spindle cells. Multinucleated giant cells are visible with small and hyperchromatic nuclei.

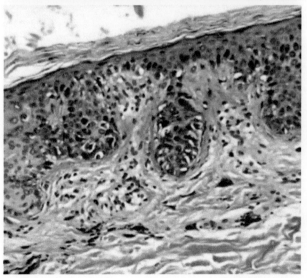

交界痣（junctional nevus）

痣细胞位于表皮深层，主要为透明痣细胞，其形态、大小基本一致，边缘整齐，细胞质内含有不等量的黑素。真皮无炎症反应。

The nevus cells are mainly clear nevus cells, located in deep epidermis with uniform size, edges shape and variable melanin in the cytoplasm. There is no inflammatory reaction in dermis.

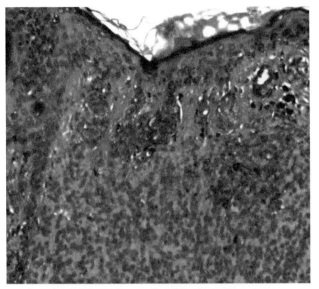

复合痣（compound naevus）

皮内痣和交界痣混合存在。痣细胞巢在表皮内和真皮内均可见到。

The dermal nevus and junctional naevus cells coexist. Nevus cell nests located in epidermis and dermis.

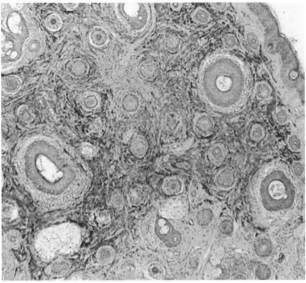

蓝痣：痣细胞大多位于真皮较深层，梭形分支，色素较多，颗粒较粗。分为普通型和细胞型蓝痣。细胞型蓝痣较多梭形平滑肌样细胞，色素较少，较易恶变。

Blue nevus: Most of nevus cells are located in the deeper dermis, spindle branches, more pigments, coarse particles. It is divided into common and cell type blue nevus, the latter contains more spindle smooth muscle-like cells, with less pigments, and more susceptible to malignant change.

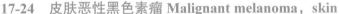

17-24　皮肤恶性黑色素瘤 Malignant melanoma，skin

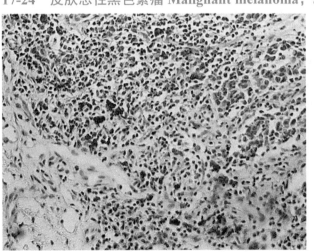

肿瘤细胞圆形、梭形，胞浆丰富，部分细胞胞浆内见黑色素。细胞核大、深染，核仁明显，呈实性片状分布。

The tumor cells are arranged in solid sheets consisted of round or spindle cells, rich cytoplasm with focally melanin, enlarged, hyperchromatic nuclei with prominent nucleoli.

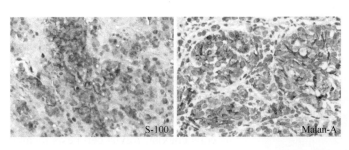

S-100　　　　　　　　　Malan-A

免疫组化显示 S-100、Malan-A 阳性，大于 10% 的肿瘤细胞有呈现强的胞质染色。

Immunohistochemical S-100 and Malan-A are positive. Strong cytoplasmic expression appears in more than 10% of tumor cells.

17-25　皮肤 Merkel 细胞癌 Merkel cell carcinoma，skin

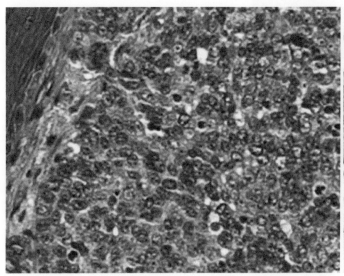

①真皮中下部弥漫性大片状密集的瘤细胞向下侵犯皮下组织及肌肉，一般不累及表皮。②癌细胞排列紧密，大小较一致，胞质较少，核深染、染色质细致。核分裂像及核碎片多见。

① Diffuse large sheets tumor cells in the middle and lower layers of dermis，infiltrating toward the subcutaneous tissue and muscles，and generally do not involve the epidermis. ② The cancer cells are closely arranged，the size is consistent，the cytoplasm is less，the nuclei are dark and the chromatin is fine. Nuclear mitosis and nuclear debris are common.

癌细胞呈浸润性生长。

Tumor infiltrating growth patterns.

第十八章 传 染 病

Chapter 18 Infectious Diseases

18-1 肺结核 Pulmonary tuberculosis

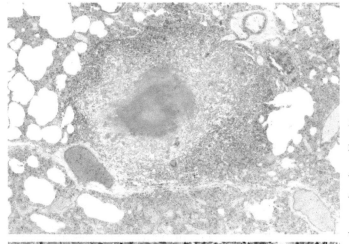

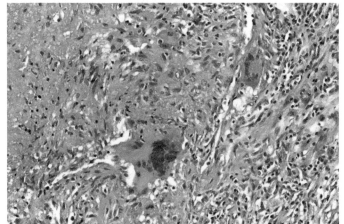

结核肉芽肿境界清楚，中心为干酪样坏死，呈红染颗粒状、无结构物质，围绕干酪样坏死物的是上皮样细胞和多核朗格汉斯巨细胞，周围有淋巴细胞浸润，或纤维增生。

Tuberculous granuloma shows well demarcated, with central caseous necrosis, esoinphilic granular, nonstructural material. The epithelioid cells and multinucleated Langhans giant cells surrounded caseous necrosis with periphery of lymphocytic infiltration, or fibrosis.

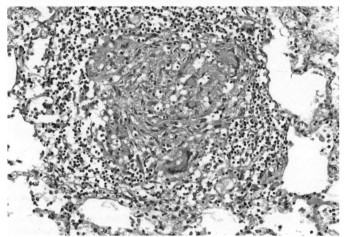

急性粟粒性结核病（acutemiliary tuberculosis）

肺中结节形态一致、表现为结核性增生（结核结节）、坏死（干酪样坏死）、炎症细胞渗出性病变。

Nodular morphology are consistent with each other in lung tissue, manifesting as tuberculosis hyperplasia（tubercles）, necrosis（caseous necrosis）, inflammatory cells exudative lesions.

慢性肺结核空洞（chronic lung cavity tuberculosis）

厚壁空洞三层结构：①内层为干酪样坏死物，抗酸杆菌染色可见大量结核杆菌；②中层为结核性肉芽肿，其中可见类上皮细胞、朗汉斯巨细胞或典型结核结节；③外层为纤维肉芽组织或瘢痕组织。

Thick-walled cavity is with three layers structure: ①The inner layer is caseous necrosis, a large number of mycobacterium tuberculosis by acid-fast bacilli staining; ② Middle layer is tuberculous granulomas, in which epithelialoid cells, Langhan's giant cells or typical tubercles are seen; ③ The outer layer is fibrous granulation tissue or scar formation.

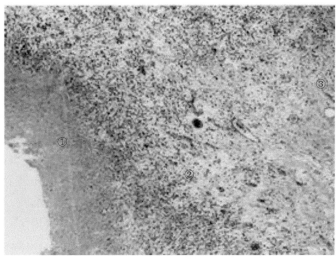

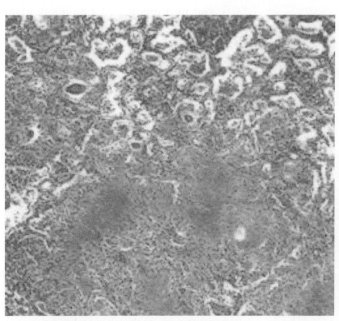

干酪性肺炎（caseous pneumonia）

肺组织广泛渗出，大片干酪样坏死。

Microscopically, amount of exudates and massive caseation necrosis are involved in portions of the lung.

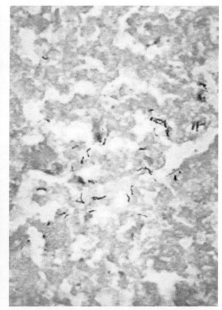

干酪样坏死物中的结核杆菌（抗酸染色）。

Mycobacterium tuberculosis in caseous necrosis（acid-fast staining）.

18-2　肺外结核病 Extrapulmonary organ tuberculosis

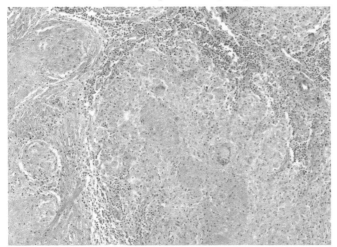

淋巴结结核（lymphomatic tuberculosis）

病变淋巴结中显示干酪样坏死和朗格汉斯巨细胞及上皮样细胞增生。

Lesions in lymph nodes display caseous necrosis and Langhan's giant cells and epithelialoid cells proliferation.

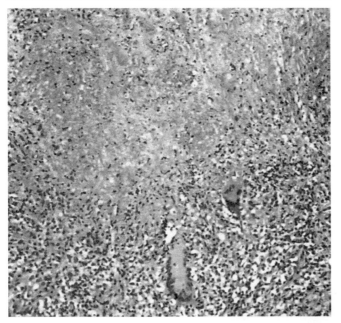

干酪样坏死和郎格汉斯巨细胞及上皮样细胞增生。

Caseous necrosis and Langhan's giant cells together with epithelioid cells proliferation.

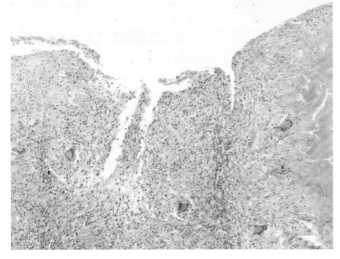

肠结核（溃疡型）[intestinal tuberculosis（ulcer type）]

溃疡一般较浅，底部有干酪样坏死物，其下为结核性肉芽肿，可见类上皮细胞、朗汉斯巨细胞或结核结节。肠浆膜面见纤维素渗出或结核结节（由结核性淋巴管炎所致）。

Ulcers generally shallow, the bottom with caseous necrosis, under which is tuberculous granuloma, showing epithelioid cells or Langhan's giant cells formed tubercle. Intestinal serosa excudate fibrin or form tubercles（caused by tuberculous lymphangitis）.

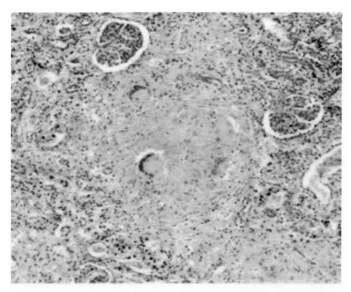

肾结核（renal tuberculosis）

肾实质中表现有结核的基本病变，结核性肉芽肿和干酪样坏死。

Renal parenchyma shows all basic lesions of tuberculosis including tuberculous granuloma and caseous necrosis.

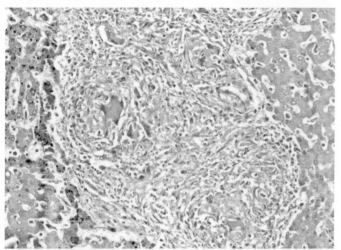

肝结核（liver tuberculosis）

肝小叶内可见弥漫分布的结核结节，系全身粟粒性结核病之肝。

There are diffuse visible tubercles distributed in liver lobule，which is liver of systemic millet tuberculosis.

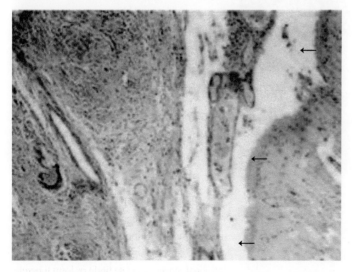

结核性脑膜炎（tuberculose meningitis）

脑室脉络丛及室管膜中有结核结节形成。

Tubercles present in choroid pleura and ependyma.

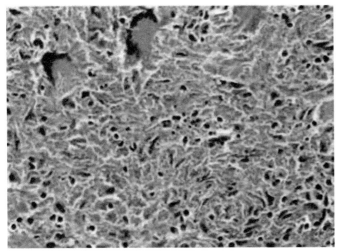

睾丸和附睾结核（tuberculosis of testis and epididymis）

结核肉芽肿中央干酪样坏死周围见上皮样细胞、朗格汉斯巨细胞和淋巴细胞浸润。

In tubercle, epithelioid cells, Langhan's giant cell and lymphocytes surround the caseous necrosis.

18-3 肠伤寒 leotyphus（Typoid fever）

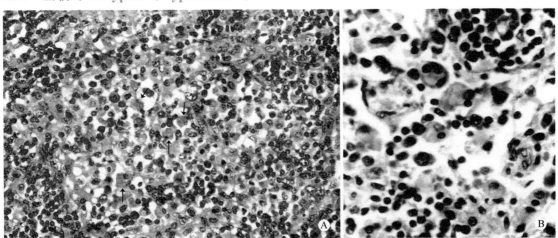

A：肠系膜淋巴结中可见吞噬有一个或多个红细胞的巨大组织细胞（噬红细胞现象，箭头）。B：伤寒细胞和伤寒肉芽肿。

A：Large histocytes stuffed with one or more red cells（erythrophagocytosis）are seen（arrows）in mesenterial lymphnode. B：Typhoid cells and typhoid granuloma.

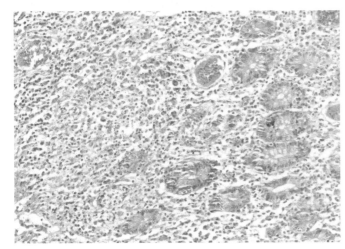

髓样肿胀期（medulloid swelling stage）

回肠黏膜下淋巴滤泡增生；增生的巨噬细胞体积大，胞浆丰富，核肾形或椭圆形，胞浆内可见被吞噬的淋巴细胞、红细胞及伤寒杆菌（需特殊染色）等，这种细胞称为伤寒细胞。

Lamina mucosal lymphoid follicular hyperplasia; hyperplasitic macrophage morphology: bulky, abundant cytoplasm, kidney-shaped or oval nuclei. The cytoplasm of these cells swallowed lymphocytes, red blood cells, and typhoid bacillus（which required special staining）etc., called typhoid cells.

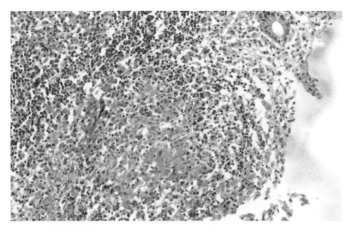

溃疡期（ulceration stage）

肠道病变边界清楚，切面上溃疡呈花坛状。溃疡中可见较多的伤寒细胞。

Intestinal lesions show clear boundary, the section are parterre-like ulcers. Here more typhoid cells are seen in ulcer.

18-4 细菌性痢疾 Bacillary dysentery

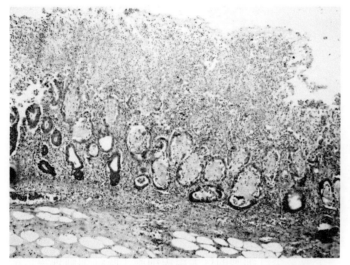

结肠黏膜高度充血、水肿，纤维素性脓性渗出。

In bacillary dysentery, the colonic mucosa is obvious hyperemic and edematous. A fibrinosuppurative exudate.

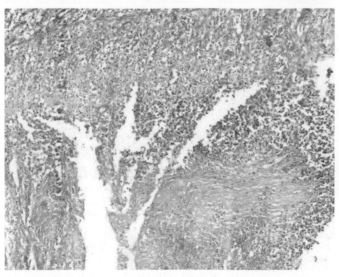

在溃疡表面被覆中性白细胞和纤维素渗出，伴有各层肠壁充血、水肿，纤维素渗出和部分小血管内可有血栓形成。

Ulcer surface is covered by neutrophils and fibrin, accompanied by all layers of the intestinal wall edema, fibrin exudation, and may have some small vascular thrombosis.

18-5 皮肤麻风 Leprosy，skin

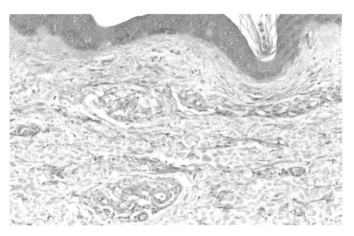

结核型麻风（tuberculoid leprosy）

皮炎和结核样肉芽肿多位于真皮浅层，极少有干酪样坏死，其外围绕有淋巴细胞及少量增生的纤维结缔组织。

Dermatitis and tuberculous granuloma present more in the superficial dermis，but few have caseous necrosis，surrounding with lymphocytes and a small amount of hyperplastic fibrous connective tissue in its periphery.

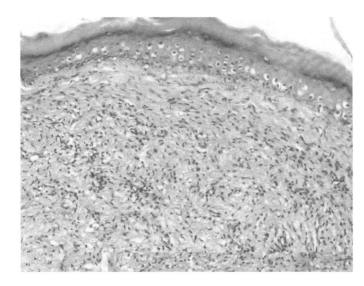

瘤型麻风（lepromatous leprosy）

①大量泡沫细胞（麻风细胞）组成的肉芽肿；②表皮基底细胞下与浸润灶之间有一层无细胞浸润的区域"透明带"；③可见病灶处表皮萎缩变平或溃疡形成，淋巴细胞少见。

① Granuloma composed of a large number of foam cells（leprosy cells）；② Between the epidermis basal layer and infiltration focal is non-invasive area as "zona pellucida"；③ Visible lesions epidermal atrophy flattened or ulcerated，lymphocytes are rare.

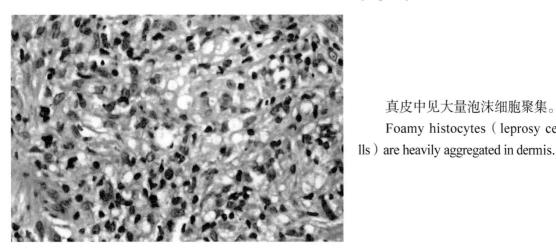

真皮中见大量泡沫细胞聚集。

Foamy histocytes（leprosy cells）are heavily aggregated in dermis.

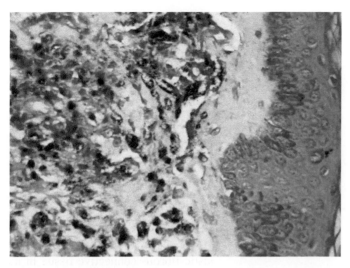

聚集在真皮浅层的泡沫细胞中可见大量红染的杆菌（麻风球）。抗酸染色。

Numerous red stained bacilli（lepra globi）are seen in the fomy histiocytes collected in superficial dermis of the skin. Ziehl-Neelsen stain.

18-6　狂犬病神经细胞中的内基小体 Negri body in neurocyte，rabies

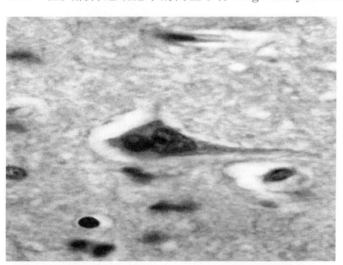

狂犬病的神经元胞浆内可见特征性的 Negri 小体，是卵圆形、嗜酸性的包涵体。

The characteristic Negri bodies found only in neurons of rabies which is eosinophilic，oval intracytoplasmic incl- usion.

18-7　淋球菌性输卵管炎 Gonococcal salpingitis

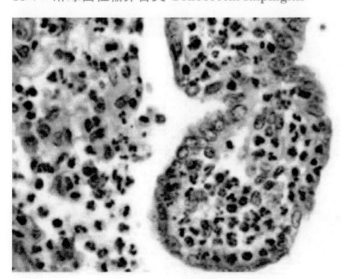

淋球菌感染引起卵巢、输卵管和宫颈黏膜的化脓性炎。

Suppurating inflammation in ovaries，fallopian tubes and cervical mucosa most commonly caused by Neisseria gonorrhoeae infection.

18-8 尖锐湿疣 Condyloma acuminatum

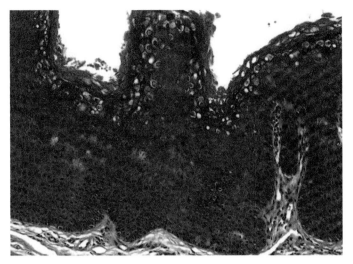

皮肤、黏膜呈乳头状瘤样增生，表皮角质层增厚，细胞角化不全，表皮浅层出现"凹空细胞"。棘层肥厚，表皮钉突增粗延长。真皮层可见毛细血管及淋巴管扩张，大量慢性炎症细胞浸润。

Skin, mucous membranes show papillary tumor-like hyperplasia, thickening of the stratum corneum, cells parakeratosis, superficial skin presents "koilocytotisis". Acanthosis thickening, epidermal spikes extended. Dermis capillaries and lymphatic dilation, a large number of chronic inflammatory cells infiltration.

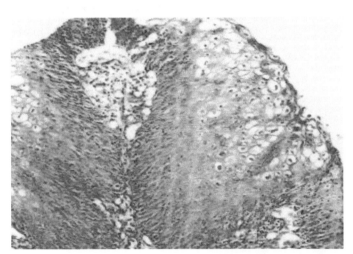

表皮角化过度和增厚（棘皮病）引起乳头状增生伴棘细胞明显空泡化（凹空细胞）。

Superficial hyperkeratosis and thickening of the underlying epidermis（acanthosis）result in the papillary epithelium with clear vacuolization of the prickle cells（koilocytosis）.

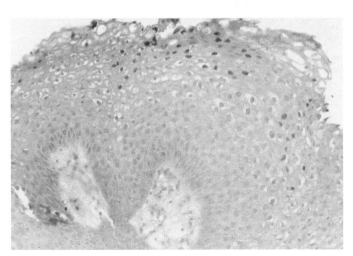

免疫组化检测凹空细胞 HPV 呈阳性。凹空细胞较正常细胞大，胞质空泡状，细胞边缘常残存带状胞质。核增大居中，圆形、椭圆形或不规则形，染色深，可见双核或多核。

Immunohistochemical detection is HPV positive of koilocytotisis. Koilocytotisis is larger than normal cells, cytoplasmic vacuoles, cell edges often remaining ribbon cytoplasm. Large nuclear located in center, round, oval or irregular in shape, stained dark, visible dual- nuclear or multi-nuclear.

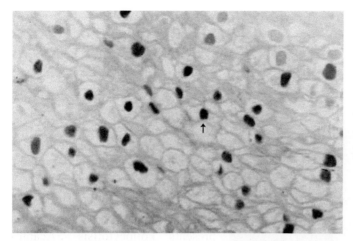

凹空细胞伴 HPV 感染的细胞核呈阳性（黑色箭头所示）。

HPV infection shows koilocytosis nuclear positive（arrow）.

18-9 梅毒 Syphilis

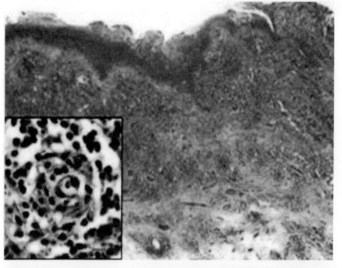

第一期下疳（primary chancre）

下疳表现为非特异性急性或慢性淋巴结炎，有明显的浆细胞浸润（左下放大图）。

The regional nodes are usually enlarged and may show nonspecific acute or chronic lymphadenitis with an intense infiltrate of plasma cells（down left magnification）.

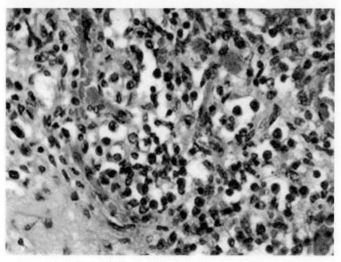

增生性动脉内膜炎伴有巨噬细胞、淋巴细胞浸润。

The proliferative endarteritis are accompaning with macrophages and lymphocytes infiltration.

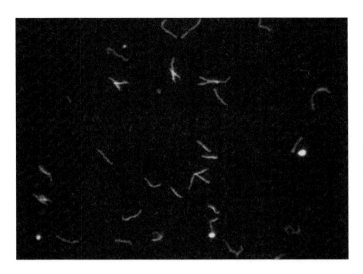

梅毒螺旋体是革兰阴性菌，呈细长螺旋状外观，鞭毛沿螺旋状原生质卷曲（暗视野免疫荧光检查）。

Spirochetes are Gram-negative, slender corkscrew-shaped bacteria with axial periplasmic flagella wound around a helical protoplasm （immunofluroescence techniques with dark-field examination）.

18-10 真菌感染 Mycotic infection

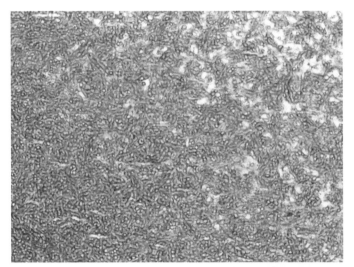

在黏液中可见曲菌感染的菌丝和孢子。细菌呈细长，略呈串珠型的分支竹节状。经 HE 染色呈紫蓝色。

Visible aspergillus fungal hyphae in the infected mucus . Fung is slender, slightly beaded type of branch bamboo-like. Aspergillosis were stained purple blue in HE staining.

18-11 曲菌感染 Aspergillus infection（Aspergillosis）

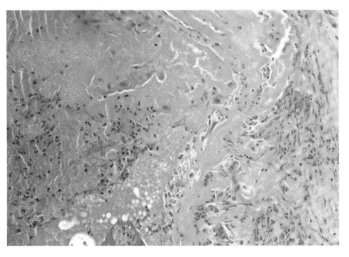

明显的出血，而炎细胞则相对较少。曲菌经 HE 染色呈紫蓝色（PAS 染色更清晰），AgNOR 染色呈棕黑色。

There is significant bleeding and relatively fewer inflammatory cells infiltration. Aspergillosis were stained purple blue in HE staining（clearer in PAS staining）, and brown and black in AgNOR.

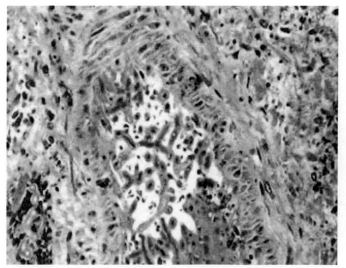

真菌性肺炎（fungal pneumonia）

曲菌感染阻塞肺动脉分支，导致感染局部肺组织梗死。

This fungus is causing pulmonary damage by occluding a major arterial branch，resulting in a surrounding infarct.

18-12 隐球菌病 Cryptococcosis

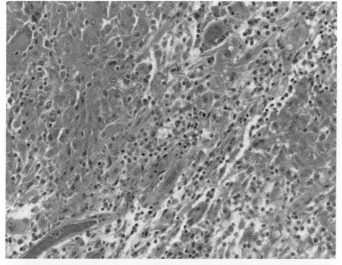

非特异性炎，大量组织细胞反应，可见隐球菌。在菌体周围形成透明的空隙，菌体若在多核巨细胞内，菌体周围的透明区就更为明显。

Non-specific inflammation, a large number of histocytes reaction, visible cryptococcosis. Around the bactoria is formed a transparent gap. If the bacteria located within multinucleated giant cells，the transparent area around bacteria is more obvious.

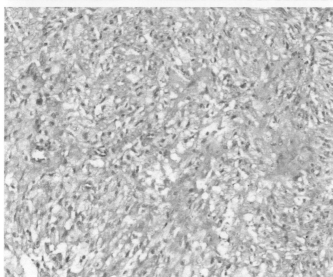

隐球菌性肉芽肿（cryptococcal granuloma）

大量泡沫细胞及多核巨细胞中可见隐球菌。

There are cryptococcosis in foam cells and multinucleated giant cells.

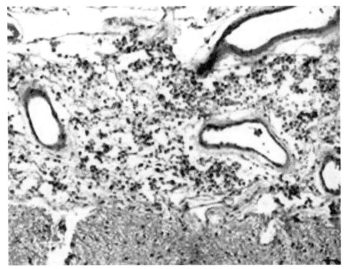

脑隐球菌病（cerebral cryptococcosis）

隐球菌病胞壁含有大量的黏液素（特殊染色呈红色）。隐球菌病经脑膜进入血管间隙，引起脑膜炎。

The wall of the cryptococcal organism contains large amounts of mucin（which special stains red）. The organisms extend through the meninges into the Virchow-Robin space caused cryptococcal meningitis.

18-13 组织胞浆菌病 Histoplasmosis

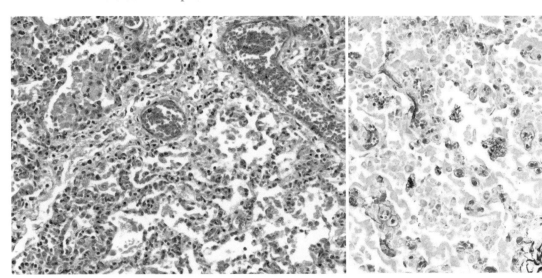

在肺组织中，菌体小，圆或卵圆形，单个芽生细胞，平均直径 1～5μm。常在泡沫细胞及巨噬细胞中，很少在细胞外。应用 PAS 和六胺银（GMS）染色，在细胞内能更清楚地看到菌体。

In lung tissue，histoplasmosis are small，round or oval，single sprouting cell，the average diameter of 1～5μm，usually locates within foam cells and macrophages. Application of PAS and methenamine silver（GMS）staining，intracellular bacteria can be more clearly seen.

右图：应用甲基绿染色在肺组织的细胞内能看到胞浆菌菌体。

Right：Application of methylgreen staining，intracellular histoplasmosis can be more clearly seen in lung tissue.

18-14　放线菌病 Actinophytosis

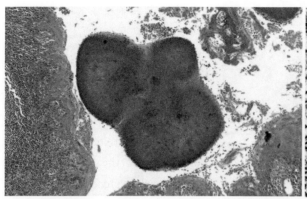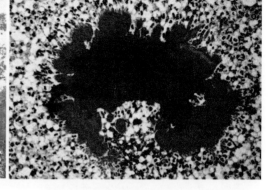

诺卡氏放线菌病，为一种机会性肺感染，多发生于免疫抑制、化疗、激素使用后，镜下呈灶性支气管炎，伴微脓肿和境界不清的肉芽肿形成。

Nocardia actinomycosis, an opportunistic pulmonary infections, occurs in immunosuppression, chemotherapy, hormone use. In microscopy, focal bronchitis is often accompaning with microabscesses and confusion of granuloma.

特征性的硫磺颗粒代表细菌克隆，大量中性白细胞围绕在颗粒周围。

A characteristic sulfur granule representing bacterial colony is seen. Numerous neutrophils are seen around the granule.

第十九章 寄生虫病
Chapter 19　Parasitosis

19-1　肠阿米巴病 Intestinal amebiasis

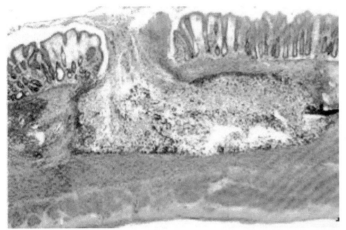

肠阿米巴溃疡（intestinal amoe-biasis ulcers）

阿米巴穿透黏膜下层且向两侧扩展，形成一个特征性的、潜掘状口小底大的烧瓶状溃疡。

The amebae penetrates the sub-mucosa and extend laterally, prod-ucing large, characteristically under-mined and a flask-shaped ulcer with a narrow neck and broad base.

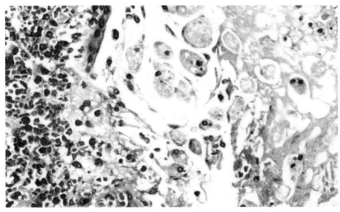

大量阿米巴滋养体，其中的一些含有红细胞。肠黏膜有局灶性溃疡。

Mumerous ameba trophozoites, some of which contain red blood cells. The intestinal mucosa is focally ulcerative.

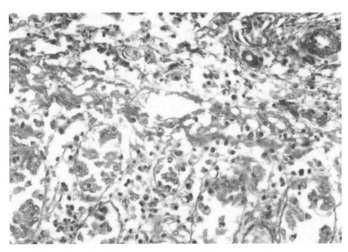

在溃疡边缘肠壁内可找到阿米巴滋养体。滋养体一般呈圆形，体积较巨噬细胞大，有一个球形的泡状核，直径 4 ~ 7μm。胞质内常含糖原空泡或吞噬的红细胞、淋巴细胞和组织碎片等。在滋养体周围常有一空隙，可能因组织被溶解所致。

Amoeba trophozoites can be found at the junction of the ulcer edge and intestine wall. Trophozoites are round, larger than macrophages, with a spherical vesicular nucleus, diameter 4 ~ 7μm. Intracytoplasmic glycogen vacuoles or phagocytosis red blood cells, lymphocytes and tissue debris are often seen. Around trophozoites often showing a gap, it may be caused by organization dissolving.

19-2　肝血吸虫病 Schistosomiasis，liver

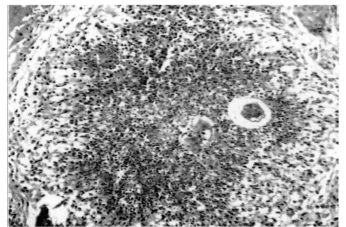

嗜酸性脓肿（eosinophilic abscesses）

急性虫卵结节，虫卵周围有大量的嗜酸性粒细胞浸润。

Acute egg's granulomas, numerous scattered eosinophills around egg.

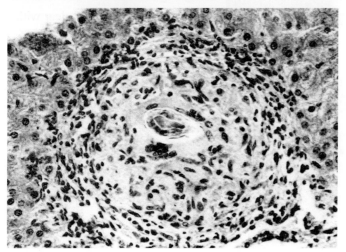

虫卵性肉芽肿。可见上皮样细胞聚集并围绕卵壳金黄色的虫卵。

It shows an egg granuloma. Epithelioid cells collections around an egg with golden-yellow shell .

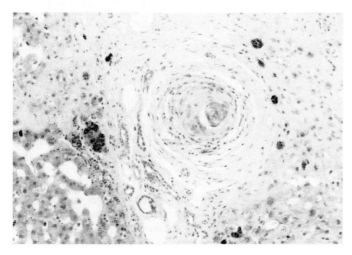

肝明显的纤维化，但肝小叶结构破坏不严重，不形成明显假小叶可与门脉性肝硬化鉴别。其中可见钙化的血吸虫卵，或围绕血吸虫卵形成的假结核结节及枯否细胞增生和吞噬的血吸虫性色素。

Though significant liver fibrosis, not serious hepatic lobule structural damage, and not significant pseudolobuli different from portal cirrhosis. Schistosome eggs calcification, false tubercles formation around schistosome egg can be seen in the liver fibrosis. Kupffer cell hyperplasia and phagocytosis schistosome pigment are seen.

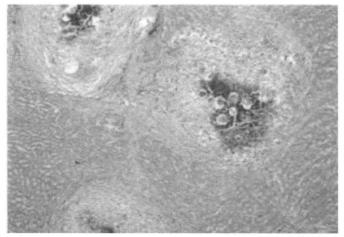

慢性虫卵结节（chronic schistosoma egg's granulomas）

慢性虫卵结节中可见上皮样细胞聚集并围绕虫卵。

There are epithelioid cells collected around some eggs.

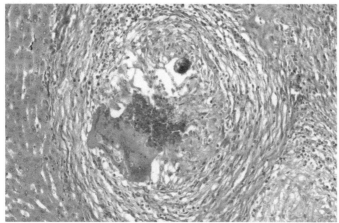

汇管区有慢性虫卵结节"假结核结节"，伴有明显的纤维组织增生。

Hepatic portal area shows chronic eggs nodules "false tubercles" accompanied by obvious fibrosis.

19-3　肠血吸虫病 Intestinal schistosomiasis

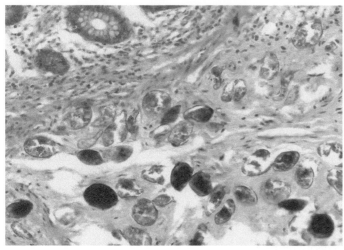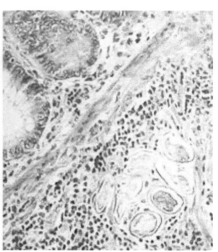

结肠各层中均见有钙化虫卵沉着，尤以黏膜及黏膜下层为著，围绕虫卵引起慢性炎症，形成虫卵结节。结节中大部分虫卵已死亡、钙化，呈深蓝色。周围有类上皮细胞、嗜酸性细胞和异物巨细胞，及肠壁组织纤维化。

All layers of colon show calcified eggs deposition, especially in the mucosa and submucosa, causing chronic inflammation around the eggs, forming egg nodules. Most of the eggs have died, calcified in the nodules, showing dark blue in the sections. It is surrounded by epithelioid cells, eosinophils and foreign body giant cells, and intestinal tissue fibrosis.

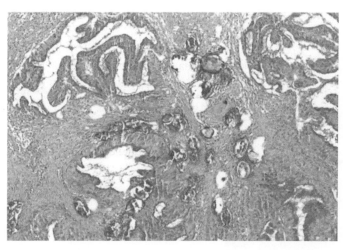

直肠黏膜上皮高级别上皮内瘤变伴血吸虫病（rectal mucosal high-grading intraepithelial neoplasia with schistosomiasis）

细胞异型，核分裂增多，腺样结构畸变，局限于黏膜上皮或侵及固有层，未浸润黏膜肌层进入黏膜下层（该病无转移的危险）。可在黏膜下层见到钙化的血吸虫卵，或围绕血吸虫卵形成的假结核结节。

Cells atypia, mitotic figures are increased, glandular structure distortion, limited to epithelial or the lamina propria, not infiltrating the muscularis mucosa into the submucosa（no metastatic risk）. Schistosome eggs calcification can be seen in the submucosa, or false tubercles formation around schistosome eggs.

19-4　几种常见肠道溃疡性病变的示意图 Comparison of several common ulcers of bowel

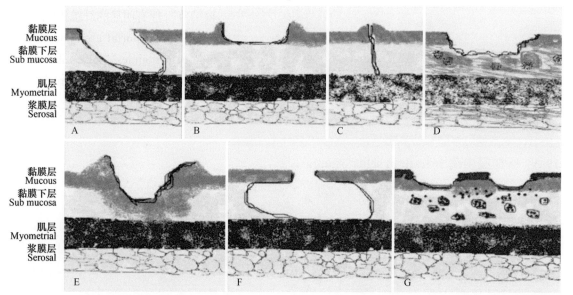

肉眼鉴别几种常见肠道的溃疡性病变。

A：消化性溃疡呈潜掘状。B：肠伤寒溃疡：与肠长轴平行呈花坛状。C：急性血吸虫性溃疡：呈浅小的丘状，肠壁增厚变硬和肠壁纤维化。D：肠结核溃疡：与肠长轴垂直呈鼠咬状。E：癌性溃疡（肠癌）：溃疡呈火山口状。F：肠阿米巴溃疡：口小底大呈烧瓶状。G：急性菌痢：呈浅表地图状。此外，克罗恩病：鹅卵石样、跳跃、裂隙状，溃疡性结肠炎：浅，沿结肠带分布，呈斑片状（无肉芽与瘢痕）。

Visual identification of several common intestinal ulcerative lesions.

A：Peptic ulcer is excavated. B：Enteric typhoid ulcer：is a kind of flower-bed ulcer, parallel to the long axis of the intestines. C：Acute schistosomiasis ulcer：is a small shallow ulcer, with thickening and fibrosis of the intestinal wall. D：Intestinal tuberculous ulcer：is a kind of ulcers perpendicular to the long axis of the intestines, with rat biting pattern. E：Cancerous ulcer（colon cancer）：ulcer is a crateriform. F：Intestinal amoeba ulcer is a flaskoid pattern. G：Intestinal ulcer of acute bacillary dysentery：a superficial map-liked. In addition, intestinal ulcer of crohn's disease：cobble, jumping, crevasse. ulcerative colitis：ulcer showed a shallow and patchy, distributing along bands of the colon（without granulation and scar）.

19-5 华支睾吸虫病 Clonorchiasis sinensis

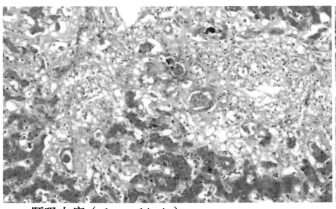
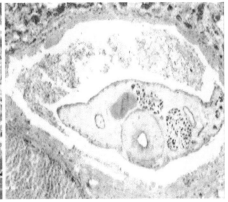

肝吸虫病（clonorchiasis）

肝内胆管扩张，腺上皮细胞增生，严重者呈乳头状、腺瘤样或不典型增生。部分胆管上皮发生杯状细胞化生或癌变。管壁有淋巴细胞、浆细胞和嗜酸性粒细胞浸润。伴有明显的纤维结缔组织增生。

Intrahepatic bile ducts dilatation，bile duct epithelial cells show hyperplasia，severe papillary，or atypical adenomatous hyperplasia. Part of epithelium cell occur in goblet cells metaplasia or canceration. There are intrawall with lymphocytes，plasma cells，and eosinophils infiltration and obvious fibrosis.

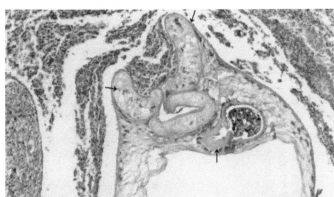
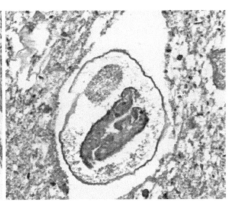

肺吸虫病（paragonimiasis）

病灶处出血和炎细胞浸润围绕在并殖吸虫虫体（箭头所示）周围并形成脓肿和囊肿。

The bleeding and infiltration of neutrophils and eosinophils surrounding worms form a cyst or abscess.

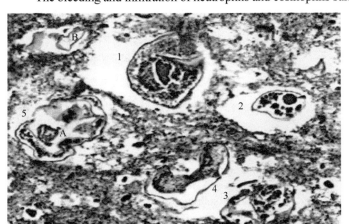

胸膜吸虫病（pleural paragonimiasis）

活检的胸膜炎病灶内见并殖吸虫成虫（数字 1～5 所示）和陈旧性虫体的残留（A 示生殖腺和 B 示输卵管）。

Sections of several adults paragonimus taken from a pleural biopsy.（Numbers 1～5 show）and old worms residual（A: Remnants of the gonad and B: uterine tubes）can be seen.

19-6 泡状棘球蚴病 Alveococcosis
（多房包虫病 Multilocular hydetid disease，或泡型包虫病 Alveolar hydetid disease）

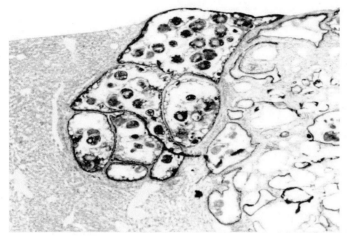

肝多房棘球蚴病（liver alveolar hydatid cysts）

肝多房棘球蚴病的许多囊肿内见大量原头蚴（PAS-苏木素染色）。

There are a large amout of procephalon protoscoleces in may cysts of liver alveolar hydatid cysts（PAS-haematoxylin stain）.

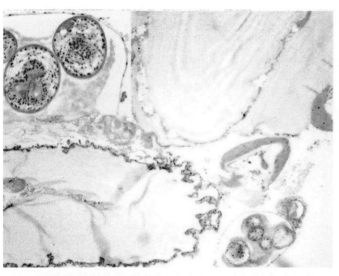

肺包囊虫病（echinococcosis pulmonum）

包囊虫囊壁组织与虫卵头节。

Cystic wall tissue and scolex of worm eggs.

19-7 蛲虫病 Enterobiasis

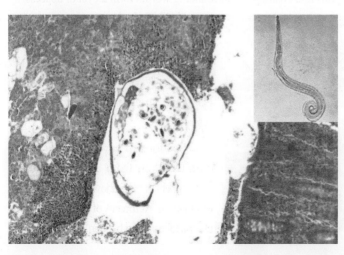

蛲虫细小，乳白色，呈线头样。虫体中部膨大，尾端长直而尖细，病理切片显示在肠壁黏膜下层可见一虫体横断面，由角化蛋白层和完整的平滑肌环绕中央的虫体内脏结构。

Pinworm small，creamy-white，line-like.Worms central dilated，rear end of the long straight tapering and histology shows cross section of a worms in intestine submucosa，composed of keratin and full smooth muscle surrounding the central visceral structure.